Animal Welfare:
Limping Towards Eden

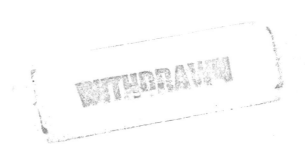

The Universities Federation for Animal Welfare

UFAW, founded in 1926, is an internationally recognised, independent, scientific and educational animal welfare charity concerned with promoting high standards of welfare for farm, companion, laboratory and captive wild animals, and for those animals with which we interact in the wild. It works to improve animals' lives by:

- Promoting and supporting developments in the science and technology that underpin advances in animal welfare

- Promoting education in animal care and welfare

- Providing information, organising meetings, and publishing books, videos, articles, technical reports and the journal *Animal Welfare*

- Providing expert advice to government departments and other bodies and helping to draft and amend laws and guidelines

- Enlisting the energies of animal keepers, scientists, veterinarians, lawyers and others who care about animals

'Improvements in the care of animals are not now likely to come of their own accord, merely by wishing them: there must be research ... and it is in sponsoring research of this kind, and making its results widely known, that UFAW performs one of its most valuable services.'

Sir Peter Medawar CBE FRS, 8th May 1957
Nobel Laureate (1960), Chairman of the UFAW Scientific Advisory Committee (1951–1962)

For further information about UFAW and about how you can help to promote and support its work, please contact us at the address below.

Universities Federation for Animal Welfare
The Old School, Brewhouse Hill, Wheathampstead, Herts AL4 8AN, UK
Tel: 01582 831818   Fax: 01582 831414   Website: www.ufaw.org.uk

Animal Welfare:
Limping Towards Eden

A practical approach to redressing the problem of our
dominion over the animals

John Webster

Emeritus Professor of Animal Husbandry, Department of Clinical
Veterinary Science, University of Bristol, UK

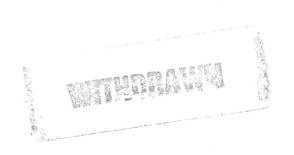

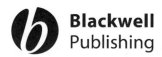

Blackwell
Publishing

© 2005 by Universities Federation for Animal Welfare (UFAW)

Series editors:
James K. Kirkwood, Robert C. Hubrecht and Elizabeth A. Roberts

Editorial Offices:
Blackwell Publishing Ltd, 9600 Garsington Road, Oxford OX4 2DQ, UK
 Tel: +44 (0)1865 776868
Blackwell Publishing Professional, 2121 State Avenue, Ames, Iowa 50014-8300, USA
 Tel: +1 515 292 0140
Blackwell Publishing Asia, 550 Swanston Street, Carlton, Victoria 3053, Australia
 Tel: +61 (0)3 8359 1011

First published 2005 by Blackwell Publishing Ltd

Library of Congress Cataloging-in-Publication Data
Webster, John
  Animal welfare : limping towards Eden / John Webster. – 2nd ed.
    p. cm.
  Includes bibliographical references and index.
  ISBN 1-4051-1877-6 (pbk. : alk. paper)
1. Animal welfare.   I. Title.
HV4708 W43 2005
179′.3–dc22   2004021358

ISBN-10: 1-4051-1877-6
ISBN-13: 978-14051-1877-4

A catalogue record for this title is available from the British Library

Set in 10 on 12.5 pt Sabon
by SNP Best-set Typesetter Ltd, Hong Kong
Printed and bound in India
by Replika Press Pvt. Ltd

The publisher's policy is to use permanent paper from mills that operate a sustainable forestry policy, and which has been manufactured from pulp processed using acid-free and elementary chlorine-free practices. Furthermore, the publisher ensures that the text paper and cover board used have met acceptable environmental accreditation standards.

For further information on Blackwell Publishing, visit our website:
www.blackwellpublishing.com

To Lizzie with love. Let us limp together . . .
the best is yet to be.

Contents

Preface

The title of this book, *Animal Welfare: Limping Towards Eden*, was agreed with my publisher on the grounds that it would attract most attention if it appeared to be a second edition of its predecessor, *Animal Welfare: A Cool Eye Towards Eden*, first published in 1993. They, who understand these things, reasoned that all books with a scientific base have a finite life span. A new edition would both attract new readers to the same important subject and help to bring old readers up to date. However, I must at the outset make it clear that *Limping Towards Eden* is not a second edition of its predecessor, *A Cool Eye*; it is an entirely new book (albeit on the same subject). Thus, so far as I am concerned, my intention is not that you should read *Limping* in preference to *A Cool Eye*. You should read them both.

Animal Welfare: A Cool Eye Towards Eden was subtitled *A constructive approach to the problem of man's dominion over the animals*. It was written at a time when the scientific approach to the understanding of animal welfare was relatively new. *Part I: How Is It For Them?* drew on science and good animal sense to categorise and analyse welfare problems perceived by the animals themselves as they seek to meet their own physiological and behavioural needs. *Part II: What We Can Do For Them* was part science, part polemic and part practical husbandry as it sought to explore specific problems arising from our determination not to leave animals well alone, but to manipulate their environment, their diet and their very constitution for our own purposes. Its main aim was therefore to set out the ground rules for understanding animal welfare and acting upon that understanding.

The last ten years have witnessed an explosion of active concern in matters of animal welfare and a smaller, though still quite impressive amount of constructive action. This has become manifest in new legislation, new codes of practice for the husbandry of farm animals, new codes of ethics for the treatment of laboratory animals, and new developments in quality-assured, high welfare schemes for food production. All this has been fed by new research and new understanding of animal welfare science. The time has come to review progress. *Animal Welfare: Limping Towards Eden* is subtitled *A practical approach to redressing the problem of our dominion over the animals*. It is a review of our halting progress towards that unachievable destination where man and animals can coexist without causing each other to suffer, written in full knowledge of the impossibility of arriving at that destination, but with the enthusiasm of one who travels hopefully and the common sense of one who carries a good map.

The first chapter examines animal welfare from a broader perspective than I have attempted previously. It addresses the role of science and the limitations of science and seeks to complement them with an analytical (dare I say scientific?) approach to practical ethics. Chapters 2 and 3 re-examine the ground rules that define animal welfare: first the nature of the challenges faced by animals and their capacity to cope, then an exploration of the fundamental basis of sentience and suffering. In Chapter 4 I introduce the central theme (the 'Big Tune') of this book: namely the development of practical, robust protocols for the assessment and control of animal welfare in real-life circumstances (e.g. on the farm) rather than within the confines of the controlled laboratory experiment. Successive chapters then examine current high-priority problems arising from our practice of using animals, individually or *en masse*, for food and clothing, for science and technology, for sport, or to be our companions. Finally, I try to assemble these pieces into a series of stepping stones on the infinitely long pathway to Eden.

At the time of writing *A Cool Eye* it was relatively easy to set down the principles that underpin our understanding of animal welfare and the practice of good husbandry, partly because the scientific and other forms of 'literature' on the subject were then in their relative infancy, and partly because most principles remain principles whatever new knowledge may accrue. It is inherently more difficult to review progress, particularly when so much has been going on. In this book I have had to be selective, both in the subjects I cover and in the sources I quote. Many references cited for further reading are reviews that provide a point of entry for readers wishing to explore matters in greater depth. I tend to cite original communications only when the material is very new or strictly necessary to support a potentially contentious assertion. I have also spared both you and me from long, comprehensive recapitulation of national and international codes of practice, regulations and legislation, not least because most of this is available free on the world-wide-web. It is, of course, essential to be aware of and act according to regulations and codes of practice. They do *not*, however, explain *why* you should do what they tell you to do, nor give much attention as to how the animal in receipt of this recommended practice might feel as a result of your actions. My aim is not to impose codes of practice on animal owners alone but to guide all us humans who care both for and about animals first towards a better understanding of how animals feel and thus towards standards of conduct more in keeping with their welfare. That would make all sentient creatures (them and us) feel better.

Acknowledgements

In my journey on the path of animal welfare I have been educated and encouraged by fellow travellers too numerous to mention. I am most grateful to you all and shall try to thank you personally when next we meet. I must, however, identify some of my closest colleagues and mark them out for special thanks both as contributors to the information that is presented in this book and as critics of my opinions. Special thanks therefore (in alphabetical order) to Nick Bell, Matt Leach, David Main, Mike Mendl, Mohan Raj and Becky Whay.

Introduction: Facts and Values

Everything should be kept as simple as possible, but no simpler.

Albert Einstein

'Man has dominion over the animals whether we like it or not.' These were the opening words of *Animal Welfare: A Cool Eye Towards Eden* (Webster, 1994). Their stark message is that any enquiry into animal welfare must start from the premise that the quality of life for most other sentient animals with whom we share the planet is largely governed by how and where we let them live and what we let them do. 'We may elect to put a hen in a cage or to create a game reserve for a tiger, but in each case the decision is ours, not theirs. We make a pet of the hamster but poison the rat.' The fact that we are in charge makes it our responsibility to get it right. Hence the subtitle: *A constructive approach to the problem of man's dominion over the animals.* The argument was presented in two parts. *Part I: How Is It For Them?* was an analysis of the nature of welfare and suffering in sentient animals. *Part II: What We Can Do For Them* was advocacy; an exposition of the main welfare problems currently faced by animals, especially farm animals, and a series of recommendations for action. It was written at a time when the scientific basis for defining and evaluating animal welfare was becoming established and the first steps were being taken to put this evidence into effect. It defined and developed the concept of the 'Five Freedoms', as a comprehensive, practical protocol for assessing the welfare of animals, whether on farm, in the laboratory or in the home. It then used this protocol to explore practical problems in animal husbandry and seek ways to resolve them. This approach was essentially pragmatic. Most matters of emotion, public concern and philosophical debate were either taken as read or simply fell off the edge of the page.

The expression 'a cool eye towards Eden' needs some explanation. Eden was presented as a simple image of that ideal state where 'the lion lies down with the lamb and a little child leads them'. When viewed with a cool eye, such a paradigm is seen to be impossibly distant. Nevertheless it is still a good direction in which to look and a good direction in which to travel. This new book, *Animal Welfare: Limping Towards Eden*, written ten years later, critically reviews our progress.

The expression 'limping towards Eden' is intended to convey the cautious optimism of one who has always accepted that the road would be long and hard. The new subtitle, *A practical approach to redressing the problem of man's dominion over the animals*, conveys the message that this second book does not seek merely to update our understanding of the problem; its primary aim is to offer solutions.

It is necessary to acknowledge at the outset that the expression 'animal welfare' means different things to different people (and other animals). The scientist defines it as 'the state of an animal as it attempts to cope with its environment' (Fraser & Broom, 1990) and gathers evidence relating to the physical and mental state of a sentient animal (i.e. how it feels) as it seeks to meet its physiological and behavioural needs. This is easier said than done. You would think me presumptuous if I were to speak with authority on how *you* feel. Thus we may both conclude that any attempt by us to define how a cow or a rat may feel is a matter to be approached with extreme caution.

For most people, 'animal welfare' is an expression of moral concern. It arises from the belief that animals have feelings that matter to them which means that they should matter to us too. The nature of this belief will obviously be governed by how we think they feel. Our perception *may* carry the authority of scientific understanding or a lifetime of practical experience with animals. It may, at the other extreme, be uninformed, anthropomorphic and sentimental. A concern for animal welfare may be considered a virtue, whether well informed or not. However, all those who express a moral position with regard to our use of animals or work actively to create a good life for animals should see it as their duty to seek a better understanding of animals so that their perception of what is good and bad for animal welfare should accord as closely as possible with how the animals feel about these things themselves.

It is necessary therefore to give due attention to animal welfare as a matter for scientific investigation, a matter for moral concern and a matter for action. Wherever possible, I use the scientific method to review the evidence as it relates to the welfare of sentient animals and, wherever possible, I use established ethical principles to review the elements that can and should define the value that we humans give to other animals. Throughout, I shall seek to distinguish analysis from advocacy. I shall also seek to make a clear distinction between scientific evidence and ethical values. However, I shall not let these stern paradigms of scientific caution and moral rigour divert me from my primary aim, which is to get things done; to work towards real, practical improvements in animal welfare. To quote Thomas Carlyle: 'The end of a man is an action and not a thought, though it were the noblest'.

One of the first steps to right action is to acknowledge that our attitude towards animals is governed almost entirely by our own self interest and, if viewed from their perspective would appear to be grossly unfair. We may be motivated to devote a great deal of care to a valuable racehorse, or a well-loved pet, almost

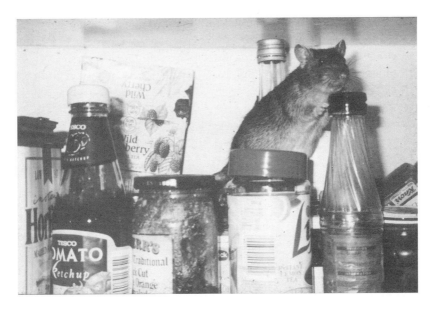

Figure 1.1   Intrinsic v. extrinsic value: Cordelia at play.

none to a time-expired hen on a commercial farm, and violent harm to a rat in a drain. Our actions towards the other animals – whether we care for them, simply manage them or seek to destroy them – is defined not by their own sentience but by how we categorise them in terms of their *extrinsic value* (i.e. their value, or otherwise, to us). This does not necessarily make us good or bad people; it is just an amoral but inescapable fact of life. In *Eden I*, I drew attention to our duty to respect the *intrinsic value* of the life of any sentient animal and illustrated the point by reference to Cordelia, the rat in the larder (Figure 1.1). When surprised by the presence of a rat in a larder, the typical, normal human response will be to categorise it as unhealthy vermin and seek to remove it 'with extreme prejudice' (i.e. to exterminate it). However, when we discover that this rat is, in fact, a well-loved pet and her name is Cordelia, our attitude changes. We now care for her (and may even, eccentrically, dedicate a book to her). While I do not subscribe to the extreme Buddhist view that we should seek to preserve the life of all animals at all times, we must acknowledge that the quality, and thus the intrinsic value of the life of a rat, or any other animal, is defined by its own sentience, not by our definition of its extrinsic value (as pet or vermin). Thus I firmly believe that we have a duty of respect to all sentient life, not just those whom we see as our friends.

In the ten years between *A Cool Eye* (*Eden I*) and *Limping Towards Eden* (*Eden II*) the animal welfare story has advanced apace. The most notable new developments are as follows:

- a huge increase in the expression of public concern for animal welfare;
- a parallel increase in the scientific study of animal welfare;
- political action for new legislation to improve animal welfare;
- development of voluntary, welfare-based quality assurance schemes for farmed livestock;
- advent of new biotechnology, which makes almost anything possible in the design of animals to suit our own needs.

It is high time to review progress. *Limping Towards Eden* sets out to review critically but constructively what advances have been made in understanding animal welfare through scientific research and clinical observations, what we have achieved in promoting animal welfare through legislation or voluntary codes of practice, how we should deal with problems emerging from the new technologies and where do we go from here. The intention is to map our progress so far and, from this, plot a bold but not foolhardy course into as yet uncharted waters.

To this end, I shall assemble four key navigational aids:

(1) Comprehensive, robust protocols for assessing animal welfare and the provisions that constitute good husbandry.
(2) A sound ethical framework which affords proper respect for the value of animals within the broader context of our duties as citizens to the welfare of society and the living environment.
(3) An honest policy of education that can convert human desire for improved welfare standards into human demand for these things.
(4) Realistic, practical, step-by-step strategies for improving animal welfare within the context of other, equally valid aspirations of society.

1.1 Husbandry and welfare

I take it as self-evident that all who are directly concerned with the management of animals have a responsibility to promote their welfare through the practice of good husbandry. This applies whether the animals are on a farm, in the home, in the confinement of a laboratory or a zoo, or in the expanse of a nature reserve. Husbandry is a good word. Whether it is applied specifically to the care of animals or more generally to care of the living environment, it readily incorporates a proper understanding and application of scientific and economic principles. Moreover, it commands us to cherish and preserve the intrinsic value of the lives over which we have dominion. A good definition of animal husbandry is 'animal science enriched by tender loving care'. This attitude may be criticised by some as paternalistic, but what else could husbandry be?

Since the primary aim of these books is to contribute, through improved understanding, to real improvements in animal welfare, it follows that much of what I write is addressed to those directly involved in the study and practical care of animals. For them I have sought to create a comprehensive structure for the analysis and assessment of animal welfare and, from this, explore ways by which the cause of animal welfare may be advanced on the farm, in the home, in the laboratory and in the wild. My secondary, equally important target audience is anyone who wishes to develop an educated understanding of the elements of good and bad welfare in animals; the aim here being to bring human perception of animal welfare as close as possible to welfare as perceived by the animals themselves. Most of the pressure for changes in the care and management of animals arises from those who have no direct dealings with animals. For the sake of the animals it is important that you get it right too.

1.2 Definitions of welfare

It is in the nature of those who study animal welfare to create their own definitions of animal welfare according to the 'Humpty Dumpty' principle that 'When I use a word, it means just what I choose it to mean, neither more nor less'. The most generally accepted single-sentence definition of animal welfare is that of Fraser & Broom (1990), i.e. 'the state of an animal as it attempts to cope with its environment'. The merit of this definition is that it recognises that the welfare state of an animal is the outcome of its impressions of incoming stimuli from the environment and the success or otherwise of its actions designed to accommodate these stimuli. Its limitations are many. It does not begin to define what the stimuli may be, whether they emerge from the external environment (like fear in the presence of a predator) or the internal environment (like hunger in the absence of food), or a combination of the two (like anxiety in the absence of a specific threat but awareness that threats exist). Moreover it makes no attempt to say what constitutes good or bad welfare. In essence, it merely says that the welfare of an animal is defined by its welfare state, which is unarguable but not very helpful.

More detailed approaches to define the welfare of an animal as the outcome of its success, or otherwise, in responding to incoming environmental stimuli have revolved around three questions. These three questions appear in Table 1.1, defined both in scientific language and common parlance. I believe that both sets of definitions are necessary to achieve a proper understanding of animal welfare and a proper empathy with animals. The simple question 'Is the animal happy?' appears particularly fuzzy and sentimental at first sight but acquires a degree of scientific rigour when based on evidence of mental satisfaction or freedom from mental distress. It is therefore the responsibility of the welfare scientist to discover reliable indices of mental satisfaction and/or distress. However, the danger with focusing on specific measurable indices is that you may see with perfect clarity the things you are looking for, but overlook things that are not actually staring you in the face. Having, for example, sought and failed to identify scientific markers of mental

Table 1.1   Key questions in the assessment of animal welfare.

Everyman	Scientific
• Is the animal living a natural life?	• Is the animal living in an environment consistent with that in which the species has evolved and to which it has adapted?
• Is the animal fit and healthy?	• Is the animal able to achieve normal growth and function, good health and to sustain fitness in adult life?
• Is the animal happy?	• Is the animal experiencing a sense of mental satisfaction or, at least, freedom from mental distress?

distress in an animal exposed to a putative source of stress, it does help to stand back and say 'Yes, but is it happy?'.

It also appears self-evident to me that the approaches to welfare assessment defined by these three sets of questions are not mutually exclusive. Indeed it is my firm belief that all three approaches are necessary to help us understand what we mean by animal welfare. However, this belief is not universal. Many advocates of animal welfare, scientific or otherwise, argue on the basis that only one of these three premises is necessary to establish a sufficient picture of animal welfare. Debates between advocates of the different positions tend to be unproductive. In order to justify the use of all three approaches it is necessary to examine the strengths and weaknesses of each when viewed in isolation.

1.2.1 The 'natural' argument

Here are three images to illustrate the 'natural' argument: the cow grazing grass in a green field, the lioness hunting on the African plains, the domestic cat asleep in front of an open fire. All these images convey a sense of good welfare because, in everyman's language, all these animals are behaving in a way that they were 'meant' to behave. In evolutionary terms, the cow and the lioness are both free to engage in behaviour that is well adapted to the environment in which they evolved. The cat that curls up before an open fire is not displaying a biological response to natural selection in the conventional meaning of the phrase, but it is obviously doing something that is very natural to a pleasure-seeking cat. Here, everyman's interpretation of the question 'Is it natural?' appears to work better than that of the scientist.

The natural argument is key to very many approaches to the design of environments to promote animal welfare. Most modern zoos and game parks seek to recreate as many features as possible of the natural environment for animals in captivity. This is, of course, partly to improve the educational/entertainment experience of the visitors, but it is also clearly intended to provide an environment that permits the animals free expression of natural behaviour (i.e. behaviour appropriate to the environments in which they evolved). The same approach was adopted by Wood-Gush, his colleagues and disciples, to the design of high-welfare environments for pigs (Stolba & Wood-Gush, 1989). They first studied the behaviour of pigs in social family groups in the natural (if rather chilly) environment of a Scottish woodland, then sought to create an artificial pig park that provided sufficient environmental resources to permit similar expression of behaviour by pigs kept for farming purposes. The key aim of this study was not to promote natural woodland environments for farmed pigs but to fabricate an environment that allowed the pigs free expression of natural behaviour within the confines of a model farm. Thus the success of the approach was defined by behaviour of the pigs rather than the exact nature of the habitat. This illustrates one of the central themes of this book. We have a responsibility to make *provision* for good husbandry, but what matters to the animal is the *outcome*, namely its own welfare state.

When assessed by outcome, rather than provision, the 'natural' argument has much to offer to the pursuit of good welfare for animals confined by man in environments very different from those in which they evolved. When we accept that it is good and natural for the pet cat to come in and lie down before the fire, we acknowledge two things: (1) it is natural for a cat to do more than simply avoid the discomfort of feeling cold; it will actually seek the hedonistic pleasure of more warmth than is strictly necessary; and (2) the cat can come and go as it pleases.

The welfare of the cat is good on two grounds. It can achieve positive satisfaction, albeit in an 'unnatural' environment; and it is free to act in a way calculated to promote its own welfare. This simple example illustrates a logic that can be interpreted more widely. Consider again the cow grazing grass in a green field. This appears, at first sight, natural and good. On further reflection it is still good because the cow has considerable freedom of expression to do natural things, graze, lie in comfort and ruminate, socialise with other cows or not, as the mood takes her. A field is a good place in which to exhibit natural behaviour, but it is not essential to these things. The welfare objective should be to make provision for as much natural, socially acceptable behaviour as is reasonably possible. If this can be achieved in the relative confinement of (e.g.) a covered straw yard with an outdoor loafing area, then this may be sufficient. However, in the case of two of the most severely criticised elements of 'factory farming' – the battery cage for laying hens and the pregnancy stall for sows – it is clear that no attempt has been made to permit animals free expression of natural behaviour. Their welfare is compromised because there is almost nothing that they can do (beyond eating and sleeping) to promote it.

The argument that animals should be kept in their natural state in order to ensure their welfare may appear to the scientific rationalist to be both superficial and sentimental. However, when it is re-expressed in terms of outcome, i.e. natural behaviour rather than natural habitat, it becomes much stronger. It is, however, a limited argument and an incomplete basis for assessing good and bad welfare. Obviously it cannot be carried to extremes. Animals on farms or in the home cannot have complete freedom to do what they like, when they like and with whom they like. In the paternalistic world of animal husbandry the keeper has to have some say in these things. More seriously, the decision to define natural behaviour as the single most important criterion for good welfare can create real problems for animals and their owners. For example, when families of sows and piglets were kept together in the Edinburgh Pig Park, the sows were free from classical behavioural disorders of sows in pregnancy stalls, such as stereotypic chewing of the bars of the cage. However, piglet mortality was higher than in conventional pig farming systems. There was also considerable evidence of bullying when different ages of piglets were kept together. I have heard welfarists argue that high piglet mortality 'is simply a production problem' which rather devalues the distress associated with dying.

Animal welfare is a complex thing. It deals with the totality of experience that determines the state of body and mind of a sentient animal. It cannot be expressed simply in terms of words such as 'natural' or 'healthy' or 'happy', when these concepts are considered in isolation, not least because these things frequently conflict. The natural death of a wild animal may be slow and painful (and this is probably worst for the predators at the top of the food chain since there is no one to put them out of their misery), the healthy bird in a cage may be suffering from extreme frustration, the chronic human smoker may enjoy smoking but fail to sustain fitness. The words of Albert Einstein are as relevant to the topic of animal welfare as they are to the general theory of relativity: 'Everything should be made as simple as possible, but no simpler'.

1.2.2 The 'fit and healthy' argument

Anyone who 'owns' an animal, whether on the farm, in the laboratory or in the home, has a responsibility of care which should, at the very least, seek to ensure that the animal is 'fit'; i.e. healthy, protected from injury and able to achieve normal growth and function. It is, moreover, reasonable to expect that this state of fitness should be sustainable. Most farmers would claim that the whole point of livestock farming is to promote good health and normal function since it would be economically foolish to do otherwise. Many will go further and claim that these things matter more, both to them and to the animals, than some fuzzy concept of happiness, linked perhaps to the freedom to exhibit 'natural' patterns of behaviour. When scientists in the European Community and Australia were asked to review the welfare of sows in pregnancy stalls, the Australians concluded that confinement stalls for pregnant sows were acceptable on welfare grounds; the Europeans concluded that they were not. The two groups had studied the same evidence but apportioned value differently. According to the Australian view, the sows in confinement stalls showed an acceptable degree of fitness and this was sufficient reason to justify the system on the grounds of animal welfare. The European view was that the denial of natural behaviour was sufficient reason to impose a ban.

While fitness is an essential element of good welfare, it is not a sufficient description of good welfare. Consider this observation, which appears in many forms:

> *I know my cows/hens are happy. If they weren't, they wouldn't give milk/lay eggs the way they do.*

This sentence does contain a partial truth. A cow or hen that fails to produce milk or eggs in the expected amounts could well be unfit and this loss of fitness could be associated with distress. Thus the animal failing to perform to target may also be unhappy. However, the implication of the sentence is that loss of fitness is not just one (important) potential source of distress, but the *only* source of distress. This view is clearly unsupportable. It is also unacceptable to use productivity in farm animals as a sufficient definition even of fitness. Commercially satisfactory production targets for a flock of broiler chickens or a herd of dairy cows are frequently associated with a prevalence of lameness that is unacceptable on welfare grounds because many individual animals are in chronic pain. I shall consider this issue in more detail in Chapters 5 and 6. In both these examples, commercially acceptable production standards for the population are not compatible with sustained fitness in individuals. Thus, even within the limited definition of 'fit and healthy', productivity can never be a sufficient description of good welfare.

1.2.3 The 'happy' argument

According to this argument, 'happiness', i.e. mental satisfaction or, at least, freedom from mental distress, is the only measure necessary to define good welfare. This argument is based on the premise that the welfare state of an animal is determined by how it feels as it faces up to the elements of its life. What matters to the animal itself is that it *feels good*. It is not concerned by its present state of health and fitness unless that lack of fitness directly impacts on the way it feels. For example, bone weakness associated with improper nutrition will predispose an animal to fractures, and thus failure to sustain fitness, but does not present a welfare problem until the weakness proceeds to the point where it starts to hurt. I accept the simple logic of this argument so far as it goes. If good and bad welfare are defined by how an animal feels, then, by definition, how it feels is all that matters. I can also accept the argument that the welfare of an animal can be satisfactory when it is profoundly unfit. The old man and the old dog in the park on a sunny day, both walking slowly and stiffly to minimise the pains of arthritis, may be profoundly unfit but feeling good. However, while one can, with perfect sophistry claim that feeling good is the only measure of how good one feels (and therefore is all that matters to the animal), I cannot accept this as a sufficient description of our responsibility to ensure the welfare of the animals in our care. Our responsibility must be to promote both their happiness *and* their fitness. Husbandry is, I repeat, a paternalistic concept. We would be in breach of our duty of care as parents if we allowed our young children unrestricted access to drugs (or even sweets). This is obviously because these things compromise their sustained fitness even though they can make the children feel extremely good at the time. Since this book is written to be read by people, not other animals, the concept of welfare must embrace not only how animals feel but also our responsibility to promote their fitness so that they may continue to feel good for the best part of their lives.

1.3 Sentience

The summary definition of animal welfare used throughout *Eden I* was that 'the welfare of a sentient animal is determined by its capacity to avoid suffering and sustain fitness'. This can be further shortened to:

  Good welfare = 'Fit and happy'

Or, if you are uncomfortable with the word happy, then

  Good welfare = 'Fit and feeling good'

This shortest of all definitions is, I believe, sufficient so long as it is clear what is meant by fit and happy. Fitness describes physical welfare, e.g. freedom from disease, injury and incapacity, and this acquires particular importance when these problems can be directly attributed to the conditions in which the animals are reared. Words like happy, feeling good and suffering describe the mental state of a sentient animal. This, of course, requires a definition of sentience. *Chambers Dictionary* defines sentient as 'conscious, capable of sensation, aware, responsive to stimulus'. This range of definitions can be taken to mean almost anything so is quite useless for practical purposes. All biologists will agree that all animals, starting with the simple amoeba, are responsive to stimuli. Most will agree that reptiles and fish are capable of sensation. Philosophers and experimental psychologists spectacularly fail to agree on what they mean by the words conscious and aware. Some argue that only humans (and possibly the higher primates) are aware. According to their particular Humpty Dumpty definition, awareness implies self-awareness; the recognition of oneself as a unique individual, and/or a conscious awareness and (more or less) rational interpretation of how one feels. By this argument, the human, using language, can say to him/herself 'I am in pain' and thus transfer the sensation into a mental concept. The 'unaware' animal, having no language, is unable to articulate pain as a concept. However, this is no reason to argue that the distress associated with pain will be either less or greater. A woman in severe abdominal pain may be aware that this pain is associated with childbirth (which should lessen the distress) or terminal cancer (which will increase it). The 'unaware' animal in a similar degree of pain but unable to rationalise it may then, according to circumstances, feel either more or less distress than the aware human. To generalise this argument, I propose that unpleasant sensations (such as pain) evoke a sense of emotional distress in a sentient animal and the existence of this distress does not depend on the ability of the animal to interpret the sensation in a conceptual way.

A sentient animal is therefore a feeling animal, where the word feeling implies much more than simply responding to sensation. A frog with its head removed but spinal cord intact will respond to a harmful 'nociceptive' stimulus to its foot by withdrawing its leg. A sentient animal, such as a rat, will respond similarly to a similarly nociceptive stimulus such as an electric shock from the floor of its cage. If these shocks are repeated, the rat will learn to associate them not only with the acute sensation of pain but also with an emotional sense of distress and will be motivated to seek ways to avoid receiving further shocks. If it is helpless to avoid repetition of the stimulus it will display anxiety which may progress to profound depression. The sentient animal therefore demonstrates both a physical reflex to the stimulus and an emotional response, i.e. distress. This emotional response is adaptive (where possible) because it leads the animal to avoid this distressing experience in the future. Whether or not this response can be called 'aware' is a truly academic question (in the worst sense of the word academic): the animal is in distress and that is sufficient cause for concern. In matters of animal welfare, the words of Jeremy Bentham must still act as our guide:

The question is not 'Can they reason? Can they talk?' but 'Can they suffer?'

Animal sentience involves conscious feelings. It also implies that these feelings matter. Marian Dawkins (1980, 1993) has pioneered the application of economic theory to the study of motivation in animals by seeking to measure how hard animals will work to achieve (or avoid) a resource or stimulus that makes them feel good (or bad). I shall discuss this approach at greater length in Chapter 3. For the moment, it is sufficient to say that it matters to a sentient animal how it feels, and some feelings matter more than others. This leads, I suggest, to a workable definition of sentience as it applies to animal welfare:

A sentient animal is one for whom feelings matter.

This definition of sentience as 'feelings that matter' recognises that animals experience emotions associated with pleasure and suffering. Many of these emotions are associated with primitive sensations such as hunger, pain and anxiety. Some species may also experience 'higher feelings' such as friendship and grief, but it would be an anthropomorphic fallacy to overemphasise their importance. However, it would be equally fallacious to underestimate the emotional distress caused to farm animals by hunger, pain and anxiety. Although these sources of suffering in animals may be called primitive that does not make them any less intense.

Freedoms and Provisions

animal welfare and to put this understanding into practice, it is not sufficient only to express the wish to see an animal fit and feeling good, but to convert this expression of good intent into a set of working rules suitable for application in the field. My approach to the practical implementation of good welfare is encapsulated in the 'Five Freedoms and Provisions' (Table 1.2), which form the basic philosophy of the UK Farm Animal Welfare Council (FAWC, 1993). The Five Freedoms identify the elements that determine the ideal welfare state as perceived by the animals (i.e. feeling *really* good). The Five Provisions define the husbandry and resources required to promote, if never achieve, this ideal welfare state.

I should explain how this concept of the Five Freedoms came about. The seminal book on farm animal welfare was *Animal Machines* by Ruth Harrison (1964), which first drew attention to the 'factory farming' of pigs, hens and veal calves in conditions of extreme confinement. Government response to public concern aroused by this powerful book was to set up the Brambell Committee (1965) of Enquiry into the welfare of animals kept under intensive husbandry conditions. In response to their specific terms of reference, i.e. the problems of extreme confinement, they proposed that all farm animals should have, at least, the freedom to 'stand up, lie down, turn round, groom themselves and stretch their limbs'. These soon became known as the Five Freedoms. At the time they were a clear exposition of the most serious deficiencies in farming systems that interpreted welfare (if they thought of it at all) only in terms of health and productivity, which, as I have indicated already, does not even equate to sustained fitness. The Brambell recommendations, for the first time, extended the definition of animal welfare to include the need for farm animals to perform natural behaviour.

This was a great step forward and, as we shall see, is eventually having a major impact on minimum standards for the farming of hens, pigs and veal calves. It is right that animals should have the freedom to 'stand up, lie down, turn round, groom themselves and stretch their limbs'. Nevertheless this does not begin to be a complete description of welfare. It is not even a sufficient description of natural

Table 1.2 The Five Freedoms and Provisions.

(1) *Freedom from thirst, hunger and malnutrition* – by ready access to fresh water and a diet to maintain full health and vigour.

(2) *Freedom from discomfort* – by providing a suitable environment including shelter and a comfortable resting area.

(3) *Freedom from pain, injury and disease* – by prevention or rapid diagnosis and treatment.

(4) *Freedom from fear and distress* – by ensuring conditions that avoid mental suffering.

(5) *Freedom to express normal behaviour* – by providing sufficient space, proper facilities and company of the animal's own kind.

behaviour since it only refers to behaviours related to the maintenance of physical comfort and excludes, for example, social behaviour. Nevertheless these aspects of maintenance behaviour did (and still do) tend to dominate welfare discussions, and thus welfare legislation, to the exclusion of all the other factors that might contribute to the sustained fitness of an animal and its sense of feeling good. However, the Five Freedoms is a memorable phrase, and affords animals one freedom more than Franklin Roosevelt promised the American people, so it would be a pity to lose it. Within FAWC therefore, I proposed that the phrase be retained but reinterpreted to encompass all the factors likely to affect the welfare of farm animals whether on the farm itself, in transit or at the point of slaughter.

The Five Freedoms may appear to describe an ideal but unattainable state ('Eden'). However, they should not be interpreted as an absolute standard for compliance with acceptable principles of good welfare but as a practical, comprehensive check-list of paradigms by which to assess the strengths and weaknesses of any husbandry system. The first four freedoms (Table 1.2) describe freedoms *from* potential sources of stress, the fifth describes the freedom *to* express natural behaviour. They should certainly not be taken to imply that all animals should be free from exposure to any stress, ever. The aim of good husbandry is not to eliminate stress but to prevent *suffering*. Suffering does not equate with stress. It may occur when an animal fails to cope (or has difficulty in coping) with stresses (1) because the stress itself is too severe, too complex or too prolonged or (2) because the animal is prevented from taking any constructive action it feels necessary to relieve the stress.

Table 1.3 illustrates the practical application of the Five Freedoms to the evaluation of alternative husbandry systems for laying hens. I shall develop this approach in much greater detail throughout the book. For the moment, I have simply considered three alternative systems – the conventional battery cage, the

Table 1.3 An outline comparison of the welfare of laying hens in the conventional battery cage, the enriched cage and on free range.

	Conventional cage	Enriched cage	Free range
Hunger and thirst	Adequate	Adequate	Adequate
Comfort			
thermal	Good	Good	Variable
physical	Bad	Adequate	Adequate
Fitness			
disease	Low risk	Low risk	Increased risk
pain	High risk (feet and legs)	Moderate risk	Variable risk (feather pecking)
Stress	Frustration	Less frustration	Aggression
Fear	Low risk	Low risk	Aggression Agarophobia
Natural behaviour	Highly restricted	Restricted	Unrestricted

'enriched' cage, improved to EU Council Directive 99/74/EC (1999), which sets out minimum standards for laying hens to include more space and environmental enrichment (e.g. a perch and a nest box), and the 'free-range' system – and ranked them according to the Five Freedoms. Thus:

- Adequate freedom from hunger and thirst can be achieved in all systems.
- Thermal comfort can be maintained in all cage systems. On free range it will be variable. However, since hens can choose whether to be indoors or out, then thermal comfort is likely to be satisfactory most of the time.
- Physical comfort is unacceptably bad in the conventional barren battery cage when space allowance for hens is only $450\,cm^2$. To give two examples only: the birds damage their feet on the wire floors and they are unable by virtue of restricted space and the barren environment to perform natural comfort behaviours such as wing flapping, grooming and dust bathing. In the enriched cage, which provides a perch, a scratching surface and more space, some of these comfort behaviours become possible. Outdoors, on free range, the bird has both the freedom and the resources necessary to perform comfort behaviour, provided of course, that it has the courage to go outside.
- Control of bacterial and parasitic infections is easier in cages, mainly because the birds are kept out of contact with their excreta, and that of passing seagulls.
- Osteoporosis leading to chronic pain from bone fractures is likely to be a problem with all laying birds in the extreme confinement of the barren cage stocked at $450\,cm^2$ per bird. This is because one of the major predisposing factors to osteoporosis is extreme, enforced inactivity. The enriched cage permits more movement and some increase in bone strength. Active birds on free range have denser bones but are at greater risk of damage, e.g. to the sternum or keel bone as they fly to roost.
- There is good evidence that laying hens experience extreme frustration in the barren cage; most especially, the frustration associated with their inability to select a suitable nesting site prior to laying their daily egg. The enriched cage and the free-range unit are both equipped with nest boxes which avoids this source of distress, provided, of course, that there are enough nest boxes to go round.
- A laying hen is probably less likely to experience fear when confined in a group of three or four birds within a caged system than when in a group of 4000 birds on a free-range unit. This fear may result from its experience of aggression, or it may simply experience agarophobia, i.e. fear of open spaces. Note, however, that while this fear may be a stress, it may be adaptive rather than a source of suffering, especially if the bird can take appropriate action to stay out of fearful situations. It does not pay to be brave if you are a chicken.
- According to the fifth of the freedoms, the freedom to express normal behaviour, the free-range unit wins by a distance.

I shall deal with the welfare of the laying hen in much more detail in Chapter 5. These examples are presented here in brief only to illustrate the central logic of the Five Freedoms. The welfare of animals in any system must be assessed according to all the paradigms (which add up to rather more than five). It is not sufficient to claim that the free-range system is superior simply because the birds are free to express normal behaviour. If mortality, preceded by a period of malaise (i.e. feeling unwell), on a free-range unit is shown to be significantly greater than in a caged system, then this must be taken into account, not just on economic grounds, but also because it is an important measure of poor welfare. There are those (and I do not include myself in this group) who will claim that the freedom to express natural behaviour is so important that it overrides any of the other freedoms (the first four freedoms *from* potential sources of stress). Where they and I differ in this regard is in the way we *value* these different elements of welfare. It is only natural that different individuals should rank the five freedoms differently according to their own sets of values when passing judgement in matters of animal welfare. However, an overall judgement on the welfare of animals in any particular system is not acceptable if it omits reference to any of the freedoms, whether through ignorance or design. The ideal judgement will be one that assesses the importance of the different freedoms in a way that most closely approximates to the animal's own measure of these things. This is why the study of motivation (what matters to an animal and how much it matters) is so central to the science and practice of animal welfare.

Another diagnostic role for the five freedoms is to identify and characterise risk factors for poor welfare. Many individual abuses of animal welfare are obvious. These include sins of commission (the imposition of direct harm) and sins of omission (such as starvation and neglect). The latter can usually be ascribed to poverty, ignorance or neglect, features of poor stockmanship which, like the poor, will be with us always. The main concern of scientists, welfarists and legislators should be for those elements of poor welfare that cannot be attributed to obvious individual cases of cruelty or neglect but to problems that may occur wherever animals are kept, on farms, in the laboratory or even in an animal refuge, and which can be linked directly to intrinsic features of the system. To paraphrase Ruth Harrison, 'If one individual causes one animal to suffer through a direct act of cruelty he is liable for prosecution. If thousands of individuals cause millions of animals to suffer as a direct consequence of the system in which they are reared then this becomes accepted as standard practice'.

A quick scan through the Five Freedoms for evidence of potential systematic abuse to welfare reveals the following examples:

- *Hunger or acute metabolic disease* – through improper feeding and/or breeding.
  Example: the high-yielding dairy cow.
- *Chronic discomfort* – through bad housing, loss of condition, etc.
  Example: pigs on concrete floors.

- *Chronic pain or restricted movement* – due to distortion of body shape or function.
  Examples: lameness in broiler chickens and dairy cows.
- *Increased disease* – through overwhelming exposure to pathogens, pollutants and/or diminished immunity.
  Example: post-weaning diarrhoea in pigs.
- *Chronic anxiety or frustration* – through improper housing, stockmanship or social contact between animals.
  Examples: tail-biting in pigs, feather-pecking in poultry.
- *Metabolic or physical exhaustion* – due to prolonged, excessive productivity.
  Examples: 'spent' laying hens and dairy cows.

This list introduces an important further element, not included within the Five Freedoms, namely the concept of exhaustion; the suffering experienced by animals that once could cope but now can cope no more. The nearly-spent hen and the emaciated dairy cow do not suffer because they are killed at an early age (death is the end of suffering). They suffer because *they are not killed*. They are made to continue production when they appear, *and feel*, physically worn out.

1.5 Ethics and values in animal welfare

I have already argued that we have a moral duty to respect the intrinsic value of any animal in our care, independent of its extrinsic value to us. However, this moral judgement and any action consequent upon this moral judgement cannot be made in isolation. We should also give due respect to other sentient beings directly or indirectly involved in our use of animals. These include the farmers who produce our food, consumers who cannot afford expensive high-welfare food and, not least, those individuals who owe their life and health to the results of experiments with laboratory animals. We must also consider the overall impact of any decision on the living environment. When we acknowledge our duty of respect to animals, farmers and those in need of medical care, we recognise the intrinsic value of these parties. We should also acknowledge that we are powerfully motivated by self-interest. Thus our actions with regard to these other parties is likely to be heavily influenced by what may be described pedantically as our perception of their extrinsic value or more bluntly as 'what it takes to make us feel good'. This can manifest in many ways. The gourmand and the vegan will have very differing views on the production of food from animals. The gourmand is motivated primarily by the venial love of good food and the vegan (perhaps) by an ascetic sense of moral righteousness. Both parties may be able to marshal a rational defence of their point of view. However, both parties should, if they are honest, concede that their motivation is linked to the primitive emotional need to feel good about ourselves.

Practical solutions to complex moral issues in the real world require coherent rules of practical ethics. Mepham (1996) has proposed an 'ethical matrix' for the analysis of ethical issues relating to food production. This matrix recognises our ethical responsibility to have respect for all concerned life forms, in this case, farmers and their animals, consumers and the living environment. This respect is considered in relation to three principles of ethics outlined by Beauchamp & Childress (1994):

(1) *Beneficence*: a utilitarian respect for the aim to achieve the greatest good (and least harm) for the greatest number of all concerned parties.
(2) *Autonomy*: a respect for the rights of each individual, e.g. to freedom of choice.
(3) *Justice*: a respect for the principle of fairness to all.

The ethical matrix creates a formal structure for identification of the parties worthy of respect and for analysis of the reasons why they are worthy of respect. It formally identifies the complexity of all ethical decisions relating to life forms and so avoids the fallacy of the single-issue argument. It recognises that animal welfare is important but not all-important.

Table 1.4 illustrates the application of the ethical matrix to the production of food from animals. The utilitarian principle of the greatest good, and least harm, for the greatest number suggests that we should afford respect to populations of farmers, farm animals, consumers and the living environment. The classic free market argument first put forward by Adam Smith (1776) infers that, in a fair society, the welfare of the consumer is best served not by regulation but by the 'invisible hand of the market', since we are all consumers. However, there is a clear moral case for regulation to afford special protection to farm animals since they are not stakeholders in the free market, but merely resources. Conservation of the environment is also a utilitarian imperative even within the limited context of the human species, since it is essential to the welfare of future generations. It can be

Table 1.4 The ethical matrix as applied to the production of food from animals (after Mepham, 1996).

Respect for	Beneficence (health and welfare)	Autonomy (freedom/choice)	Justice (fairness)
Treated organisms	Animal welfare	'Telos'	Duty of care
Producers	Farmer welfare	Freedom to adopt or not	Fair treatment in trade and law
Consumers	Availability of safe, wholesome food	Choice and labelling	Affordability of food
Living environment	Conservation	Biodiversity	Sustainability of populations

argued that farmers need no special protection since they are consumers too; thus their overall needs should also be protected by the invisible hand of the market. However, if we, the majority who do not earn our living from the land, value farm animals and the living environment, we must do more than simply preach the moral principle of respect for these things. We must give direct support to those responsible for putting these principles into practice; and that means the farmers.

The matrix acknowledges the practical strengths of utilitarianism as applied to animal farming systems but recognises that our actions should also be motivated by the principles of autonomy and justice. Autonomy implies that we have a duty of respect to other living creatures, and the living environment by virtue of their very existence. This principle is most simply expressed by the phrase 'Do as you would be done by'. We should give respect to other individuals because we would expect them to respect us. Application of the principle of autonomy to other people, the consumers and producers of food from animals, is relatively straight-forward. Individual consumers should have the right to select their food on the basis of knowledge (or at least trust) of those things that matter to them: price, quality, safety and maybe (if they wish) production methods. Farmers should have the freedom to adopt, or not adopt, production methods of which they may or may not approve, such as hormone implants in beef cattle or genetically engineered crops.

Respect for the autonomy of a non-human animal is a more difficult concept since it cannot be reciprocated (we may assume that animals feel no moral obli-gation to us). Nevertheless, the principle encourages us to recognise the *'telos'*, i.e. the fundamental biological and psychological essence of any animal; in simple terms, 'the pigness of a pig'. It is an insult to the autonomy of a pig to deny it the freedom to express normal behaviour even if we cannot demonstrate on utilitar-ian principles any physical or emotional stress. It would be a far greater insult to the telos of a pig to destroy its sentience, e.g. by genetic engineering to knock out genes concerned with its perception and cognitive awareness of its environment. Once again, a strictly utilitarian argument could be marshalled to defend such a practice since it could be argued that the less sentient pig would be less likely to suffer. I offer this example in support of the argument that, even when consider-ing non-human animals, utilitarianism is not enough.

The principle of justice implies fairness to all parties. In the context of farm animal welfare the principle of justice imposes on us the duty of care. All those who keep farm animals and all those who eat their products should accept that these animals are there to serve our interests. Their 'purpose' is to contribute to our own good. It is therefore only fair to do good to these animals in a way that is commensurate with the good they do for us.

The ethical matrix operates in practice as a check-list of concerns, an aid to diagnosis. Its power comes from the fact that it creates a rational, analytical (i.e. scientific) approach to morality and I shall use it throughout this book whenever tempted to introduce value judgements concerning the use of animals by man, whether for production of food, for science and medicine, or for sport and recreation.

1.6 Human attitudes to animal welfare: desire and demand

Animal welfare, when viewed as an expression of human concern, is a topic that generates a great deal of emotion. Some may devalue this emotion on the grounds that it is uninformed and lacking in reason. This criticism is unjust. One does not need a degree in animal welfare science to get the feeling that some things just are not right. Emotion and righteous indignation are powerful weapons for attracting public attention. While I consider the lunatic fringe of the animal rights movement to be both mad and bad, I have a great respect for those who have used the weapons of emotion and indignation to arouse public awareness of real problems in animal welfare; the good people who have been putting the passion into compassion. Passionate advocacy is a highly effective way to highlight a problem. Evidence and reason are the better tools for its resolution. Both have their parts to play. The passionate advocate draws attention to the concern, and the cautious scientist seeks a workable resolution to the concern, the advocate returns to see that this resolution is put into effect. As President Harry Truman once said, having heard in private a well-reasoned case from a lobby group, 'That sounds like a very good proposal. Now go out and put pressure on me'.

I am therefore in complete sympathy with those who feel powerful concern for the welfare of animals. It is, unequivocally, a good thing. However, for most of us who can afford the luxury of middle-class morality in a stable society, it can also be an easy thing. It is easy to ride the philosophical cable car to fashionable areas of the moral high ground (third-world poverty, animal welfare) and make impeccable judgements without losing a bead of metaphorical sweat when these are made at little or no personal cost to ourselves. It becomes much more difficult for those who are directly involved in the use of animals for food or science in the service of medicine, since any action designed to benefit the animal has to be weighed against the potential cost to the other concerned parties. In the matter of food from animals this includes all human parties in the food chain from the farmer and his family to the mother trying to support her family on a meagre budget. In the matter of science and medicine it includes both those who do the science and those who need it to stay alive. It has been said that 'the lesser the knowledge, the stronger the convictions, the greater the understanding, the greater the caution'. In this context, I would point out that it requires very little knowledge to care passionately *about* animals. It requires a great deal of understanding to care properly *for* them.

The key to improving welfare standards for animals is, of course, improving human attitudes and human behaviour, since it is we who have dominion. The first is relatively easy, the second extremely difficult. Much of this book will deal with farm animals since theirs is the biggest problem. The average British citizen who reaches the age of 70 years will have managed to consume in his or her lifetime: 550 poultry, 36 pigs, 36 sheep and 8 oxen. In contrast, the new science that underpins the surgery and medicine necessary to sustain the average citizen to this age will have demanded the modest price per head of approximately two mice and half a rat.

There is undoubtedly a powerfully expressed public *desire* for improved standards of farm animal welfare. Unfortunately this desire is not matched by *demand*. When a British public is faced by an admittedly loaded question such as 'Is factory farming cruel?', more than 90% will reply in the affirmative, yet more than 90% of food from animals is purchased without regard to considerations of animal welfare. We eat less red meat (beef and lamb) but more poultry, which is, to say the least, inconsistent with our perceptions of the relative welfare problems of lambs and broiler chickens. Food scares, most conspicuously bovine spongiform encephalopathy (BSE) in cattle and its link to new variant Creutzfeldt-Jakob disease (CJD) in humans, have generated an increased demand for 'natural' food, a trend that the organic movement has exploited with great success. Good welfare is an intrinsic element of organic farming, but it would be dangerously naïve to assume that people have been drawn to organic food primarily through a concern for animal welfare. It is, of course, that much more primitive emotion, fear. Food marketed strictly on the basis of improved welfare standards has, in general, not achieved anything like the market penetration of organic food. One encouraging exception to this general rule is the UK demand for free-range eggs (currently running at approximately 80 million eggs/month in the UK), almost all of which are produced according to high welfare standards as defined by the RSPCA 'Freedom Food' scheme.

Since most people do not buy high-welfare foods, it means that either they consider the price is too high or they simply buy the cheapest on offer without thinking about animal welfare at all. The value they attribute to animal welfare (at the time of purchase) is low or non-existent. I am not being judgemental here. This is simply a fact of life. At present the price of high-welfare food tends to be substantially higher than the standard product. This is partly because the mark-up needs to be higher when the total sales are less. It is also because many consumers seeking a superior product *expect* to pay more. Champagne that sold at Plonk prices would no longer be perceived as Champagne. There will always be a small niche market for expensive food that is perceived to be superior on grounds of taste, of brand and even sometimes on the grounds of better welfare. However, the production of small quantities of high-welfare food for niche markets will not do much to ameliorate the welfare of farm animals in general.

It is necessary therefore to ask what would be the real costs to farmers and to the general public of improvements to animal welfare, as if they were not simply part of a niche market, but imposed throughout an economic community, which

Table 1.5 Estimated effects of enforced animal welfare changes on costs to the farmer and the consumer (from McInerney, 1998).

Welfare change	Cost to farmer (%)	Effect at retail level		Impact on weekly food expenditure	
		Commodity	Price change (%)	Pence/person	Percentage of total food budget
Introduce BST	−8	Liquid milk	−2.56	−2.27	−0.17
		Cheese	−1.92	−0.27	−0.02
Ban hormones	+4	Beef	+1.44	−0.57	−0.04
Ban sow crates and tethers	+5	Pork	+1.19	+0.43	+0.03
		Bacon/ham	+1.30	+0.06	<+0.01
'Ban' broilers	+30	Poultry meat	+13.2	+3.60	+0.27
'Ban' battery cages	+28	Eggs	+17.9	+2.87	+0.22

could realistically be the EU or rather less realistically the World Trade Organisation. This question has been addressed by McInerney (1998). The five examples presented in Table 1.5 are:

(1) legalisation to permit recombinant bovine growth hormone (rGH or BST);
(2) a ban on the use of anabolic hormones in beef cattle;
(3) a ban on confining dry sows in individual stalls;
(4) a 'ban' on broilers (effectively an increase in age at slaughter from six weeks to eight weeks);
(5) a 'ban' on the battery cage.

Examples 1 and 2 refer to practices that are legal in the USA and approved by the World Trade Organisation (WTO). The word 'ban' in examples 4 and 5 is used as shorthand and needs explanation. It refers to recommended improvements to minimum standards, e.g. the new (1999) EU Directive 99/74/EC regarding laying hens in cages, which will (from 2012!) ban the keeping of hens in barren battery cages and require a nest, a perch, litter for dust bathing and $750\,cm^2$ space per bird.

The first point to take from Table 1.5 is that the benefits to farmers of BST or anabolic hormones are small and the benefits to consumers invisible. The only significant beneficiary is the manufacturer of the hormones. The free marketeer will argue that these products have value, by definition, because farmers buy them. However, after reflecting on the ethical (Table 1.4) and economic issues (Table 1.5), the customers for BST (both farmers and consumers) may decide that the benefits (which are trivial) are outweighed by the costs, especially in terms of consumer acceptability and animal welfare.

According to McInerney (1998), the EU recommended improvements to minimum standards for the caged layer would increase production costs by 28%, something no individual producer and no individual nation within the EU could sustain without a commensurate increase in income from a premium market. However, if the standards were imposed throughout the community the average increased cost to the consumer would be 2.87 p/week, a sum so small as to be unnoticeable in all but the poorest of families. Similar calculations for broilers and pigs indicate that radical improvements to the welfare of animals raised in Europe for eggs, pig and poultry meat could be achieved at a total cost to the consumer of less than 10 p (15 euros) per week! It is, of course, possible to argue with the details of these estimates. Yet even if they are in error by a factor of 100%, the cost to the individual consumer of imposing substantial improvements in minimal standards of farm animal welfare is still trivial, and far less than the cost to the farmer. We, the consumers, cannot lay the blame for poor animal welfare at the feet of the farmers. The problem and the solution are in our own hands.

1.7 Limping towards Eden: stepping stones

At the beginning of this chapter I outlined four elements essential to the progressive improvement of standards of welfare for sentient animals.

(1) Comprehensive, robust protocols for assessing animal welfare and the provisions that constitute good husbandry.
(2) A sound ethical framework which affords proper respect for the value of animals within the broader context of our duties as citizens to the welfare of society and the living environment.
(3) An honest policy of education that can convert human desire for improved welfare standards into human demand for these things.
(4) Realistic, practical, step-by-step strategies for improving animal welfare within the context of other, equally valid aspirations of society.

I have set the scene for what follows by defining and defending definitions of welfare and sentience, and by outlining sets of rules for the comprehensive assessment of animal welfare: the Five Freedoms and human values; the 'ethical matrix'. Chapters 2 and 3 review the science of animal welfare: 'What should we measure and what does it mean?' This section, like all scientific reviews, will raise important questions, reveal some fascinating observations, yet leave dozens of questions unanswered pending (to quote the phrase on each scientist's meal ticket) 'considerable further research in this area'. However, neither the animals nor society are prepared to wait for scientists to provide perfect answers. One of the main reasons for readdressing the matter of animal welfare at this time is that I believe that the first priority is not for further study but action now. We already have sufficient knowledge to create and implement comprehensive, robust protocols for assessing animal welfare and the provisions that constitute good husbandry for animals kept commercially in groups whether on farms, in kennels, riding establishments or in scientific laboratories.

Much of the book will therefore be concerned with specific practical welfare problems for specific animals and ways by which these may be resolved. The most direct and effective route to their resolution is to improve the actions of those directly responsible for the care of animals. This requires two things: (1) effective education to improve husbandry based on a proper understanding of the elements of good and bad welfare; and (2) effective policing to ensure that these improvements to husbandry are put into effect.

Society at large also has a major role to play in working to achieve improved standards of animal welfare. This does not require everyone to have an in-depth knowledge of all the details. One can be a good driver without an intimate knowledge of the workings of the internal combustion engine. However, 'right action' on the roads (courtesy and safety) requires first that each driver understands and implements the Highway Code and second that each driver can trust others to do the same. This is a classic example of the principle of 'Do as you would be done by'. For the majority of society, those who are not directly involved with animals, the two most important principles of right action for animal welfare are: (1) recognition that the quality of animals' lives is determined not just by those who work with them but by us all, since it is we who determine their value; and (2) demand for reliable welfare-based quality assurance and the recognition that this must be based on effective quality control.

The first step to improving animal welfare is to increase their *value* to us and this is the responsibility of us all. Only then can those who work with animals repay this added value with improved standards of husbandry. Those who do not work with animals but who derive benefit from them through food and medicines should not be expected to rely simply on assurances of good husbandry, they should demand evidence of improved standards, i.e. a properly policed policy of quality control. Evidence of good (and bad) practice or, at least, the knowledge that such evidence is available for inspection, is the best way to ensure that those of us who benefit from other animals (i.e. all of us) can *trust* those whom we contract to care for them. When society gives added value to animal welfare and can trust those who work with animals to put this into effect, then those who work with animals can feel a sense of *pride*. As for the animals, they should be fit and happy, so everybody should be satisfied.

Challenge and Response

2

A little alarm now and then keeps life from stagnation.
Fanny Burney

The welfare of an animal has been defined as its state as it seeks to cope with its environment. The environment presents challenges and the animal responds. The aim of the response is, ideally, to remove the challenge. If this is not possible, the animal seeks to accommodate the challenge through the process of adaptation. The ability of the animal to cope with challenge is measured by the success of its response in eliminating or adapting to the challenge. If it has no problems in coping, its welfare is satisfactory; when it has difficulty in coping, its welfare is compromised; when it fails to cope, its welfare is bad. At some point on the welfare continuum between compromised and bad, the animal will begin to suffer.

Table 2.1 (adapted from Dawkins, 2001) lists some of the challenges to which animals may be exposed and some of their responses. Each of these challenges presents a threat to fitness, where loss of fitness is defined in the evolutionary sense as failure to survive, reproduce and thereby pass on one's genes. Evolutionary fitness has been achieved through adaptations to the environment designed both to correct any harm (loss of fitness) resulting from an environmental challenge and to avoid exposure to harm. Corrective responses induced by exposure to challenge may be physiological or behavioural. For example, a young lamb exposed to cold will shiver and it will curl up with its legs tucked under its body. Shivering is a physiological response designed to maintain homeothermy (normal body temperature) by increasing heat production. Curling up is a behavioural response designed to maintain homeothermy by decreasing heat loss. Avoidance responses are all behavioural. Thus a litter of young pigs that have just finished drinking from their mother will return to a straw nest or heated creep area and huddle together, not because they are already experiencing cold stress but to avoid the experience. They have elected to get their 'response' in first.

A physiological corrective response such as shivering and a behavioural avoidance response such as huddling are both examples of what animals *do* when faced with an environmental challenge. Shivering and huddling are qualitative indices that simply indicate the existence (or the threat) of cold stress. We could obtain a

Table 2.1 Ways in which animals respond to challenge (adapted from Dawkins, 2001).

Challenge	Signal	Corrective response	Avoidance behaviour
Cold stress	Cold sensation	Shivering	Shelter
		Increase food intake	Huddling
		Conserve heat	
Starvation	Hunger	Eating	Searching for food
		Conserving energy	Hoarding
Dehydration	Thirst	Concentration of urine	Seeking water
		Drinking	Restricting evaporative heat loss
Incapacitating or life-threatening injury	Minor injury	Wound healing	Learned caution
	Predators	Rest	Hiding and escape
Disease	Malaise	Immune defences	Self-hygiene
		Resting	

quantitative measurement of the intensity of the physiological response to cold stress by monitoring oxygen consumption, which is a direct indicator of the increase in metabolic heat production necessary to maintain body temperature. We could obtain a less accurate quantitative indication of the intensity of cold by recording a physiological parameter such as heart rate, which reflects metabolic rate, though not precisely. Thus shivering, increased heart rate and increased oxygen consumption are all measures of a response to the challenge of cold and therefore indices that can be used to identify a threat to welfare. In this example, oxygen consumption is the most useful measure because it can quantify the intensity of the stress. It is, however, the most difficult of these measurements to make.

Other examples of challenge and response illustrated in Table 2.1 are largely self-explanatory. Hunger is the primitive but effective physiological response to the challenge of starvation. A corrective behavioural response when food supply is short is to conserve energy by reducing activity. Avoidance behaviour includes searching for food and hoarding food during times of plenty, as an insurance against times of want. This hoarding may be external (the squirrel who stores nuts) or internal (the bear that lays down fat before withdrawing to its cave for the winter). Responses to the threat of dehydration include, obviously, drinking when thirsty, drinking in the anticipation of thirst (e.g. the camel) and physiological mechanisms designed to conserve water by concentrating urine in the kidney.

Injury, whether from predators, natural hazards such as thorn bushes, or man-made hazards such as concrete floors, can be corrected by physiological wound healing but is best avoided. These avoidance behaviours may be instinctive, e.g. the monkey's instinctive fear of snakes, or acquired by experience. There is relatively little that animals can do to avoid infectious disease, although most species of mammal and bird actively avoid contact with their own faeces or that of others. The main response to the threat of infection is physiological: activation of the immune system. This, like all corrective physiological responses, imposes a cost on the animal and the cost is a measure of how hard it must work in order to cope.

This chapter is primarily concerned with challenge and coping with challenge to physical fitness. I shall consider the scientific evidence as it relates to: (1) the physiological and behavioural mechanisms used by animals in response to environmental challenge; and (2) the qualitative and quantitative measurement of these responses to environmental challenge. This evidence will be used to determine and develop the approaches used to identify and quantify causes of stress and poor welfare in animals. However, I must re-emphasise that both the physiological and behavioural responses merely indicate what animals *do* in order to cope with challenge. Perhaps the most important question 'Do they suffer?' depends on how they *feel* as they seek to cope with challenge. One can only guess at how animals feel from observations of what they do. The direct assessment of how they feel requires a different experimental approach and will be addressed in Chapter 3, Sentience, Sense and Suffering.

2.1 Stress, adaptation and exhaustion

I have now to address the concept of 'stress', a word much used and much abused both in common parlance and in the scientific literature. When someone says that 'I am suffering stress' whether through overwork or the loss of a loved one or the continued presence of a once-loved one who will not go away, we all know what they mean. They are having difficulty coping with a physical or psychological challenge and become tired and emotional. When most biological scientists use the word stress they mean much the same thing. Manser (1992) has defined (biological) stress as follows: 'A state of stress occurs when an animal encounters adverse physiological or emotional conditions which cause a disturbance of its normal physiological and mental equilibrium'. In the sciences of physics and engineering, however, 'stress' is used to describe the imposition of an external force upon an object (the challenge) and 'strain' used to describe its consequences. A harassed physicist would be more inclined to describe him- or herself as under strain.

Amongst welfare scientists 'stress' has become a portmanteau word used either to describe poor welfare in general or within phrases such as 'weaning stress' or 'transport stress'. The obvious problem with this use of the word is that it lacks specificity. One is no closer to resolving a problem in animal welfare by pronouncing an animal to be under stress than one is to the resolution of a medical problem by pronouncing it to be sick. More information is required. In *Eden I*, I illustrated this point by posing the question 'Is it stressful to wean piglets from their mother at three weeks of age?'. To answer this question it is necessary to identify the specific sources of potential stress:

- an abrupt change in diet, possibly leading to hunger, indigestion or food allergies;
- a move from warm, bedded accommodation to a cold cage;
- increased exposure and reduced immunity to infectious microorganisms, especially those associated with gastroenteric disease;
- fear and threat of aggression resulting from exposure to pigs from other litters;
- withdrawal of the mother's contribution to security and normal development through education.

You will notice, I hope, that in drawing up this list of potential stresses I have systematically adopted the structure of the five freedoms. It should be equally apparent that each of these different sources of stress will require different solutions.

2.2 The General Adaptation Syndrome

The word stress can, however, be used in a specific sense to define the 'General Adaptation Syndrome' (GAS), a concept pioneered by Hans Selye (1950) to describe common features of the physiological response of animals to a wide range of physical or psychological challenges which he called 'stressors'. Selye argued that the first response of an animal to a physical stressor such as cold or a psychological stressor such as the appearance of a predator will be one of *alarm*. Whatever else may happen, the acute presence of the stressor will stimulate the hypothalamus/pituitary/adrenal axis (HPA) and evoke a standard physiological response measurable typically as an increased release of adrenocorticotrophic hormone (ACTH) from the anterior pituitary, which stimulates the release of 'stress hormones', the glucocorticoids, cortisol or corticosterone, from the adrenal cortex. This alarm response will prime the animal to other responses, like mobilising fat reserves when faced by the need to shiver or to run away from the predator. It may be possible to eliminate the stressor and remove the stress during the alarm phase. However, if the challenge persists the animal will proceed to the stage of adaptation. Selye argued that in this stage of the general adaptation syndrome the HPA response, together with other physiological changes more specific to the stimulus, would increase resistance to the original stressor, but may, at the same time, reduce resistance to other stressors. Thus the animal chronically exposed to cold may mobilise energy reserves to increase heat production and blood flow to the skin to reduce heat loss, and this will have the consequence of making it feel less cold. However, this will come at a cost, which may, for example, involve some degree of suppression of the immune system leading to an increased susceptibility to disease. If the intensity and duration of the stress exceed the capacity of the animal to adapt then the response will proceed to the third stage, that of *exhaustion*, when resistance to the initial stressor and all others progressively fails and, unless the stressor is withdrawn, the animal will fall into a decline and die.

Figure 2.1 which is adapted from Broom & Johnson (1993) illustrates with two examples a more current view of the GAS. In Figure 2.1a the animal has been exposed to an acute environmental challenge such as fear resulting from the appearance of a predator, or introduction to a novel experience such as transport in a lorry. This has induced an alarm response, quantifiable to some degree by measuring some physiological element of the HPA response (e.g. an increase in plasma cortisol concentration). During this time, which may last minutes or hours, the animal will be in 'fight or flight' mode, with its metabolism directed towards catabolic (energy consuming) processes by hormones from the adrenal cortex (e.g. cortisol) and medulla (e.g. adrenaline). In the first case, appearance of a predator, the 'fight or flight' response is entirely adaptive. In the second case, transport on a lorry, the 'fight or flight' response is not adaptive, unless, of course, the animal manages to escape. This is an illustration of a general truth, which is that the alarm response is frequently inappropriate for domesticated animals (including humans) and this, itself, is a potential source of stress.

In the example of the GAS illustrated in Figure 2.1a the stress response does not outlast the alarm phase. Either the physiological and behavioural responses evoked during the alarm phase have been sufficient to eliminate the challenge or the challenge itself has gone away. However, the hormonal redirection of metabolism towards 'fight or flight' mode and away from 'rest and digest' functions such as growth and repair of tissues, and maintenance of the immune system, potentially causes a reduction in overall fitness, by increasing susceptibility to other challenges. A popular (and almost entirely misguided) example of this concept is the folk belief that one can 'catch a cold' by staying out in the rain. This belief, re-expressed in scientific terms, would imply that the alarm response to an acute cold stress suppressed the immune response to an infectious *Rhinovirus* to the extent that exposure proceeded to clinical disease.

The other extreme of the GAS is illustrated in Figure 2.1b. In this case the challenge outlasts the period of the alarm response. The animal proceeds to the phase of adaptation. A sustained response is required to counter the disturbance to its normal physiological and mental equilibrium. This response may still involve increased activity of the HPA system, although probably not to the extent occurring during the alarm phase. In this sense and at this stage, the animal may be said to have adapted and is 'coping' with the sustained challenge. However, this adaptation imposes a lasting physiological cost and this is likely to cause a loss of fitness. If the challenge persists then the animal may in time proceed to the stage of exhaustion either because it cannot sustain the continuing cost of the response or because it succumbs, through loss of fitness, to a separate challenge such as infection.

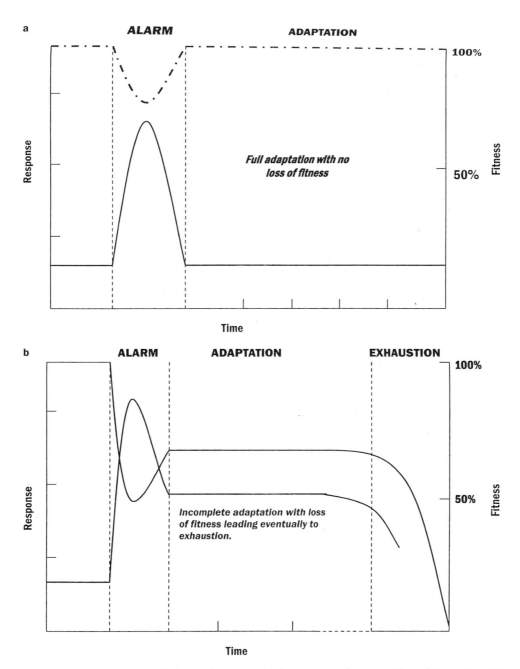

Figure 2.1 Responses to challenge: the General Adaptation Syndrome. **a** Alarm followed by full adaptation with no loss of fitness. **b** Incomplete adaptation with loss of fitness leading eventually to exhaustion.

The examples illustrated in Figure 2.1 describe the two extremes of the GAS. I shall give just two examples of the infinite variety of acute and chronic challenges and possible responses that can occur within these two extremes:

- Wild mammals and birds are exposed to chronic challenge from cold during the northern winters. They adapt to this cold with a variety of physiological and behavioural responses. This comes at a metabolic cost. For those that survive in good health, this is a cost they can bear with no apparent loss of fitness. Those that fail to survive usually succumb to exhaustion of energy reserves rather than acute hypothermia during the alarm phase.
- Many animals may be exposed not to chronic challenge but to a succession of acute challenges. A cruel experimental model of this form of repeated stress is the exposure of laboratory rats to repeated electric shocks. This will trigger a succession of alarm responses and, in severe cases, the animal may proceed to exhaustion without ever achieving an effective degree of adaptation.

2.3 Physiological stress: the alarm response

It is now necessary to examine the alarm response in more detail. How can we measure it and what do these measurements mean? In particular, what can they tell us about the welfare of animals exposed to challenge? The first thing to say is that activation of the HPA system is a constant feature of the acute alarm response to any environmental challenge. Indeed, if there is no activation of the HPA axis, there is (by definition) no acute stress. The second thing to say is that measurement of HPA activation is extremely easy (indeed dangerously easy). An elevated concentration of glucocorticoids (cortisol or corticosterone) in the peripheral blood of an animal following a putative physical stress such as cold or emotional stress such as isolation is a reliable indicator that the animal has activated a physiological response to that stimulus.

From here on matters can become confused. The first problem is that the HPA axis can be aroused by all sorts of environmental stimuli. If a young calf is exposed to an acute physical stimulus such as cold, plasma cortisol concentration will increase and the size of the increase will reflect the perceived intensity of the cold stimulus. A young calf exposed to the emotional stimulus of handling and transportation from its farm of origin to a rearing unit will also display an increase in plasma cortisol concentration. It is, at first sight, reasonable to assume that this is an indicator of transport stress and that the magnitude of the increase is a measure of the magnitude of the stress. However, when I used to put my dog and/or young children in the car and drive them to the seaside all became very excited and this excitement will have undoubtedly been associated with an increased release of both glucocorticoids and catecholamines (adrenaline and noradrenaline) from, respectively, their adrenal cortex and medulla. My dog and children were highly aroused, but their welfare was in no way compromised. They were antici-pating a good time. The dog, knowing that it was approaching the seaside, was going through a very different experience from the calf loaded onto a lorry for the first time. It would, however, be impossible to deduce from measurements of plasma glucocorticoid concentration taken in isolation whether my dog was in a state of delight or of terror. Measurements of glucocorticoids can do more than provide a semiquantitative indication of acute arousal. They do not indicate whether this state of arousal is an indicator of bad or good welfare. This becomes critical when one cannot assume *a priori* from other indices whether the stimulus is good or bad, e.g. in the study of social responses between animals. The second problem with measuring the concentration of glucocorticoids in plasma is that the procedures used for collection of the sample (isolation, restraint and bleeding) themselves may constitute a greater stress than the challenge one is seeking to measure. Ways to overcome this sampling problem include the measurement of glucocorticoids in saliva (which involves restraint but no bleeding) or sampling from catheters previously installed in a suitable vein such as the jugular. This method can be further refined by the use of remote sampling devices carried in a pack on the back of a completely unrestrained animal.

Table 2.2 presents some of the measurements used to measure the acute ('alarm') response to acute environmental challenges. These include indicators of activation of the HPA axis and indicators of the physiological response to activation of the HPA axis. The most commonly used indicator of *activation* is obtained by meas-uring the concentration of glucocorticoids in plasma or saliva. When interpreted in the context of the environmental challenge and other (behavioural) responses, this can give useful evidence relating to both the existence and intensity of acute stress. Concentrations of catecholamines in plasma are less useful because they are rapidly removed or metabolised after release into the circulation. Measurement of catecholamine metabolites in urine can provide a useful indicator of the intensity

Table 2.2 Physiological indicators used to measure the acute ('alarm') response to acute envi-ronmental challenges.

Category	Indicator
Activation of the HPA axis	Increased concentration of glucocorticoids in blood and saliva
	Increased concentration of catecholamines in blood and urine
	Increased concentration of ACTH (or β endorphin) in blood
	Brain function (electroencephalogram, neurochemistry)
Direct response	Heart rate
	Metabolic rate (oxygen consumption)
	Respiratory rate and body temperature
	Metabolites in blood (e.g. glucose, free fatty acids)
	Enzymes (e.g. lactic dehydrogenase)

(and to some extent the duration) of the alarm response. Adrenocorticotrophic hormone (ACTH) released from the anterior pituitary into the peripheral blood can be used to measure alarm, although when employed simply as a measure of the alarm response, it adds little to the information that can be derived from glucocorticoids alone. It is also possible to use β endorphin as a marker but pointless to measure both β endorphin and ACTH since they are released together as fragments of the same peptide.

The alarm response, for example to the sudden appearance of a predator, is mediated through the HPA axis but triggered by an increased state of mental arousal, i.e. it starts in the brain. When I write 'The animal becomes consciously aware that there is a problem', this sentence will be entirely clear to anyone except a philosopher who has extreme difficulty with words such as consciousness and awareness (see Chapter 3). Since all conscious feelings involve not only that psychological concept 'the mind' but also that physical entity the brain, it is entirely proper to consider the use of neurosciences, techniques for the study of the brain, when investigating how an animal feels as it responds to challenge. However, when planning any scientific procedure with animals there is a moral imperative (and in the UK a legal obligation) to use a method that provides the necessary information at least cost to the animal measured in terms of pain, suffering, distress or lasting harm. There is a special moral dilemma attached to experiments that impose such costs in the pursuit of increased understanding of animal welfare. It is possible to record the electroencephalogram (EEG) as a non-invasive marker of the alarm response in lightly restrained animals. The presence of theta waves at 4–7 Hz has been used as an indicator of the alarm response to indicate, for example, what does and does not alarm farm animals in the period immediately preceding stunning and slaughter (see Gregory, 1998b). Here the mild cost (of the EEG) to the individuals in the experiment can be justified by the potential benefit to millions through the development of more humane procedures in the abattoir.

For the most part, however, I suggest that direct measurements of the electrophysiology and/or biochemistry of the brain are seldom justified when used simply as evidence of a physiological response to a stressor, whether used in the stage of alarm, adaptation or exhaustion. When used to assess the acute activation of the HPA axis, the measurement of a brain chemical such as corticotrophin releasing factor imposes a greater cost, yet provides no more information than the measurement of glucocorticoids in peripheral blood. However, neuroscience does have an important role to play in the interpretation of how animals feel when presented by challenge and I shall consider this in Chapter 3.

Recordings of heart rate, respiratory rate, body temperature and oxygen consumption have been much used in the study of stress *responses*. The first three have the merit that they are non-invasive and can be recorded or telerecorded from unrestrained animals. Heart rate responses are rapid and sensitive, but, in common with glucocorticoids, they can be confusingly non-specific since they can indicate either pain or pleasure. Respiration rate and body temperature can be helpful in assessing heat and cold stress but are not much use otherwise. It is possible with modern apparatus to make precise measurements of oxygen consumption in lightly restrained or free-ranging (but trained) animals. Oxygen consumption is a direct measure of the overall metabolic cost of responding to any challenge and, as such, it can be highly valuable.

2.4 Physiological responses to challenge: the cost of adaptation

A sudden perturbation to the environment will elicit the alarm response from an animal. This response is non-specific because the animal cannot, at once, be expected to marshal the most appropriate physiological and behavioural response. The first priority is to prime itself for action. If the challenge outlasts the period of the alarm response, then the animal must proceed to the phase of adaptation and this adaptation must be appropriate to the specific nature of the challenge. Table 2.3 lists three categories of measurement used to measure adaptive and other physiological responses to persistent or repeated environmental challenges. The first category involves measurements of the direct costs of the physiological response. These include increase in metabolic rate (measured as an increase in oxygen consumption), reduction in growth and food conversion efficiency and changes in body composition, e.g. a redistribution of body reserves between protein and fat. The second category involves measurement of the cost to the animal in terms of loss of fitness. Measures include impaired reproductive performance, increased morbidity and loss of appetite. The third category encompasses a list of physiological 'markers' that may be used as indices of the cost of

Table 2.3 Indicators used to measure adaptive and other physiological responses to persistent or repeated environmental challenges.

Category	Indicator
Direct cost of adaptive response	Increased metabolic rate (oxygen consumption)
	Impaired function: growth rate, food conversion efficiency
	Changes in body composition
Direct indices of loss of fitness	Impaired reproductive performance
	Increased morbidity
	Reduced appetite
Indirect 'markers'	Concentration of glucocorticoids in blood and saliva?
	Increased response to ACTH
	Suppression of anabolic hormones
	Neurobiological markers (neuropeptides)
	Immunosuppression; antibody and cell-mediated responses; neutrophil : lymphocyte ratio

adaptation or loss of fitness. Indices of the HPA axis are used as putative markers of the cost of adaptation. Indices of immune status are used as putative markers of loss of fitness. These can involve measures of antibody and cell-mediated responses to exposure to specific antigens (Bateman *et al.*, 1989). The heterophil: lymphocyte ratio (essentially the ratio of polymorphic 'white cells' to lymphocytes) has also been used as a marker of activation of the immune system (Gross & Siegel, 1983).

It is obviously most useful to be able to measure the physiological costs of adaptation or loss of fitness directly by recording the impairment in, e.g., fertility or food conversion efficiency. However, such measures are expensive, time-consuming and rely on large population numbers. It is therefore proper to explore the extent to which quicker, cheaper (but indirect) markers may be used as a measure of physiological stress during the adaptation period. However, this approach has been generally unsuccessful for the good reasons that the adaptation response, unlike the alarm response, is (1) specific to the challenge and (2) governed by its own success in meeting the challenge.

These points are well illustrated by the results of an elegant study in which growing chicks were exposed to one or more of a combination of seven potential challenges (stressors) over a seven-day period (McFarlane *et al.*, 1989a–c). Significant responses were observed to four of these stressors: chronic exposure to ammonia and heat, infection with *Coccidia* and repeated exposure to electric shocks. These effects are summarised in Table 2.4. These four stressors all significantly impaired weight gain, food intake and food conversion efficiency. Their combined effects were approximately additive, i.e. there was a sustained cumulative cost of coping with this combination of physiological, pathological and psychological stressors. Moreover, the measurements of weight gain, food intake and food conversion efficiency taken over a seven-day period were able to integrate these cumulative costs. However, corticosterone (the main glucocorticoid in chickens) did not differ from controls. Heterophil:lymphocyte ratios were highly significantly elevated by heat stress, just significantly elevated by electric shock and ammonia, but unaffected by infection with *Coccidia*, the one challenge that might

Table 2.4 Effects of multiple stressors on chicks (from McFarlane *et al.*, 1989a–c).

Stressor	Ammonia	*Coccidia*	Heat	Electric shock
Weight gain (7-day)	−−−	−−−	−−−	−−−
Food intake	−	−−−	−−−	−−−
Food conversion efficiency	−−	−−−	−−−	−−−
Body fat:protein ratio	n.s.	−−−	n.s.	n.s.
Heterophil:lymphocyte ratio	+	n.s.	+++	+
Corticosterone	n.s.	n.s.	n.s.	n.s.

Significance of effects is indicated thus: reduction: $P < 0.05$ by −, $P < 0.01$ by −−, $P < 0.001$ by −−−, increase: $P < 0.05$ by +, $P < 0.01$ by ++, $P < 0.001$ by +++; n.s. not significant.

be expected *a priori* to affect the immune system. The message from Table 2.4 is that while non-specific markers may be used to measure the non-specific alarm response, they are seldom of use in assessing the cost of coping during the adaptation phase. Here the measures need to be specific to the challenge and they need to integrate the extent to which the animal is, or is not, succeeding over time in reducing or even eliminating the challenge.

2.5 Adaptation to cold stress: an example of habituation

To illustrate the nature and consequences of the adaptation response I shall briefly consider adaptation to cold, an informative stressor for research purposes since it is measurable, repeatable and non-destructive. An animal is said to be in a thermoneutral state when its metabolic heat production is unaffected by air temperature (it is not having to produce extra heat simply to keep warm). The lower limit of the thermoneutral zone is defined by the *lower critical temperature*. Below this air temperature, the animal must increase heat production in order to maintain homeothermy. The increase in heat production is a measure of the physiological cost of adaptation. Many years ago my colleagues and I carried out a series of trials with cattle kept both indoors and outside during very severe winter conditions in Alberta, Canada (Webster *et al.*, 1970). Mean air temperature in January was −24°C. In these animals cold adaptation was achieved in part by increasing food consumption, which directly increases both heat production and energy supply for heat production, and in part by growing a thicker coat. However, there was also a major change in their perception of cold. As they adapted they became progressively tolerant of low skin temperatures. This enabled them to conserve heat by reducing blood flow to the skin to the absolute minimum necessary to maintain the integrity of the tissues. The effect of this decreased sensitivity to cold was to reduce, and for most of the time eliminate, the metabolic cost of coping with cold. The lower critical temperature (the temperature below which the animals began to increase heat production through shivering) was, by February 20°C lower in those animals adapted to living outside than in those adapted to life indoors at +18°C (Figure 2.2a). Moreover, the upper limit of the zone of thermal comfort also shifted downwards to the same extent, with the result that animals adapted to living outside during the winter became intolerably hot when reintroduced to a 'comfortable' environment. This is illustrated in Figure 2.2b. When (trained) cattle were taken from outside in February and tethered in a byre at +18°C, there was a period of one hour while the snow trapped in their thick coats melted. Within one more hour they were showing signs of severe heat stress; elevated body temperature and respiration rate 180/minute. For these cold-adapted animals, 0°C was right in the middle of their comfort zone, 20°C was far too hot. What these animals were experiencing was *habituation* to cold. A generic definition of habituation is:

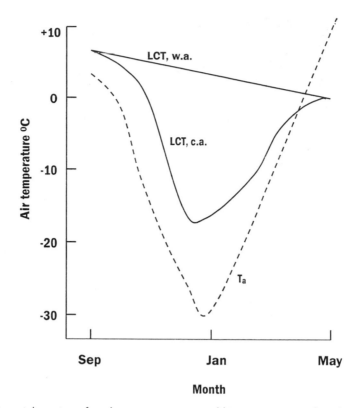

Figure 2.2a Adaptation of cattle to severe winter cold in western Canada. Changes in lower critical temperatures (LCT) of inwintered and outwintered cattle.

Gradual loss of conscious perception of or response to a repeated stimulus that permits an animal to disregard stimuli that it perceives to be irrelevant.

In this example, habituation, the psychological decision to tolerate lower skin temperatures, was a major factor in reducing and for much of the time eliminating the challenge of winter. As we shall see, the concept of habituation is more commonly used to describe adaptive responses to stimuli to the special senses. A simple example is the decision by the conscious brain 'not to hear' the constant (but unthreatening) ticking of a clock. An example more relevant to animal welfare is the habituation of farm animals to the sights and sounds of normal farm activities. At first, these sudden sights and sounds may induce an alarm response, but this will diminish and probably disappear as the animal discovers through experience that they are irrelevant because they pose no threat.

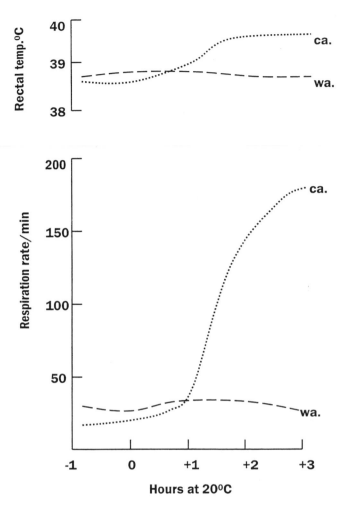

Figure 2.2b Responses of inwintered and outwintered cattle to exposure to an air temperature of 20°C. *w.a.* Warm acclimated or inwintered; *c.a.* cold acclimated or outwintered; T_a weekly average air temperatures.

2.6 Exhaustion

The aim of the adaptation response is to reduce, or ideally eliminate the challenge; in other words to 'cope'. However, the animal may fail to cope because the challenge is too severe, too complex or too prolonged, and/or because it is prevented from making an appropriate response. If so, the GAS will proceed to the stage of exhaustion (Figure 2.1b). In this stage it is common to record both severe impairment of the HPA axis and profound immunosuppression. However, I suggest that by this stage it should be obvious even to the most stubborn experimental scientist that the animal is failing to cope. Furthermore, it should be possible to predict

Table 2.5 Fat and energy reserves of beef calves, lambs and red deer calves at eight months of age (from Simpson *et al.*, 1978).

	Cattle	**Sheep**	**Red deer**
Body weight (kg)	220	36	46
Body fat (kg)	30–40	4.4–5.2	0.5–1.9
Energy stored as fat (MJ)	900–1400	220–280	20–75
Energy reserve (days) when expenditure = 1.2 intake	180–270	230–280	13–52

the time to exhaustion for a number of specific physiological stressors without recourse to inhumane severity of experimentation. I illustrate this point with another example from my studies on cold stress. The biggest problem faced by large grazing/browsing animals compelled to live outdoors during a long cold winter is not (I repeat) hypothermia resulting from acute exposure but the exhaustion of energy reserves. One of the major determinants of winter tolerance therefore is the extent of energy reserve laid down as fat at the beginning of winter.

Table 2.5 compares the fat and energy reserves of lambs, beef calves and red deer calves at the end of their first summer (Simpson *et al.*, 1978). Using conventional rules for scaling energy exchanges in animals of different size it is possible to predict the extent to which the three species of young animal could withstand chronic, moderate cold exposure, namely when energy expenditure as heat exceeds by 20% their intake of metabolisable energy in food. Table 2.5 shows that both cattle and sheep typically enter their first winter with substantial energy reserves whereas the deer calf is far less well equipped to withstand a prolonged period of cold weather. These figures provide a sufficient explanation for the practical observation that winter mortality in deer calves can be very high on the Scottish moors. There is absolutely no need to carry out experiments that expose deer to chronic cold stress to provide further 'objective' confirmation of something that is entirely predictable from first principles.

2.7 Behavioural responses to challenge

The function of normal behaviour in an animal exposed to challenge is to modify the external or internal environment in such a way as to achieve or restore the optimal (or desired) state. Taking shelter modifies the external environment, eating modifies the internal environment. All animals have some capacity to make a behavioural response to an environmental challenge. The most primitive amoeba will move away from a potentially toxic chemical. Thus behavioural responses are not the exclusive preserve of sentient animals. However, when a sentient animal is exposed to a potential environmental challenge, it is not simply programmed to a

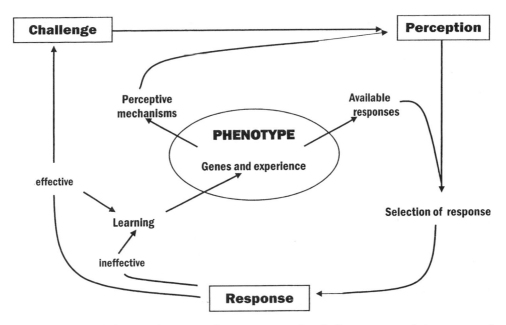

Figure 2.3 The behavioural response of a sentient animal to challenge; impact of phenotype and experience.

reflex response like an amoeba or a frog whose brain has been destroyed. It is able to make a choice from a range of potentially appropriate responses or, indeed, choose not to respond at all.

The nature of the behavioural response of a sentient animal to environmental challenge is illustrated in Figure 2.3. The animal may perceive the challenge both consciously and unconsciously according to the nature of the challenge and its own mechanisms of perception. These mechanisms of perception are first set out by the animal's genetic construction, then modified and developed by its experience. This combination of nature and nurture defines the unique neurobiological phenotype for each individual. Having perceived and, to some degree, interpreted the challenge, the sentient animal will select a behavioural response from the options available. Thus a cow caught out in the rain may shelter under a tree, but it cannot build a nest. If the behavioural response (taking shelter) can be achieved without the expenditure of too much effort, this will be the preferred choice. If shelter is available but not close to hand, the cow may choose to stand out in the rain and shiver (i.e. invoke the physiological response to cold). If the behavioural response to the challenge is effective, then the challenge will be removed or, at least, contained. The response may, on the other hand, be unsuccessful. In either event the animal will learn from the experience. When presented again by a challenge to which it has failed to mount a successful response, its perception of the challenge will be modified and it may (or may not, depending on the extent of its cognitive abilities) modify its response. If this too fails, then its welfare may be seriously compromised.

The extent to which the behavioural responses of an animal to environmental challenge may or may not be informed by cognitive processes (i.e. reasoned thinking) is a matter of great uncertainty and debate among ethologists and experimental psychologists and I shall return to this topic in Chapter 3. However, my primary concern is animal welfare not animal cognition. In this context, I am with Bentham to the last letter: 'The question is not "Can they reason?" but "Can they suffer?"' When a sentient animal is exposed to a potential stressor it feels threatened. The intensity of this feeling is a measure of the perceived threat and determines the nature of the response. The success or lack of success of the response will modify how it feels next time the threat returns. Thus the conscious response of a sentient animal to challenge is, at least in part, an emotional response, i.e. behaviour directed by *how it feels*. Whether or not this involves intelligence has no direct bearing on whether or not it suffers.

It follows from all this that sentience, the 'emotional' interpretation of incoming stimuli in terms of feelings (good, bad or indifferent), is a powerful driving force for evolution, since it helps to promote fitness both for the individual and for the species. The behavioural response of a sentient animal to an environmental challenge usually imposes less of a cost than the physiological response. The sentient animal selects from the available range behaviours intended both to correct the problem posed by the challenge and to avoid it in future (Table 2.1). Darwin considered it axiomatic that emotions, and behaviour consequent upon emotions, were not the exclusive property of humans but are present in many orders of the animal kingdom. The UK Animals (Scientific Procedures) Act (1986) formally acknowledges sentience as defined by the capacity to feel pain, suffering or distress in all vertebrates and some invertebrates (e.g. squid and lobsters).

So far I have only considered appropriate behavioural responses to environmental challenge. However, all animals (including ourselves) can exhibit a wide range of inappropriate or distinctly abnormal patterns of behaviour when under severe challenge or unable to mount an effective response. The most obvious example of 'inappropriate' behaviour when exposed to severe challenge is panic. When sheep are herded with care by an experienced, well-controlled sheep dog they respond appropriately and without obvious signs of stress. When sheep are 'worried' by a dog out of control they are liable to panic and may injure themselves by running into hedges (or over cliffs!). However, the fact that sheep behave inappropriately when in a state of panic does not make them stupid. So do we. The skill of the shepherd lies in understanding the natural appropriate behaviour of the animals in his or her care when in the presence of a perceived threat such as a dog or man, and adapting his or her behaviour (and that of his/her dog) in such a way as to minimise stress for all parties.

The other category of abnormal behaviour is that which may develop when an animal has been unable, through its actions, to resolve the difference between the

Table 2.6 Behavioural indices of good and bad welfare.

Welfare status	Category of behaviour	Examp
Measures of good welfare	Full expression of normal behaviour (ethogram)	Maintenance behaviour Social behaviour Rest and play
	Expression of pleasure	Play Hedonism
Effective coping behaviour	Maintenance behaviour	Rest, grooming Seeking food and water
	Orientation and startle responses	Alertness Response to novel objects
	Normal defence behaviour	Flight, fight, freezing Ritualised responses
	Avoidance behaviour	Shelter Avoiding perceived threats
Abnormal behaviour	Abnormal body posture and movement	Lameness 'Dog-sitting'
	Injurious behaviour	Tail biting (pigs) Feather pecking (hens)
	Stereotypies	Bar chewing (pigs) Weaving and box walking (horses)
	Redirected behaviours	Sham dust bathing (hens) Sham ruminating
	Suppression of normal behaviour	Inappetence Learned helplessness

environment as it exists and that which it desires. In these circumstances an animal may exhibit one or more patterns of abnormal behaviour that are at least pointless and, in some cases, positively harmful. Examples of abnormal behaviour are listed in Table 2.6. Whether or not these activities help an animal to cope with stress arising from the frustration of normal responses to environmental stimuli (or lack of stimuli), their very presence should alert us to the existence of a welfare problem.

2.8 Behavioural indices of good and bad welfare

Since behaviour is what an animal does to cope with challenge and promote its welfare, it follows that observations of behaviour are central to the evaluation of its welfare. This applies especially to those measures of behaviour that may indicate that an animal is having difficulty in coping or failing to cope with environmental challenge. Table 2.6 lists three categories of behaviour that may be used to indicate the welfare status of an animal. The first category comprises the natural, functional patterns of behaviour that may be associated with the expression of good welfare in a good, low-stress environment. One of the core routines of ethology is to draw an *ethogram* for the species under investigation. The ethogram describes the full repertoire of major activities identified by the observer (e.g. eating, drinking, resting, grooming, socialising) and the relative amount of time allocated to each. Approaches to measuring the ethogram are described by Martin & Bateson (1993). It should be self-evident that such measurements should extend over the full 24-hour cycle. The ethogram measured in a 'natural' environment that presents challenges, but challenges with which the animal can cope, can act as a yardstick against which to compare patterns of behaviour in an environment that may present a welfare problem, either because it presents difficult challenges or because it restricts the expression of natural behaviour. This latter criterion needs to be assessed with care. Some elements of the ethogram may reflect a powerful internal drive that exists independent of external circumstances. The existence of sham dust bathing in caged hens is an illustration in point. Other behaviours may be specific to the environment, for example pigs wallow only when they perceive the need to cool down. A 'normal' ethogram indicative of satisfactory welfare should include, at least, the full expression of normal patterns of maintenance and social behaviour. An example of the former is grooming. If an animal is unable to groom itself, or fails to groom itself, through injury or apathy, this suggests poor welfare. An example of the latter is 'correct' social behaviour, i.e. the expression and performance of appropriate, non-injurious social interactions. Other expressions of satisfactory welfare in a low-stress environment include rest and play (for those species and ages that indulge in play).

It is also appropriate to look for indices of positive welfare in animals or, if you will excuse the expression, pleasure. While play may be interpreted by many stern ethologists as no more than a learning activity, e.g. training predators for the hunt, it is, I believe, practically impossible to avoid the conclusion that kittens or lambs or otters at play are having fun. It is positively mulish to suggest that the cat that purrs as it is stroked in a warm lap is experiencing anything other than the pleasure of pure hedonism.

The second category comprises those behaviours that indicate that an animal is coping with challenge (Table 2.6). These include appropriate patterns of maintenance behaviour designed to restore comfort and vigour, e.g. extra grooming after exposure to dirty conditions, or rest following exertion. They also include appropriate responses to the presence of a potential source of alarm. These include a constructive degree of alertness and response to the appearance of a novel object or novel experience. When the threat is both real and understood such as that presented by the appearance of another animal, the animal can select an appropriate response from its repertoire. The most obvious forms of this response involve fight, flight or freezing. However, most sentient animals faced by repeated exposures to potentially threatening contacts with other animals, especially those of their own species, develop a series of ritualised behaviours that serve to avoid physical damage (or too much loss of face) to either party. The stable hierarchy that ensues (the 'pecking order') not only reduces stress, but also saves effort. It is relevant to point out here that the signals used by animals in stable groups to remind each other of their place in the pecking order may be very subtle and can be missed even by the most diligent ethologist.

The third category comprises those abnormal patterns of behaviour that may be used as indices of poor welfare. The Commission of the European Communities (CEC, 1983) identified the following types of behaviour as likely to 'indicate severe abnormality or disturbance':

- Abnormal body posture and movement indicative of pain or discomfort, e.g. lameness, 'dog-sitting' in sows and cattle in stalls.
- Injurious behaviours, e.g. tail biting in pigs, feather pecking in hens, self-mutilation in dogs.
- Stereotyped behaviours: fixed patterns of behaviour performed repetitively and having no obvious function, e.g. bar chewing in sows, crib-biting and weaving in horses.
- Redirected behaviours performed with abnormal frequency or intensity in the absence of an appropriate substrate (environmental resource), e.g. sham dust bathing in hens, sham rumination in veal calves.
- Apathetic behaviour: apparent loss of interest in positive or negative environmental stimuli, e.g. inappetence, 'learned helplessness'.

The interpretation of abnormal patterns of behaviour, such as stereotypies or injurious feather pecking, in terms of how the animals actually feel is a complex and uncertain business that can be left to subsequent chapters. To give one example: feather pecking leading to cannibalism in poultry may appear at first sight to be a simple case of unnatural aggression. In fact, it is in most cases more likely to be a non-aggressive 'mindless' expression of investigatory behaviour (Chapter 5). However, whatever may be the motivation, the existence of feather pecking in a flock of birds denotes bad welfare for the simple reason that birds are being injured or killed.

2.9 Integration of measures: triangulation

The purpose of this chapter has been to outline the physiological and behavioural measurements that can be used to assess the welfare of an animal as it seeks to cope with the challenges of life. Each animal has a range of reflex, instinctive and conscious responses. The sentient animal can (up to a point) select conscious behavioural responses from its available repertoire according to how it feels. We,

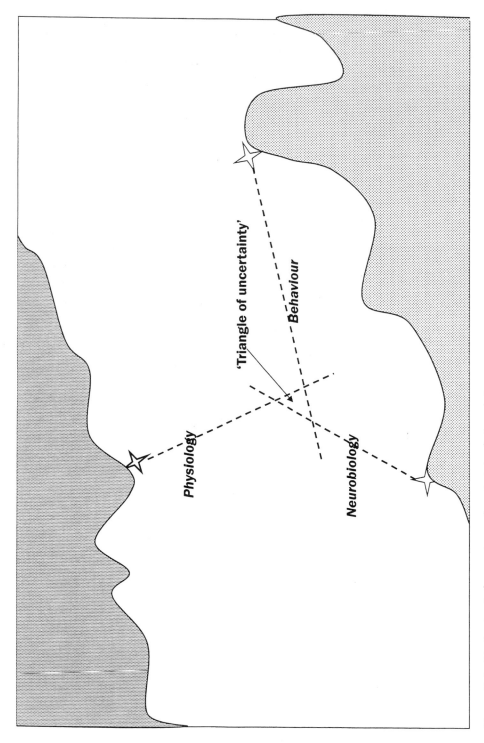

Figure 2.4 Navigation in fuzzy science: the principle of triangulation.

the human observers, make measurements of its physiological and behavioural responses and from this seek to draw conclusions as to its welfare state. However, the measurements described in this chapter allow us to do no more than make an educated guess as to how an animal feels. The assessment of welfare state from measurements of physiology and behaviour is therefore a 'fuzzy' science in which nothing is certain.

When faced by an area of fuzzy science that is built upon a long list of measurements, none of which can be assumed to be precise, it is good practice to adopt the technique of *triangulation*. Figure 2.4 illustrates this by reference to my favourite recreation, offshore sailing. In the days before satellite navigation made it all too easy, it was necessary to estimate one's position by obtaining bearings on fixed marks, either from a visual signal (e.g. a lighthouse) or from a radio signal. The former are moderately reliable, the latter much less so. Now a bearing on a single mark gives only a position line. Bearings on two marks close to one another or close to 180° apart do not add to the available information. Bearings on two marks that give two position lines (ideally intersecting at about 90°) give one an apparent fix, but one cannot be certain of its accuracy. However, if one takes bearings from three judiciously selected marks one can create a 'triangle of uncertainty' (Figure 2.4). The more accurate the bearings, the smaller the triangle.

Estimating one's position in welfare science carries a similar degree of uncertainty. In Figure 2.4 I have identified three scientific bearings that may be used to estimate both the welfare state of an animal *and* how it feels. None of the approaches is inherently better or worse than any other. For example, measurement of a physiological marker such as glucocorticoid concentration in plasma is sometimes called 'objective' and thereby considered more 'scientific' than the subjective observation of behaviour. This notion is seriously flawed. The measurement of cortisol concentration is neither more nor less objective than the measurement of time spent in stereotypic behaviour. Both are simply observations. It is pointless to stack up physiological measurements of stress and poor welfare (cortisol, acute-phase proteins, etc.) since they come from the same source so will do no more than confirm the position line. This chapter has mainly considered the assessment of welfare state by taking bearings on two beacons, physiology and behaviour. These beacons are relatively easy to spot and, when used together, can give an approximate impression as to welfare state. However, if we really wish to explore how an animal feels we have no option but to seek a bearing on a third beacon within the mind and within the brain. This will be the theme of the next chapter.

Sentience, Sense and Suffering 3

Beasts are engaged in thought and reason as well as men. Reason is, and ought to be, the slave of the passions, and can never pretend to any other office than to serve and obey them.

David Hume (1711–1776)

The previous chapter, 'Challenge and Response', described the scientific approach to understanding how animals respond to challenge from the environment, either through behaviour (taking action) or by modifying their physiology. This approach is sufficient to identify threats to animal welfare and indicate their severity in terms of their outcome, namely the degree of difficulty experienced by an animal in coping with challenges to its well-being. If we accept that we have a moral responsibility to protect animals in our care from welfare abuse, then evidence that an animal is having difficulty in coping with a threat to its welfare is sufficient reason for action designed to remove or at least reduce that threat. Most of the readers of this book will, I am sure, take this principle as self-evident. It is, moreover, enshrined in the 1911 Protection of Animals Act that it is an offence to 'cause unnecessary suffering [to any animal] by doing or omitting to do any act'. This establishes in law the fact that when we impose a sufficient insult to the welfare of an animal, that animal suffers. The 1911 Act has served us well, but is ripe for review. Two of its greatest deficiencies are that: (1) the expression 'any animal' has usually been interpreted in an anthropocentric manner to focus on those species that have been allotted a high extrinsic value by humans; and (2) no offence occurs until unnecessary suffering has been established (whether through a sin of commission or omission). Despite its title, the 1911 Act does not require owners to make provision to protect their animals from the risk of incurring unnecessary suffering.

I discuss the present and future evolution of animal welfare law in more detail in Chapters 10 and 11. The key question at this stage is: '*What is suffering?*' This begets a family of more specific questions.

- How do animals feel as they interpret incoming information from the external environment (e.g. the appearance of a predator) and sensation from the internal environment (e.g. pain)?

- How are the nature and intensity of their feelings determined by their inherited genetic constitution and their individual experience?
- How much do these feelings matter to an animal?
- Can we infer that when non-human animals feel bad, they actually experience suffering?

These questions are central not only to the legal interpretation of the meaning of unnecessary suffering but also to the whole moral basis for our treatment of animals. In this sense, they are philosophical questions. If we accept the principle of autonomy or 'Do as you would be done by', then if we can show that feelings matter to an animal they should matter to us too. History has shown us that most problems first identified by philosophers have been well served (if not entirely resolved) by the application of good science. The rules of good science, the 'scientific method', are as follows:

- Comprehensive, unprejudiced review of the evidence.
- Creation of a logical hypothesis based on all the available evidence (not just a selection of the favourable evidence).
- Challenge of the hypothesis by experiments designed not to support it but to test it to destruction.
- Confirmation and development, or rejection and modification of the hypothesis on the basis of the evidence and irrespective of previous convictions.

Many of those most passionately committed to honourable causes such as animal welfare, environmental protection, the brotherhood of man, tend to view science and scientists as powerful and dangerous enemies. Undoubtedly scientific knowledge confers power and all power can be dangerous, not least because scientific knowledge does not confer a monopoly of the truth. Moreover, *scientists*, as people, are no more or less venial and inadequate than anyone else. Nevertheless, when it abides by these rules, the scientific method is an intelligent, honest and unprejudiced way to advance knowledge and seek the truth. The consequences of applying science may be good or bad for reasons attributable to good or bad intentions, or simply unforeseen. Nevertheless, the scientific method *per se* can be seen as a moral virtue. The cautious, evidence-based virtue of the scientific method becomes especially important when addressing an issue so emotionally and morally fraught as suffering in animals.

3.1 A sentient view of the world

I have already defined sentience as 'feelings that matter'. Figure 3.1 presents a more detailed conceptual (though not anatomical!) picture of how I believe a sentient animal interprets the stimuli and sensations it receives and what motivates it to respond. The 'control centres' of any animal (the central nervous system or CNS)

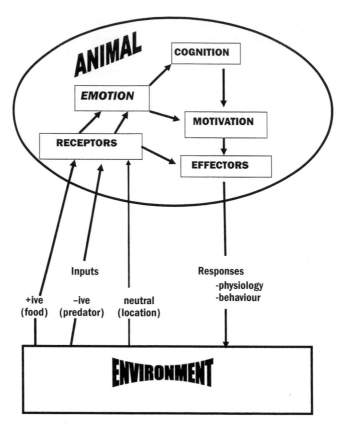

Figure 3.1   Sentience: an emotional view of the world.

are constantly being fed with information from the external and internal environment. Much information, e.g. our proprioceptive perception of how we stand and move in space, is processed at a subconscious level. Having learned to walk, we are able to control our limbs without recourse to thought or emotion. However, any stimulus that calls for a conscious decision as to action must involve some degree of interpretation. This interpretation may or may not involve a cognitive element leading to a reasoned response. Classical Darwinian theory requires that in all sentient animals (including humans), conscious interpretation of incoming sensation and the motivation to respond must have an emotional component. Indeed, I would argue that this is implicit in the word sentience*. The two quotations from David Hume that preface this chapter deftly illustrate his views as to the limits of pure reason.

---

* Experimental psychologists tend to avoid use of the word 'emotion', preferring 'affect'. Apparently they consider the former word to be too emotional. Personally, I consider the latter to be too affected.

To illustrate this point, let us consider the interpretation of a primitive and ubiquitous sensation, namely hunger. The centre responsible for control of appetite and satiety (which can be located with some precision in the brain) will respond to an internal stimulus such as a low concentration of glucose in the blood, a natural external stimulus in the form of a meal, or a conditioning external stimulus (e.g. the bell that preceded the meal for Pavlov's dogs). A wide range of signals, sights, smells and sounds will impact on receptors within the CNS. This information will be modulated by other information from within the CNS acquired partly from experience and partly from innate signals that identify, for example, an appetising smell. Information will pass downstream from this processing centre defined within the general category of 'food'. At the next processing centre the information will be interpreted in an emotional way. If the animal is hungry but no food is available it will experience a negative emotion (i.e. feel bad to a lesser or greater degree). When an appetising meal appears, it will experience a positive emotion, i.e. it will feel good.

This psychological concept of mind makes a clear distinction between the reception, categorisation and interpretation of incoming stimuli. Although it may appear abstract it has received strong support from classical physiology. Keith Kendrick (1998), for example, has made recordings from single neurones within the brains of sheep presented with external stimuli, or photographic images of external stimuli. A wide range of images (e.g. sacks of grains, bales of hay) triggers signals in a family of neurones that may be said to convey the generic information 'food'. A second set of stimuli or images, e.g. dogs and men, are categorised within the first processing centre and passed to a family of neurones that indicate 'predator'. Once again this categorisation of incoming information as 'predator' will be modulated by other inputs from within the CNS, whether innate or based on experience. The innate fear of snakes in humans and other primates is a case in point. When this information reaches the second processing centre it stimulates a family of neurones that transmit a negative emotion (feeling bad). In this simple example a wide range of stimuli has been first categorised as information, then interpreted as a positive or negative emotion. However, if the sheep is now presented with a picture of a human carrying a sack of food, two categories of information (food and predator) are passed to the emotion centre, evaluated and passed on as a single, unconfused emotional message, namely 'good'.

The animal's decision as to how (or indeed whether) to respond is therefore determined by how it feels, good or bad. Moreover, in a sentient animal (as distinct from, perhaps, an insect) the interpretation of information as good or bad is not a simple yes/no decision. The intensity of its feelings will vary. It will, for example, feel more or less hungry, more or less afraid, and this will determine the strength of its motivation to respond in positive or negative fashion. Thus by studying the strength of motivation of an animal to seek or avoid the feelings it associates with certain sensations and experiences we can obtain a measure of how much these feelings matter.

The classic but outdated Pavlovian stimulus/response concept of animal psychology held that most non-human animals simply react to stimuli that directly or indirectly predict a reward or punishment, e.g. a bell that presages the arrival of food or an electric shock. This permits animals to learn what is good and bad for them, but it does not require any degree of reasoning leading to a considered response. While this deliberate rejection of higher intelligence in animals can now be put down to ignorance on our part, I suggest, with the benefit of hindsight, that many of the subtler experiments based on the stimulus/response hypothesis do identify elements of the strength and persistency of response that can only be interpreted as strength of motivation or strength of feeling. In other words, they recognise sentience.

There is now abundant evidence that mammals and birds can employ cognition to interpret incoming sensation in reasoned fashion. One of the first and best proofs of this ability was the demonstration that rats will accumulate spatial information, e.g. routes through a maze, whether or not that information presents any immediate reward. Tolman (see Roitblat, 1987) introduced rats to mazes with two exits. In one group, a food reward was provided at one exit only. After an average of 12 trials almost all rats unerringly took the route to the exit where food was provided. In the other group, no reward was offered, in the first instance, at either exit. Unsurprisingly the rats showed no consistent preference as to route. However, when these rats were subsequently offered food at one exit only they learnt the correct route after only three to four trials. The only convincing explanation for this is that during the first stage of the trial they had, in the absence of any reward, been gathering spatial information for interpretation and use at such time as they might need it.

In Figure 3.1, I include a category of incoming information as 'neutral'. This obviously includes spatial information. It also includes other things such as time of day. Neither of these things can be directly categorised as good or bad; they are simply information. However, they may be interpreted, whether cognitively or through simple stimulus/response, in emotional fashion. Thus the approach of five o'clock can signal the excitement of tea-time as well to a dog as it can to an aunt.

The nature and extent of the cognitive abilities of animals is a fascinating topic of research and morally important to improve our understanding of the animals that we choose to exploit for our own ends. For an introduction to further reading see Roitblat (1987) and Shettleworth (1998). However, it would be a mistake to infer that the capacity of an animal to suffer is proportional to the extent of its cognitive ability (its intelligence). I have already noted that pain, for example, is a physical and emotional phenomenon. Rational interpretation of the sensation of pain can make things either better or worse. However, if welfare is determined by how an animal feels, it is the emotional response that matters. The strength of motivation of a sentient animal to respond to its impressions of incoming stimuli

Table 3.1 A sentient perception of stimulus and response: sequence of events.

(1) Perception of incoming stimuli as categories of information.

(2) Interpretation of information categories:
- positive and negative emotions
- stored information.

(3) Motivation or aversion (the measure of behavioural need).

(4) Measured response from repertoire of available behaviours.

(5) Emotional (and possibly cognitive) assessment of effectiveness of action.

(6) Modification of mood and understanding in the light of experience.

and sensations will always be directed by emotion, sometimes, possibly, reinforced by cognition (Mendl & Paul, 2004). Some animals may have the mental capacity and the stored information to choose a 'reasoned' response. However, all sentient animals, and this list includes humans, will always be motivated, at least in part, by emotion. The only beings that to my knowledge are completely devoid of emotion are the Vulcans, as epitomised by Mr Spock. However, as all Star Trekkies will appreciate, this may be life but not as we know it.

Table 3.1 summarises the steps involved in the process whereby a sentient animal perceives and interprets incoming sensation and information, how this motivates it to respond, how it evaluates the consequences of its actions and how this evaluation influences its subsequent mood, understanding and behaviour. Having evaluated incoming sensation in emotional, and possibly cognitive, fashion, the animal makes a measured response, reflecting the extent to which it feels this to be a 'behavioural need'. The aim is to manipulate the environment and so adjust the inputs in such a way as to make it feel better. Having acted, the animal then assesses, emotionally and possibly cognitively, the effectiveness of its response. If the response is successful this will modulate its subsequent perception and interpretation of incoming sensation in a way that accentuates the positive and eliminates (or reduces) the negative. In consequence it will feel better. If its response is ineffective or if it is prevented by environmental or other constraints from behaving in a way designed to improve how it feels, then it is likely to feel worse.

This evolution of mood (emotion or affect) in the light of genotype and experience will have long-term consequences for welfare since it will be a key indicator of the animal's success, or otherwise, in coping with stress. When we observe the behaviour of an animal faced by an environmental challenge we can only measure the effectiveness of its response, we cannot know how it feels. However, if we seek to measure the motivation and strength of motivation of an animal to meet its behavioural needs in the light of its own genotype and experience, then we are getting close to measuring the strength of its feelings.

3.2 Motivation: the analysis of behavioural needs

Having defined sentience as 'feelings that matter' it is now necessary to consider how we can discover what things matter to a non-human animal and measure how much they matter. Paradoxically, it is probably easier to get reliable information from animals as to the strength of their desires and aversions than it is from humans, since animals seldom cheat and never delude themselves. I discuss elsewhere the huge gap that exists between the overwhelming majority of folk who express a *desire* for improved welfare standards for farm animals and the underwhelming minority who actually *demand* food produced to high welfare standards. In the study of motivation, what we say can be an irrelevance and a distorting one at that. What matters is what an animal (or human) is prepared to *do* to obtain, or avoid, some element of the environment to which it is exposed.

Table 3.2 outlines the most common approaches to the measurement of motivation and behavioural needs in animals. I shall briefly consider each of these in order. The study of motivation has become a complex field of experimental psychology. For those who wish to explore this in more detail I recommend Dawkins (1990), Houston (1997) and Mason *et al.* (1998). I shall keep this section fairly simple and

Table 3.2 Measurement of motivation and behavioural needs.

Motivational priorities
- Preference tests:
  short term, e.g. food selection
  long term, e.g. food v. rest, comfort v. companionship

Strength of motivation
- What will I pay:
  to achieve, e.g., space, a nest?
  to avoid, e.g., cold, isolation?
- What will I sacrifice:
  to achieve, e.g., comfort, security?
  to avoid, e.g., pain, fear?

Consequences of denial
- Altered behaviour
  Redirected behaviour, e.g. displacement activity
  Rebound behaviour
  Stereotypic behaviour
- Altered mood
  Altered strength of motivation
  Altered 'awareness' of environmental stimuli
  Learned helplessness

seek only to illustrate ways whereby motivational experiments can be used to assess the behavioural needs of animals, with particular emphasis on one key element of experimental design, namely 'Does the animal understand the question?'

3.2.1 Motivational priorities

The conventional approach to measuring motivational priorities in animals is through the *preference test*. An animal is presented with a choice. A cat, for example, may be invited to make a choice between two (or more) sorts of food; a hen may be invited to choose between different varieties of floor surface (e.g. wire v. sand v. wood shavings). Such experiments are simple but can be valuable when interpreted with care. Some preferences may be trivial, e.g. children offered a choice of identical-tasting chocolate buttons prefer red to blue. However, if a large majority of cats show a preference for a particular food flavour, this information is worth millions to a pet food manufacturer. If an overwhelming proportion of hens show an aversion to standing on wire floors (or a particular design of wire floor) then that floor is demonstrably unsatisfactory.

A classic tool for preference testing is the 'T-maze'. This has three compartments: a 'start box' and two 'goal boxes' that differ in the resource they provide. A rat, for example, may be presented with two goal boxes, one a barren cage, the other an enriched environment with bedding, secure shelter and 'malleable substrates' (things to do). The rat is placed in the start box. When the door is opened, the rat (being a rat) will explore, turn both left and right, discover both goal boxes and, in this example, probably choose to spend more time in the enriched environment. This can be interpreted as a clear preference, although the rat (being a rat) will almost certainly continue to visit the less-favoured environment – just in case.

The T-maze would appear to be soluble by the simplest of minds. For rats it is a piece of cheese. However, even so simple an experiment can go awry. It is routine experimental design to randomise the position of the goal boxes to overcome any directional preference (e.g. right turn preferred to left). However, the T-maze remains a profoundly unnatural experience. The animal is removed from the security of its home pen, isolated, placed in strange surroundings, then expected to explore options in its new environment in order to indicate a preference. In such circumstances (and in my experience) a hen may fail to explore because it is alarmed by the novelty, a broiler chicken may fail to explore because it hurts to move, a cow because it simply cannot be bothered. Training may or may not overcome these problems. Another problem is that the animal may interpret the experience in a quite unforeseen way. Two examples (which shall be nameless) are of note. Mice, offered a variety of 'enriched' compartments at the end of tunnels of plastic tubing chose to spend much of their time in the tunnels. Horses invited to select a preferred bedding type in two adjacent boxes spent much of their time in the passage between. In each case the animals demonstrated a preference for something the experimenter had not foreseen. In the former case, the mice presumably preferred the security of the narrow tunnels to the more exposed goal boxes. In the latter case, the horses clearly preferred to stand in the interconnecting passage because they could obtain a limited view out into the yard.

3.2.2 Strength of motivation

In her books *Animal Suffering* (1980) and *Through Our Eyes Only* (1993), Marian Dawkins pioneered the application of consumer demand theory to the measurement of motivation and behavioural needs in animals. Her approach is to measure the value of a particular resource to an animal in terms of the work it is prepared to perform, or the other resources that it is prepared to sacrifice, in order to achieve that resource. The strength of motivation is a measure of how much that resource *matters*. In its simplest form a rat may be asked to press a button repeatedly in order to obtain a resource such as food, warmth or the company of another rat. Alternatively a hen may be compelled to work harder by pushing against heavier and heavier doors or walking further and further to achieve a desired goal such as a nest box. It has been demonstrated quite beyond dispute that the motivation of hens to seek a nest box (or something they perceive to be a nest box) in which to lay their eggs is almost independent of the amount of work they must perform to reach it. In the jargon of consumer demand theory, this motivation is 'price-inelastic'. A positive result such as this is convincing proof that the presence of a suitable nesting site for laying hens is a clear behavioural need, indeed a necessity of life.

At the other end of the spectrum of behavioural needs defined by experiments that measure strength of motivation are those commodities and resources that the animal will use if they come at little or no cost, but will not work hard to achieve. These may be termed completely 'price-elastic' or, in common parlance, luxuries. In between the extremes of complete price elasticity and inelasticity it is possible to draw (or devise) an almost infinite variety of cost–demand curves for different resources and interpret them in an almost infinite variety of ways (Mason *et al.*, 1998; Kirkden *et al.*, 2003). In the context of this book, whose main goal is to achieve practical improvements in animal welfare, the distinction between a necessity and a luxury assumes considerable political importance. It is, for example, central to new legislation to define minimum acceptable environmental standards for caged hens. I shall consider this specific debate in detail in Chapter 5.

There are, however, a number of generic problems associated with the interpretation of experiments in which animals are invited to do work to achieve a specified resource. Where the results are unequivocal then the interpretation is easy. Laying hens, for example, are clearly motivated to seek a nest box. However, many strength of motivation experiments tend to be more ambiguous. I shall illustrate this with a simple example. Trained chickens have demonstrated their motivation to push through an increasingly heavy door in order to get to food. As expected, the motivation for food is very price-inelastic. Suppose now that these or other chickens are repeatedly put through the same experimental procedure but where the 'reward' is not food but the presence of another chicken; the hypothesis being that one chicken might be highly motivated to seek the company of another (e.g. for security, companionship or sex). In this trial, let us say, the chickens will push through the door only if it involves little or no effort. The straightforward interpretation of these results is that access to a conspecific (another chicken) is more price-elastic than access to food, and this could be interpreted politically as a less important behavioural need. This is indeed one possible explanation, but there are others. For example: (1) the chicken simply does not visualise the existence of other animals in their absence. In other words, 'out of sight, out of mind'. If this is so, the bird may not remember from former trials that the door leads to a companion. Thus its only motivation to press through the door is curiosity in the absence of a specific goal, and this curiosity is very price-elastic; or (2) if the prime motivation to join a companion animal is one of security, the animal, may, in the strange environment of the test chamber, feel more secure if it simply does nothing until it is released.

The motivation to search for food is an innate part of the genetic blueprint for survival in any animal. Thus the sensation of hunger will obviously motivate an animal to seek food in its absence. Indeed, the longer the absence, the greater the motivation. However, I can think of no evolutionary reason why one animal should possess such a powerful innate motivation to seek the company of another that it will perform unnatural acts (e.g. pushing through heavy doors), except, of course, for sex. However, the observation that an animal does not perform positive (and unnatural) tasks to seek the presence of a conspecific does not necessarily imply that it would not experience distress (without necessarily understanding the cause of its distress) when separated from other animals, whose presence it may value whether simply for security or owing to a more subtle awareness of the benefits of companionship.

In general, I would suggest that strength of motivation experiments, involving the performance of tasks not obviously linked to their goal, are most valuable when they address internal drives, such as those related to nutrition and reproduction. They are less successful when they are applied to external sources of motivation and aversion, often because the animal fails to make the association between the problem it is set and its own perception of how to address its behavioural needs. Communicating with animals is like communicating with foreigners. We should not assume that because they fail to understand us, it is they who are unintelligent.

3.2.3 The Octagon: an approach to the measurement of shifting motivational priorities

I am only too aware of the superficiality of this discussion of motivation research, but this is a book on animal welfare, not animal behaviour. However, before I leave the subject, I wish to describe a facility designed for the study of motivation and aversion of farm animals to elements of their external environment which was developed by my colleague Christopher Wathes at the Silsoe Research Institute. His Octagon consists of eight chambers, structurally identical and each with provision to supply food and water. The chambers can be isolated or linked by doors through which an animal such as a pig or chicken can move at will. Each chamber is independently ventilated and the thermal environment can be controlled by the use of infra-red heaters. Animals enter the octagon and may stay there for weeks. Thus it becomes their home territory.

The first experiments we carried out in the Octagon were designed to explore whether pigs are aversive to concentrations of atmospheric ammonia similar to those they may encounter on commercial farm units (Jones et al., 1999). We had previously used conventional approaches (preference tests, bar-pressing tests) in an attempt to discover whether (or at what point) the smell of ammonia was sufficient to overcome the motivation of pigs for food. Not entirely surprisingly, these initial experiments were inconclusive. In the Octagon, however, pigs were able to express their preferences simply by moving from one area of their home territory to another (no unnatural acts were involved). The choices they were offered included access to warmth (from the infra-red heaters), access to a companion (another pig) and exposure to concentrations of ammonia ranging from 0–40 parts per million (ppm). Their choices were subtle but important. In general, the pigs showed no aversion to entering compartments at ammonia concentrations up to 40 ppm. Furthermore, for the most part they preferred a compartment that provided the comfort of an infra-red heater or another pig (another excellent source of warmth) even at 40 ppm ammonia to a compartment that provided fresh air but none of the other creature comforts. However, consistently, after about 40 minutes in a preferred compartment at high ammonia concentrations, pigs would leave and spend a period of time in fresh air (0 ppm ammonia). We concluded from these experiments that pigs show no significant aversion to the smell of ammonia and, most of the time, any aversion to ammonia was overridden by the more powerful motivation for warmth and/or the presence of another pig. However, notwithstanding these primary drives, the pigs did display a delayed aversion to living in a high ammonia concentration, and so, from time to time, expressed a secondary motivation to seek fresh air.

These experiments illustrate several important points. The first, practical conclusion is that pigs like fresh air, not all the time, but from time to time. Thus accommodation that may have a smelly bedding area but access to the outdoors is likely to be more in accord with the pigs' behavioural needs than one that offers no choice. The second conclusion is that it was not the smell of ammonia that they sought to avoid but, probably, an increasing sense of malaise associated with prolonged confinement in a polluted environment. There are also several generic lessons for motivation studies. Wherever possible, motivational experiments should be conducted over extended periods in an environment that the animals perceive as home. Moreover, they should not require the animals to perform any actions that they would not normally perform at home.

Another merit of relatively long-term experiments of this sort is that they can reveal elements of secondary motivation that may be missed in short term preference (or strength of preference) trials. To give a crude but convincing illustration of what I mean; a simple record of the time spent by humans in two 'goal boxes' (bedroom and lavatory) during normal sleeping hours would conclude that we are far more highly motivated to spend time in the former. However, when the secondary motivation to visit the lavatory manifests itself, it can override everything else.

3.3 Altered and abnormal behaviour

3.3.1 Consequences of denial: altered behaviour

Another approach to the assessment of behavioural needs in animals is to observe the behavioural consequences of denying an animal the resources necessary to perform a natural function. Table 3.2 identifies three categories of altered or abnormal behaviour: redirected behaviour, rebound behaviour and stereotypic behaviour. Evidence of such activities may be used to support the argument that an animal is lacking the environmental resource (commonly called 'substrate' by experimental psychologists) for certain normal patterns of behaviour. However, once again I must stress that observations of what animals do cannot directly reveal how they feel. More subtle experiments are necessary to address the nature of animal mood (or affect).

3.3.2 Redirected behaviour

When an animal is aroused by an intense stimulus, then denied the opportunity to make a satisfactory response it will frequently embark on a pattern of *displacement behaviour*, activity that appears purposeful but which is not directed towards the main stimulus. A typical example of this may be observed in the sequence of events when two male animals confront one another. After a fight, or more likely a ritual of threatening activities designed to establish dominance, the subordinate animal will withdraw and typically embark at once on an intense bout of self-grooming. A human animal may storm off to wash the car (or the pots). We assume (without proof but by analogy with ourselves) that animals use such displacement behaviour to reduce the intensity of acute unpleasant feelings; in this case frustration of the primary reward.

The motivation behind more chronic forms of redirected behaviour is less clear. Feather pecking in hens presents a major obstacle to the development of welfare-improved alternatives to the battery cage. Much time and money has been invested in the study of the motivation underlying feather pecking on the basis that if we knew why hens did it, we would be better equipped to prevent it. The theory that feather pecking is an expression of aggression has been largely discounted and many would now describe it as redirected ground pecking behaviour, the implication being that if one could provide the 'correct' substrate then injurious feather pecking would cease to be a problem. I shall discuss this in more detail in Chapter 5. In the present context, however, I suggest that we cannot, by defining feather pecking as redirected behaviour, conclude that the bird doing the pecking is expressing frustration at the denial of an essential behavioural need. There is clearly a welfare problem for the birds that get pecked, but, so far as the peckers are concerned, it is quite as valid to suggest that the behaviour is completely mindless. Using feather pecking as a specific example of a generic condition, I can accept that chronic redirected behaviour may well signify the absence of a desirable environmental substrate (resource). I do not believe that, taken in isolation, it can be cited as evidence of distress arising from frustration.

3.3.3 Rebound behaviour

If an animal is prevented from performing a particular action designed to satisfy a behavioural need, then it may devote an unusually long time to that action when, once again, it becomes possible. This is called rebound behaviour. To give an obvious example: an animal abnormally deprived of food will overeat when its food supply is restored unless, of course, it has become weak from starvation. This is a simple expression of adaptation to (or exhaustion by) the stress of hunger. Lorenz (1966) suggested that the motivation of animals to a wide range of behaviour patterns such as exploration and hunting builds up during periods of denial, expresses itself during deprivation as displacement activity and thereafter as rebound behaviour. Although the Lorenz 'Hydraulic Model' of motivation has been largely discounted as a general hypothesis, the search for rebound behaviour in animals may be used to investigate certain welfare problems, in particular the frustration that may arise from close confinement (denial of space) in farm animals such as the pregnant sow or laying hen.

3.3.4 Stereotypic behaviour

Animals in barren environments with 'nothing to do', i.e. little opportunity to make a constructive contribution to the quality of their own existence, may, over a period of weeks, months or years, develop stereotypic patterns of behaviour. A *stereotypy* is defined as the repetitive, invariant performance of an activity that is apparently purposeless because it is not directed towards any obvious reward. Stereotypies may be loosely categorised as *movement* or *oral*. Rodents confined in barren environments (e.g. *Clethrionomys glareolus*, the bank vole) may develop movement stereotypies such as 'looping' (similar to turning somersaults). Dogs may obsessively chase their tails. Children confined in barren homes may show stereotypic rocking and 'head-banging'. Sows confined in barren stalls may develop the oral stereotypy bar-chewing. Stabled horses can display both movement stereotypies such as weaving and box-walking and oral stereotypies such as crib-biting and wind-sucking. I shall consider these in more detail when discussing the welfare of farm, companion and laboratory animals. At this stage I am only considering in general terms the extent to which the appearance of stereotypic behaviour can be used as an index of poor welfare. It is clear that certain stereotypic behaviours can compromise fitness. Weaving horses lose body condition. Wind-sucking in horses (swallowing air) is associated with colic, although cause and effect are in dispute (Chapter 10).

The conventional (and uncontroversial) interpretation of stereotypic behaviour is that it is a mechanism for coping with a lack of the resources necessary for normal behaviour. This may be extended to the assumption that it is a response to the denial of behavioural needs and therefore an indication that welfare has been compromised. However, once again, we cannot directly infer what animals feel from what they do. The zoo elephant, observed to be weaving or pen walking, may be expressing frustration at the general absence of environmental enrichment, or engaging in displacement activity as it hears its keeper arrive with the next meal. In both cases it is fair to conclude that it is acting to manipulate its state of arousal. However, in the former instance, it may be seeking to cope with chronic frustration in a barren environment, in the latter to cope with (or even wind up) acute excitement prior to a meal. The welfare implications of these two suggested motivations are very different.

3.3.5 Consequences of denial: altered mood

If we are to achieve a proper understanding of the welfare consequences of denying animals access to resources assumed necessary for normal behaviour, then we need to explore the direct effects of denial on their mood, i.e. how they feel. The study of animal mood (affect) is in its infancy relative to the study of animal behaviour, yet it is inherently more relevant to my primary aim, which is not to refine our understanding of animal behaviour, but to discover ways in which we can help animals to feel better.

Table 3.2 identifies three expressions of altered mood: altered strength of motivation, altered awareness of environmental stimuli and learned helplessness. It is reasonable to hypothesise that any or all of these changes in mood could result from chronic denial of the resources necessary for a normal life. Elegant experiments have been devised to test this hypothesis. For example, Cooper & Nicol (1991) measured the motivation of *Clethrionomys glareolus* to select an enriched environment in preference to a barren environment following prolonged confinement in barren cages. Some of the animals had developed stereotypic 'looping' behaviour in consequence of confinement and these individuals showed a reduced motivation to seek environmental enrichment when it eventually became available (as one choice in a T-maze). This is clear evidence of a change in motivation associated with prolonged denial of environmental resources and the development of stereotypic behaviour. It is not possible to say whether these stereotyping individuals had become less aware of the difference in environmental quality between the enriched and barren goal boxes, or whether the difference no longer mattered. In either event, it is fair to conclude that their emotional interpretation of incoming stimuli (Figure 3.1) had become distorted.

The expression 'learned helplessness' has been coined by experimental psychologists to describe an extreme loss of responsiveness to stimuli in experimental animals, after prolonged exposure to conditions in which they have been denied the opportunity to perform constructive actions designed to achieve satisfaction (e.g. food) or avoid pain (e.g. electric shocks) (Overmier, 2002). This is sometimes defined as an adaptive response, an interpretation that I find chilling. By analogy with the Selye concept of the General Adaptation Syndrome to describe the physiological response to stressors (alarm, adaptation, exhaustion), learned helplessness should be interpreted not as a sign of adaptation but as one of psychological exhaustion. It is the state of mind of an animal that has given up. I shall continue to interpret it as hopelessness.

3.4 Mind and brain: the neurobiology of sensation and emotion

Sentience and suffering are properties of the mind: that which 'thinks, knows, feels and wills'. However, the mechanisms that inform and drive these processes involve the structures and chemistry of the central nervous system in general and the brain in particular. The scientific disciplines of ethology and experimental psychology are of central value to the study of animal welfare because they can teach us a great deal about what an animal thinks, knows, feels and wills, i.e. they are tools for the investigation of 'mind'. It is also important to consider what contribution to the understanding of animal welfare may emerge from neurobiology, i.e. the mechanistic study of the functions of the brain.

Figure 3.1 presented a schematic conception of the perception, categorisation and interpretation of sensory information within the central nervous system of a sentient animal. Essentially this is a highly simplified model of how the mind responds to incoming sensations and information. However, it recognises specific data handling units within the physical brain for the reception, characterisation, integration and interpretation (emotional and cognitive) of incoming stimuli. The outcome of this physical and chemical processing of sensation and emotion is *motivation* and this drives specific motor pathways in the central nervous system to generate behaviour. Neurobiology is merely a new word that embraces the classical, integrated disciplines of anatomy and physiology, the study of form and function, as they apply to the central nervous system. Almost all studies in neurobiology can be placed in one or both of the following categories: (1) construction of anatomical road maps that identify the pathways and processing centres for sensory information, interpretation and integration, and motor function; and (2) compilation of a physiological/biochemical dictionary of the language used for communication between neurones and other cells within the brain.

I have not the space (nor the competence) to review in detail the neurobiology of sensation and emotion in animals. It is, however, valid to ask what can the science of neurobiology contribute to our primary aim which is to understand the feelings and behaviour of animals, in particular their capacity to experience suffering and pleasure. The traditional approach to the study of neurobiology was based on the classical techniques of stimulation and ablation, i.e. observing the consequences of stimulation or destruction of specific nerves or areas of the brain. Some of this was experimental, but much came from studies of the behaviour of people with localised brain damage. This approach was augmented by the use of electrophysiological recordings from individual nerves to identify specific pathways. In recent years, more refined, less invasive (or non-invasive) techniques have been developed to 'map' the brain. These include the histological identification of specific pathways (e.g. c-fos pathways) 'lit-up', and the use of scanning techniques to observe (e.g.) increased blood flow in regions of the brain 'turned on' by specific stimuli. I have already cited the work of Keith Kendrick as an example of how electrophysiological recordings from individual neurones within the brain have been used to demonstrate the routes whereby incoming sensation is characterised and interpreted as an emotion within the brain of the sheep (Kendrick, 1998). Such science, though invasive, has made a significant positive contribution to our understanding of sentience (and therefore animal welfare). It has the merit of linking a mechanistic approach to the function of the brain with an ethological (and sympathetic) approach to the construction of questions designed to discover what matters to a sentient animal.

As a general rule therefore, experiments that combine neurobiology and behaviour can help us understand the nature of animal sentience and animal suffering, but conclusions should never be based on anatomical studies of the brain when considered in isolation. Later in this chapter I shall discuss in detail a serious example of this fallacy, namely the argument that fish cannot feel pain because they do not possess sites in the cerebral cortex shown to be associated with the perception of pain in mammals. Since all or nearly all the evidence points in the opposite direction, the neuroanatomical defence can no longer stand. It now becomes the responsibility of the neuroanatomist to seek out sites in the fish brain that *do* respond to painful stimuli.

The physiological study of the chemical language used for communication between neurones and other cells within the brain can be highly relevant to our understanding of sensation, sentience, mood and suffering since emotion is mediated by chemistry. Here, again, the study of brain biochemistry (or the pharmacological manipulation of brain biochemistry) is most likely to be relevant when it is linked to appropriate studies of animal motivation and behaviour. Fundamental studies of neurotransmission in the CNS have identified families of chemical neurotransmitters associated with pain, consciousness and emotional state. This fundamental work has had a huge impact on the quality of human life (and the income of the pharmaceutical companies) through the development of analgesic, anaesthetic, tranquillising and otherwise mood-altering drugs. While I am not suggesting that we should adopt a pharmacological approach to promote the welfare of animals in our care, there is a great deal to be learnt from experiments that use neuropharmacology to modulate the motivation and behaviour of animals in response to stimuli suspected of causing animal suffering (e.g. pain, fear, frustration, depression). I shall give specific examples of this approach later in the chapter. In essence it is simply a chemical version of the approach of the classical physiologists: stimulate or ablate and observe what happens.

3.5 More triangulation: design and interpretation of studies of animal feelings and motivation

In Chapter 2, I reviewed approaches to the study of physiological and behavioural responses of animals to stimuli that threaten their welfare. In this chapter, I shall consider experimental approaches to the more difficult yet more important question 'How do they feel?' Throughout the book, I shall present examples of how these elements of science have been used, or may be used, to help us identify and understand problems of animal welfare. In concluding this section, I must emphasise, once again, that animal welfare is a complex and fuzzy science that cannot be interpreted using the language of any single scientific discipline, however modern, sophisticated or expensive. Triangulation must always be the order of the day. Those who seek to understand animal welfare through science must recognise (and mostly do) that the study of behaviour cannot be interpreted without parallel studies of sensation and motivation. New discovery of anatomical and physiological/biochemical functions of the brain cannot directly enlighten us as to the workings of the sentient (emotional) mind. However, we do have good knowledge of the impact of (e.g.) analgesics and tranquillisers on the emotional responses of humans to the sensations of pain and anxiety. Where the chemistry is the same in humans and other animals it is entirely valid to use these drugs in the study of the responses of sentient animals to stimuli likely to be associated with the emotions of suffering or pleasure.

3.6 Sources of suffering

Our duty to those animals over whom we have dominion is to seek to ensure that they get a fair deal: a reasonable quality of life and a quiet death. I repeat: this does not imply that their life should be entirely free of stress. Animals are well equipped to respond and adapt to challenge. Our responsibility in law is to protect them from unnecessary suffering; in justice it is to minimise all suffering, from whatever cause. Suffering occurs when an animal fails to cope, or has difficulty in coping, with stress (1) because the stress itself is too severe, too complex or too

Table 3.3 Possible sources of suffering to sentient animals.

Hunger and thirst	Fear and anxiety
Heat and cold	Boredom and frustration
Pain	Loss and loneliness
Malaise (feeling ill)	Depression
Exhaustion	

prolonged, or (2) because the animal is prevented from taking the constructive action it feels necessary to relieve the stress.

Table 3.3 lists possible sources of suffering. These include primitive but no less intense stresses such as hunger and thirst, heat and cold, pain, fear and exhaustion, which may reasonably be assumed to be present to some degree in all sentient animals. They also include elements that would certainly be included in any list drawn up for humans, i.e. frustration and boredom, loneliness and depression; these may be more difficult to discern in other species (e.g. farm animals). If we wish to minimise suffering from any cause then we have a duty to include them as possibilities, though we should not take them for granted.

McFarland (1989) developed a conceptual model of motivational priorities and the nature of suffering in animals (Figure 3.2). In *Eden I*, I referred to this as 'McFarland's Egg' and began my description as follows: 'Try to imagine the state of mind of the animal as a multidimensional egg that exists as an island of serenity within a sea of suffering (any problems so far?). Stimuli and stressors from the internal and external environment will tend to move the state of mind of the animal towards the circumference (shell) of the egg. These stress responses include hunger, thirst, heat and cold, fear, pain and exhaustion.' As these increase in magnitude or duration, the mind of the animal is moved through state-space closer to the shell, the point at which stress reaches the threshold for suffering. Multiple stressors may operate simultaneously and their effects may be additive (recall Table 2.4).

The upper right-hand quadrant of Figure 3.2 illustrates the motivation of an animal such as a cow to respond to two potential sources of distress, namely hunger and exhaustion. At point H on the hunger dimension, but point zero on the exhaustion dimension, a cow will be motivated more to eat than to rest. After eating for some time, she moves towards zero on the hunger axis but away from zero towards R on the exhaustion axis, at which point the motivation to rest overtakes the motivation to eat and she lies down. The curve H–R exists well within the comfort zone of state-space and no suggestion of distress is involved. This would be typical for a beef cow grazing summer pasture. However, when her metabolic demand for food is very high (e.g. in the case of the high-yielding dairy cow) or when the food is very sparse (e.g. in drought conditions), then the cow may be unable to cope or have difficulty in coping with the stress of hunger without incurring the stress of exhaustion (curve H″–R″).

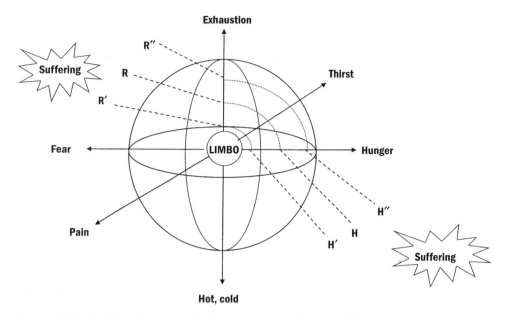

Figure 3.2 McFarland's Egg: motivational priorities, suffering and limbo.

The McFarland model is based on the premise that a sentient animal is positively motivated to adjust its state of mind away from a state of suffering. It does not incorporate any positive motivation towards achieving a state of pleasure. However, it does imply that any environmental constraint on its ability to make a constructive contribution to the quality of its own existence may itself be a source of suffering, even if it is presented with no obvious environmental stressor. Consider, finally, curve H'–R' in Figure 3.2. This could illustrate the state of mind of a sow confined in a solitary stall. She is regularly provided with all the food she needs (if not all she desires) in a form that can be eaten quickly. She can satisfy hunger with minimal effort and is protected from heat, cold or any other serious form of environmental challenge. She will never approach a state of exhaustion since all she has to do is stand up and lie down. In these circumstances she may enter what McFarland calls limbo, a state where, according to conventional measures of state of motivation, all behavioural needs are zero. McFarland then asks the question 'Does the animal suffer in limbo?' This question can be rephrased as 'Are animals positively motivated to behave so as to move out of a state of limbo?' Speaking personally, I consider boredom to be a profoundly unpleasant experience and demonstrate by my behaviour both my motivation to escape limbo and my thoroughly disturbed behaviour when this motivation is frustrated. If an impartial observer were to record similar behaviour from a pig in limbo, this could be used in evidence. However, as a general rule, such evidence is hard to find. Stereotypic behaviour is generally accepted to be an adaptation to the absence of environmental stimuli, but it does not necessarily signify an animal in a state of limbo with no significant motivational drives from either the internal or external environment. The sow in a stall may be powerfully motivated to forage, the horse in a stall powerfully motivated to run. These animals are not bored, but frustrated. The two sensations are not the same (see below).

In *Eden I*, I devoted whole chapters to the topics of hunger and thirst; heat and cold; pain and sickness; friends, foes and fears. I shall not repeat in detail what I wrote then. The main aim of this chapter is to review scientific approaches to the discovery and understanding of what animals feel and what causes them to suffer. I shall therefore concentrate on two issues: (1) identification of risk factors with potential to cause suffering and (2) proof of the existence and nature of suffering.

3.6.1 Improper feeding

The Five Freedoms and Provisions (Table 1.2) state that 'freedom from thirst, hunger and malnutrition should be achieved by ready access to fresh water and a diet to maintain health and vigour'. Hunger or thirst may arise, self-evidently, from an absolute lack of food or water. Malnutrition arises from a lack of specific nutrients usually when animals are confined and restricted to food provided by owners with inadequate knowledge of their nutrient requirements. This problem is more likely to be experienced by pets, especially exotic pets, than by animals professionally reared for commercial purposes. Severe osteoporosis, involving almost complete demineralisation of bone, is not uncommonly diagnosed in limp and immobile tortoises and other *Chelidae* presented at veterinary surgeries. The typical history of such unfortunates is that they have been fed almost exclusively on a diet of lettuce and other green vegetables, which are rich in calcium but seriously deficient in phosphorus. Freedom from hunger depends on feeding the right amount of the correct balance of nutrients specific to the species and the metabolic state of the individual (e.g. maintenance, growth, lactation). This requires expertise. However, the phrase 'a diet to maintain health and vigour' implies more than provision of the right nutrients.

A good diet should meet the following criteria:

- provide energy and specific nutrients for metabolic needs;
- ensure normal digestion;
- promote the sustained integrity and health of the cells and tissues of the body;
- provide oral satisfaction;
- do no harm.

Animals in their natural habitats have evolved foraging strategies that seek to meet all these criteria. Many of these behaviour patterns are unconscious. Those that 'did the right thing' became the fittest and so survived. This is the evolutionary basis of animal behaviour and assumed by some to be a sufficient explanation for almost everything that animals do. Nevertheless it would be fatuous to conclude that sentient animals select the right food through a conscious wish to ensure the survival of their offspring. Their prime motivation, as always, is to feel good and avoid feeling bad. When they are in the 'right' habitat and have control over their own actions, the choices that make them feel good tend to be the choices that favour survival. When man takes control of the habitat, then animals may suffer (or at least feel bad) as a result of improper feeding for reasons that cannot simply be ascribed to starvation or malnutrition. For example:

- Dairy cows that have been genetically selected for very high milk yield may be unable to meet their metabolic hunger for nutrients to support milk production without experiencing distress from overloading the digestive system. The diet fails to reconcile the objectives of correct nutrient supply and good digestion.
- Adult broiler breeder chickens that have been genetically selected for high growth rate (consequent on high appetite) cannot meet their appetite for food without seriously compromising their fitness. Left to their own devices they will eat themselves to death. The diet fails to reconcile oral satisfaction with sustaining the integrity and health of the cells and tissues of the body.
- A stabled horse that is fed largely on pelleted food, supplemented with a small quantity of dusty hay, may consume sufficient energy and specific nutrients to meet its metabolic requirements but develop oral stereotypies from a lack of oral satisfaction, and chronic broncheolitis ('heaves' or 'broken wind') through inhalation of allergic substances in the hay. Here the diet has failed to meet the criteria 'provide oral satisfaction' and 'do no harm'.

3.6.2 Pain

Pain, as perceived by humans, is 'an unpleasant sensory and emotional experience associated with actual tissue damage and described in terms of such damage' (Iggo, 1984). This definition recognises that, for us, pain is more than a sharp sensation; it is likely to have a profound impact on our mood, causing us to experience (e.g.) fear or depression. According to the model illustrated by Figure 3.1, stimuli arising from physical or chemical damage are transmitted by sensory nerves to the CNS, where they may elicit an unconscious reflex action (dropping a hot plate), but also, in a sentient animal, modulate both emotion and cognition in a way that will, at first, seek to cope with the unpleasantness, but if that fails, cause the animal to suffer.

At first sight, pain is an obviously useful element of sentience since it is a powerful signal designed to direct the behaviour of animals so as to avoid injury and promote recovery from injury. Bateson (1991) gave the following 'reasons' for pain. It is necessary:

- to distinguish between harmful and non-harmful stimuli;
- to provoke animals to give high priority to escape or to remove harmful stimuli;
- to teach animals to avoid harmful stimuli in future, or to decide what degree of pain (or harm) is acceptable in the pursuit of information or reward;
- to inhibit activities likely to delay recovery from injury.

All these reasons can be applied as well to sentient animals as to man. However, none of these responses necessarily implies that pain in animals is associated with a state of emotional distress. Since pain is so obviously a source of suffering in humans it would appear inhumane to presume that other animals do not suffer from pain too. Yet it is proper to ask questions that seek to discover the extent to which their experience of pain is similar to ours. Table 3.4 identifies a number of behavioural signs and other phenomena associated with pain in animals and considers how far they may be interpreted as indices of pain as we understand it in ourselves, 'a profoundly unpleasant sensory and emotional experience'.

Immediate reaction

Reflex withdrawal of a limb from a stimulus such as heat or pressure is an indication that the stimulus is potentially damaging or 'nociceptive'. It does not, however, signify a conscious perception of pain since it occurs in animals whose brains have been destroyed above the level of the spinal cord. Expressions of alarm, vocalisation and attempts to escape when a conscious animal is presented with a nociceptive stimulus (e.g. the response of a cat to a painful injection) indicate that the sensation has reached the level of consciousness and elicited what looks like an emotional response. However, that is still some way from demonstrating that the cat feels pain the same way we do.

Modified behaviour

The natural response of animals to the experience of pain is to modify their behaviour so as to reduce the intensity of current pain and/or reduce the risk of

Table 3.4 Pain: how do we know it matters?

Immediate reaction
- Reflex withdrawal: no evidence of conscious sensation
- Conscious alarm and escape: sensation but no evidence of an emotional response

Modified behaviour
- Rest and locomotor changes: evidence only of adaptation to an unpleasant sensation
- Learned avoidance: evidence of memory of an acute emotional response
- Reduced positive behaviour (e.g. grooming, exploration, play): possible evidence of chronic change in mood

Altered mood
- Apathy, reduced appetite, reduced strength of motivation or aversion to common stimuli: probable evidence of depression

Response to analgesics
- Externally administered: only indicates acute relief at absence of unpleasant sensation
- Self-selected: strong evidence of persistent motivation to avoid pain

its recurrence. A cow with a sore foot will limp or hold its foot off the ground. A broiler chicken with seriously distorted locomotion associated with 'leg weakness' will also show extreme reluctance to stand. These animals have modified their locomotor and resting behaviour so as to reduce the pain (i.e. make them feel better). When the damage is relatively minor this adaptation to behaviour may be sufficient to remove the sensation of pain and thus avoid emotional distress. When damage is more severe, animals may be extremely reluctant to move at all. If forced to move, they may cry out (vocalise) and exhibit signs of acute distress. However, hardening my heart, I cannot necessarily assume that these signs of acute distress will outlast the moment of enforced (and, to the animal, inappropriate) activity.

Anyone who has experienced the behaviour of cats or dogs in a veterinary surgery will know that these animals remember experiences or situations associated with pain, show distress and try to escape when next they are dragged into the waiting room. This is a clear demonstration of 'learned avoidance', a conscious emotional response, acquired as a result of previous experience. This is quite strong evidence that pain matters to sentient animals.

Altered mood

Further evidence that pain may be affecting mood can be obtained by studying normal patterns of maintenance behaviour, particularly those aspects of behaviour that involve parts of the body that are undamaged and can be moved without apparent pain or associated with comfort and pleasure, such as grooming and eating. Broiler chickens with moderate to severe locomotor disorders show a significant reduction in the performance of such activity. This substantially strengthens the case that pain is an emotional experience that matters to broiler chickens since it implies not just an adaptation to an unpleasant sensation but also a mood shift towards a state of depression.

Response to analgesics

Administration of analgesic (pain-killing) drugs, whether local or systemic, can have a spectacular effect on the behaviour of animals, provoking an apparently complete return to normal behaviour and mood. This can, of course, be dangerous if it is necessary for the animal to rest, say, a broken limb. This evidence, considered in isolation, indicates that animals such as dogs and horses do not possess our cognitive awareness of the long-term prognosis for a broken limb and the risks involved in exercising it normally as soon as the pain stops. It implies that pain matters only so long as it lasts and is not a powerful argument in support of the case that other sentient animals experience pain in a similar way to ourselves. A much more powerful, indeed clinching, piece of evidence is provided by observations of the behaviour of animals allowed to self-select analgesic drugs in their food or water. The motivation of the laboratory rat to self-select analgesics when in pain has been an invaluable model for the pharmaceutical industry seeking effective analgesics for human and veterinary use. The Bristol team secured their argument that pain associated with 'leg weakness' matters to broiler chickens with the convincing demonstration by Danbury *et al.* (1999) that birds showing any degree of lameness, from slight to severe, preferentially selected food containing the nonsteroidal anti-inflammatory, analgesic drug carprofen. Birds that displayed no evidence of lameness preferred the food that contained no drug. The pain of lameness mattered to these birds to the extent that birds selected a food that they otherwise avoided in order to avoid 'feeling bad'.

My discussion of the evidence that may be used to assess how pain matters to a sentient animal has given special emphasis to the work of my colleagues at Bristol who have been studying the problem of pain associated with 'leg weakness' in fast-growing broiler chickens. This is partly because the work is very thorough, partly because they are my colleagues and partly because in *Eden I*, I described the problem of leg weakness in broilers as 'the single most severe, systematic example of man's inhumanity to another sentient animal'. I shall discuss the halting progress of the industry in its attempts to deal with this problem in Chapter 5. For the moment I can confidently conclude that pain matters just as much to a chicken as it does to a rat or a dog.

There is also new evidence that many of the criteria that we use to define the importance of pain in mammals and birds can be applied equally well to fish (Sneddon *et al.*, 2003). Fish possess pain receptors. When noxious substances are injected under the skin in the mouth, the fish show prolonged distress, learned avoidance and (possibly) alterations in mood. Experiments involving self-selection of analgesics have yet to be published, but I would bet on a positive result. Thus a powerful portfolio of physiological and behavioural evidence now exists to support the case that fish feel pain and that this feeling matters. In the face of such evidence, any argument to the contrary based on the claim that fish 'do not have the right sort of brain' can no longer be called scientific. It is just obstinate.

3.6.3 Fear and anxiety

Fear is an emotional response to a perceived threat that acts as a powerful motivator to action designed, where possible, to evade that threat. It is also an educational experience since the memory of previous threats, the action taken in response to those threats and the consequences thereof ('was it less bad than I feared or worse?') will obviously affect how the animal feels next time around. Thus fear, like pain, is an essential part of sentience. These emotions have evolved as key elements for survival. An animal that has no sense of either pain or fear, for itself or its offspring, is at a profound disadvantage in the struggle for existence.

The concept of fear as a stress to which animals may adapt, or fail to adapt, is illustrated in Figure 3.3. This identifies three main threats that may induce a fear response. These are novelty, innate threats and learned threats. Neophobia, or the fear of novelty, is a common although not universal feature of sentient animals.

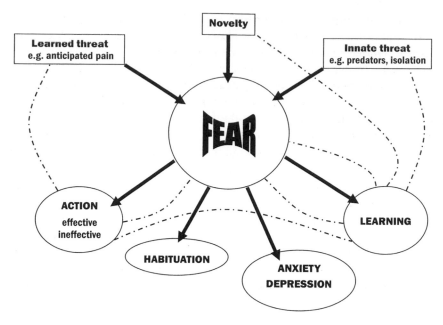

Figure 3.3 Fear: threats, reactions and consequences.

Success in life depends on achieving the right balance between curiosity (to develop survival skills) and caution (to avoid danger). At birth, novelty is all since nothing is known. Newborn mammals and birds appear to begin life with little sense of fear but a great deal of curiosity. This motivates the young animal to explore the environment under the watchful eye and protective cover of a devoted parent. The developing animal learns the skills necessary to promote its welfare and optimise its chances for survival. Among these skills is the ability to distinguish between threats that are real or imaginary. As it builds up its store of experience in its natural habitat, the chances of it encountering new experiences become less and less and this reduces the 'need' for curiosity. At this stage of development, neo-phobia, or at least a healthy caution in the presence of novelty, acquires a greater survival value than curiosity.

Innate fears, or the innate perception of specific signals as threats, are those that have been genetically inscribed into the data files of the emotional brain. Most humans, and chimpanzees, have an innate fear of snakes. Sheep have innate fears of isolation and dogs. The expression of this innate fear may not be present at birth but develops during the process of maturation. A sheep sees a dog, or the image of a dog. Even if it has no previous experience of a dog, this image is matched with a like image pre-programmed into its emotional centres. If the match is close, the animal experiences the emotion of fear. The neurobiology of this phenomenon is poorly understood. However, it would appear to be good evidence for the slow but ultimately successful vertical transmission through successive generations of genetic information conducive to survival: a small but convincing demonstration of cultural wisdom. However, it is slow. Penguins, for example, have an innate fear of predatory sea mammals such as seals but no innate fear of man notwithstanding several generations (for them) of bloody encounters. Fear of a learned threat is self-evidently one that is acquired by experience. The most primitive of all learned fears is the fear engendered by situations that have in the past led to pain, i.e. the repeat visit to the vet. The dog that is taken back to boarding kennels prior to the annual family holiday may display a rather more advanced form of learned fear; that of desertion by key members of its social group.

There are two more categories of potential fear not illustrated in Figure 3.3. These are fear engendered by the appearance of fear in others, and fear of the future. Most species that have evolved to live in groups recognise and interpret the escape or hiding behaviour of other animals when faced by a threat. They can also interpret more subtle signals communicated by sight, sound or scent. Some of this fear will be innate (e.g. distress calls or alarm pheromones), some learned.

In *Eden I*, I quoted Robert Burns' *Ode to a Mouse* to draw a clear distinction between humans and other animals:

> *thou art blest, compared with me!*
> *The present only touches thee.*
> *but forward tho' I canna see*
> *I guess and fear!*

This makes the assumption that only humans fear problems they may face in the future, e.g. financial ruin and the certainty of death. This is convenient since it frees us from guilt at the prospect that farm animals may anticipate the prospect of slaughter. However, we should not take this absolute difference for granted. It is entirely reasonable to assume that (most) non-human animals do not construct cognitive maps of their future careers. However, sentient animals clearly have some image of the immediate future. The phenomenon of learned avoidance is evidence that an animal visualises a particular situation and concludes 'If I do this, or am forced to do this, then I am likely to experience harm'. How far it can extend this image into the future may tell us something about its cognitive abilities, but it does not tell us anything about the intensity and duration of its anxiety, i.e. the degree to which it suffers. Separation anxiety is a disturbingly common behavioural disorder of dogs left alone in the house while their owners go out to work (Chapter 10). Such dogs may express extreme distress, five days a week, every week of their lives. These dogs may not be very bright but their distress is real enough. The expression separation anxiety implies that present distress at the disappearance of a loved one will extend into the unforeseeable future. An animal that lacks the ability to visualise far into the future may be more anxious rather than less because it cannot forecast the end of its distress.

Anxiety may be defined as a sense of fear that is not related to a specific immediate cause. It is therefore, by definition, a fear of what *might* happen, i.e. a fear
of the future. There is clear evidence that non-human animals not only display fear
responses to immediate threats but also can experience chronic states of anxiety.
The causes of this are partly genetic and partly acquired by experience. Scientists
have, for example, bred 'high-anxiety' strains of rats, mice and quail. The
intensity of expression of their anxiety can be greatly increased by repeatedly presenting them with situations that stress their capacity to cope. These animals are
anxious for their future. They may not be advanced enough to fear the inevitabil-
ity of death and its consequences (hell or non-existence), but it may still *feel* like
hell.

We have so far considered the sources of fear. Figure 3.3 also illustrates the consequences of fear as a learning experience. An animal that experiences fear, induced
by a threat of any sort, will, if it can, initiate some sort of action intended to
remove, or at least cope with, the threat (e.g. escape, hiding). This action may
prove to be effective, ineffective or unnecessary:

- *Effective:* A rat, sensing the remote presence of a cat by sight or smell, safely
  returns to its burrow.
- *Ineffective:* A dog discovers that it is powerless to prevent its owners leaving
  it alone all day in the house.
- *Unnecessary:* A feral cat, initially alarmed by the appearance of humans, even
  though they bring food, allows itself, over time, to become domesticated and
  eventually solicits human company for the hedonistic pleasure of being stroked
  by the fireside.

When animals are confined by man on the farm or in the laboratory, their
opportunities for effective action (e.g. escape or hiding) may be restricted or non-
existent, in which case they have no option but to wait and hope that the perceived threat will either go away or turn out not to be a problem. Whatever
the circumstances, the nature and outcome of the threat will both be stored in the
brain as an experience. If the animal learns that it can cope effectively with the
threat, or if the imagined threat turns out not to be real, the animal will habituate to these threats and the overall experience of fear will diminish. If the animal
discovers that there is nothing it can do to control the threat, then the acute, adaptive emotion of fear will escalate to the chronic non-adaptive state of anxiety (e.g.
separation anxiety) or depression. These are emotional indices of a failure to cope
and therefore sources of suffering.

The Department of the Environment, Food and Rural Affairs (DEFRA) Codes
of Recommendations for the Welfare of Livestock recommend that animals 'should
be exposed to the normal sights and sounds of farm activity'. This recognises that
for an animal that can neither hide nor escape, all novelty is a potential threat. In
these circumstances they have to learn that the presence of the farmer or the noise
of a tractor should pose no real threat and may indeed prove a source of pleasure

in the form of food. This habituation is an essential part of good husbandry. However, animals such as turkeys or veal calves reared on intensive units in near darkness and given little or no opportunity to experience life can panic at the slightest alarm. This arises from a failure to habituate and is hugely magnified by their innate (unmodified) recognition of the signs of fear in others. Mob panic in intensive poultry houses (hens and turkeys) is not just a welfare problem, it can be a killer.

3.6.4 Malaise

Ill-health is self-evidently a welfare problem because it is the antithesis of fitness. Malaise or 'feeling ill' is a source of suffering because it is the antithesis of feeling good. Our concern for the welfare of a sick animal should therefore extend beyond actions intended to remove the cause of the sickness (e.g. treating bacterial infections with an antibiotic); we have a further responsibility to minimise suffering while the disease and convalescence are in progress. Gregory (1998a) reviewed the physiological mechanisms that cause an animal to feel ill as it mounts an inflammatory and immune response to an infection or other source of tissue damage. The immediate 'acute phase response' to infection typically involves fever, recruitment of phagocytic blood cells to scavenge bacteria, and redirection of protein synthesis away from normal tissue maintenance and growth towards manufacture of the elements necessary for an effective immune response. These mechanisms are triggered by cytokines, which may be considered as the hormone-like messengers of the immune system. Cytokines may be good for you, but they can make you feel bad too.

Behavioural responses to the acute phase reaction to infection include increased sleep, loss of appetite, social isolation and mental confusion. These have a survival advantage for the individual and the population. Increased rest and loss of appetite favour the redirection of body resources away from normal digestion and development towards the immediate needs of the immune response. Social isolation can reduce the risk of transmitting the disease through the population. These behavioural changes reflect, of course, a shift in the motivational state of the animal as a consequence of feeling ill. We can answer the question 'When, and in what circumstances, will an animal suffer as a consequence of feeling ill?' according to the golden rule, by saying 'When it fails to cope, or has extreme difficulty in coping with the change in its emotional state'. Struck down by a heavy cold, my personal motivation is to retire to bed with a hot whisky. This can turn feelings of lassitude and mental confusion into a highly rewarding experience. Similarly, with a digestive upset, I am not likely to suffer unless in pain, or alternatively obliged to go through the motions of 'enjoying' a social dinner. In the former example I have coped successfully; in the latter, I have been prevented from carrying out a successful coping strategy.

These principles can and should be used to guide our approach to nursing animals through periods of sickness. Their need for rest and quiet can be met by the provision of a comfortable, well-bedded hospital pen. Hospital pens for farm animals are usually sited remote from the main housing area. This can reduce the risk of cross-infection and ensure peace and quiet for the sick animal(s). However, my clinical impression is that one should try, if possible, to avoid total isolation. In the 1980s I was closely involved in developing strategies for the prevention and control of infectious diseases in young calves. The policy of some of the very best stock keepers was to isolate sick calves in well-bedded hospital pens where they could rest without disturbance and receive individual care. However, these pens were within sight, sound and smell of groups of healthy calves in the main rearing pens. It was the belief of these farmers that by not compounding the stress of disease with the further stress of total isolation, the morale of the calves was improved and they stood a better chance of recovery. I am impressed by this argument. It is unproven, because these were farms that tended to do most things right. What I can say is that there was no suggestion that this policy of retaining social links at a distance carried a significant penalty in terms of increased spread of disease.

Fever *per se* is a potential source of suffering. It involves a resetting (upwards) of the body thermostat. In the early stages of fever the animal seeks to elevate heat production and reduce heat loss; the former by shivering, the latter by vasoconstriction. Thus the extremities of a fevered animal may feel cold even though its body temperature is elevated. During this phase the animal feels cold and will suffer if the environment is such that it has difficulty in achieving the new set point for its thermostat (e.g. in cold air, draughts or with inadequate bedding). In the extreme circumstances of a severe fever, body temperature may rise to a life-threatening degree. In this case it becomes essential to cool the animal down with antipyretic drugs and/or application of cold water.

This section has dealt briefly and specifically with malaise as a potential source of suffering, the message being that suffering can be reduced or eliminated through a proper understanding of the physiological and motivation changes that accompany the mobilisation of the defence mechanisms of the body. I discussed the relief of sickness in some detail in *Eden I* and shall not repeat myself here. The summary of my argument is given in Table 3.5.

3.6.5 Frustration and boredom

It is necessary to make a clear distinction between frustration and boredom. Frustration occurs when an animal is denied the opportunity to act according to its motivational needs in order to achieve a desired reward. Thus the laying hen denied access to a nest box is frustrated. The billy goat denied access to sexually receptive nearby females is profoundly frustrated (and lets the world know it!). Frustration of specific needs is clearly a potential source of suffering and examples of this will crop up many times during the latter course of this book. Boredom may be defined as a sense of unease associated with the absence of any specific motivational need. It is the state of mind of an animal in McFarland's Limbo (Figure

Table 3.5 Examples of the use of medicines and nursing for the relief of suffering associated with sickness in animals.

Clinical sign	Medical remedy	Nursing remedy
Fever	Antipyretics	Thermal comfort
Pain	Analgesics	Physical comfort (bedding)
	Anti-inflammatory drugs	Rest
		Reduced stress at damage site
Inappetence	Tonics during convalescence	Oral titillation ('treats')
Fluid loss	Intravenous rehydration	Oral rehydration
Lethargy and mental confusion	Unnecessary	Discreet social isolation from harassment by other animals or fussing humans

3.2). I shall not spend time on the question 'Is boredom a source of suffering for sentient animals?' because I simply do not know. It is reasonable to assume that very many animals 'in our care' have very little to do. The list includes pregnant sows in 'factory farms' and pet rabbits in a hutch at the bottom of the garden. These animals may well experience boredom. However, I am not convinced that there is good evidence to suggest that boredom (as distinct from frustration) is a cause of real distress in such animals. Since this book seeks to concentrate on the things that matter most, I shall leave it at that.

3.6.6 Satisfaction and pleasure

This chapter has concentrated on sources of suffering ('feeling bad') as welfare problems for animals, since our primary concern must be to minimise suffering in any form, whether 'necessary' or 'unnecessary'. In the absence of suffering, it is reasonable to conclude that the welfare of the animal is satisfactory. However, it is also reasonable to suggest that we should, where possible, provide sentient animals with the opportunity to experience positive welfare or 'pleasure'. I have often been presented with the argument that while non-human animals may have the mental capacity to suffer, they are unable to experience pleasure because they lack self-awareness. I challenge anyone to watch a tom cat reduced to a state of drooling abandon by discreet stroking and tummy tickling and then insist that animals cannot experience pleasure. They may not be *aware* that they are feeling good but they *are* feeling good nonetheless.

Pleasure may be a powerful need in some animals, some of the time. It may also, some of the time, simply be a bonus that comes along with sentience and the capacity to suffer. In an article entitled *'Pleasures'*, *'Pains'* and Animal *Welfare*, Fraser & Duncan (1998) reviewed how 'motivational affective states' may drive an animal to both avoid pain (in the broadest sense of the word) and seek pleasure. The phrase 'motivational affective state' implies that motivation is a consequence of how an animal feels and drives behaviour designed to modify how it feels. This is simply another way of describing the model of the emotional brain illustrated in Figure 3.1. However, the Fraser & Duncan approach is novel in that it does not assume that pain, indifference and pleasure simply reflect stages along one continuous dimension from 'negative to positive affect' (emotion). They suggest that the motivation to seek pleasure may operate independently of any motivation to move away from a state of pain or distress. The motivation of young animals to play is frequently (and very boringly) cited as evidence of a need to develop hunting skills necessary for survival. It is true that carnivores with complex and physically demanding hunting strategies are those that tend to play the most as cubs or kittens. It is also true that the cost of play is less for these animals when they do not need to eat and are in no danger. I must also restate what should be a blinding glimpse of the obvious: namely that young animals are not motivated to play by the desire to increase the fitness of their genes; they do so because it is good fun.

It is thus impossible to deny that sentient animals have the capacity to experience pleasure and are motivated to seek it. Behaviours associated with this motivation may be most apparent in young animals and in carnivorous species (e.g. kittens and lion cubs). However, having accepted this point, it is not possible to avoid the conclusion that less demonstrative creatures such as cows and lambs both seek and enjoy pleasure when they lie with their heads raised to the sun on a perfect English summer's day.

Husbandry and Welfare on the Farm: Assessment and Assurance

4

Sed quis custodiet ipsos custodes? [but who is to guard the guards themselves?]

Juvenal (Satires)

In the last two chapters I have reviewed how scientists have sought to study the elements that define the welfare of animals as they respond to the challenges of life and how the animals feel as they do so. However, if science is to be of practical service to animal welfare, it must do more than just study it. If our past and current research is to have meaning for the vast populations of animals used by humans for our own ends, then we must take it out of the confines of our own laboratories and into the world where these animals actually live. In Chapter 1, I identified four elements essential to the progressive improvement of standards of welfare for sentient animals. The first of these was the development of comprehensive, robust protocols for assessing animal welfare and the provisions that constitute good husbandry in 'real life' situations whether on farms, in laboratories, zoos and wildlife parks, kennels and riding establishments or in rescue centres run by welfare charities. This chapter will address the development of protocols for welfare assessment and control on the farm.

I have also drawn attention to the increasing expression of public desire (if not public demand) for quality assurance in relation to standards for food production. Shoppers set their own standards for qualities of food such as appearance, availability, taste and price, and adjust their buying habits accordingly. However, there are other standards that they are unable to judge directly for themselves and are increasingly reluctant to take on trust. The most powerful and universal consumer concern is, of course, for food safety. This is motivated by very reasonable self-interest and diligently reinforced by government legislation. Other concerns relate to system of production (e.g. organic), country (or farm) of origin and animal welfare. These concerns are motivated largely by a sense of justice and are thus, unfortunately, less universal and less likely to attract government backing. It is a sense of justice that generates the questions: 'Is the food I buy produced according to a system that is (respectively) fair to the environment, fair to local farmers or fair to the animals?'

The growth of these concerns has been identified, and indeed exploited, by producers and retailers who have developed Quality Assurance (QA) schemes that 'guarantee' standards of production, provenance and hygiene. UKROFS (the United Kingdom Register of Organic Food Standards), the RSPCA 'Freedom Food' scheme and a number of other 'British' schemes (e.g. the 'Red Tractor', Assured British Pigs) set out in great detail quality standards for production, all of which incorporate concerns for animal welfare. The image conveyed to the general public who do not read the fine print is that food produced to these standards is, respectively, organic, high-welfare or British. Throughout the developed world, a myriad of other standards are emerging. These inevitably have much in common, yet most seek to 'give an edge' to the producer/retailer, either by giving an assurance of added value and thereby commanding a premium price, or through the assertion that by improving animal welfare farmers can reduce costs associated with lack of 'fitness' in their animals. Both these arguments contain elements of truth. However, sometimes they fail to tell the whole story and sometimes they tell rather more than the whole story. It is reasonable to claim that farmers can profit from those improvements to welfare through reduction of disease and injury (if the costs of prevention and treatment are not too high). However, many elements of improved husbandry as perceived by the public (and the animals), such as increased space allowances and an enriched environment, can only be achieved at a cost to the producer. Production systems that claim to be high-welfare must address both elements, fitness and feeling good, and these will only be able to compete if they can attract a premium. This inevitably means that they will be aimed at a niche market that is willing and able to pay the premium. This can put a strain on all parties. Those who promote premium foods to the shopper on the basis of genuine added value (e.g. high-welfare or environmentally friendly farming) often feel the need to oversell their products on the basis of unjustified claims as to taste and/or healthy eating. Farmers may choose to improve their standards of husbandry and increase their costs to attract premium prices for goods sold into developing niche markets. In time, however, these markets tend to become saturated, the premium shrinks and the added value to the farmer disappears. So far as the animals are concerned, the problem with niche markets is that only a small minority stands to benefit.

Before any QA system can guarantee its aims and so be worthy of public trust, it must incorporate an effective system of quality *control*. It is not sufficient simply to give assurance that a farm is operating in compliance with organic, 'Freedom Food' or even British(!) standards and assume in consequence that all is well. Specifically, any QA scheme that claims to operate to high standards of animal welfare must incorporate an effective audit to ensure that these standards are being met and to remedy specific problems as they occur. It is thus essential to the success of welfare-based Farm Assurance schemes (as viewed by all parties, consumers, farmers and their animals) that we develop comprehensive, robust, *trusted* protocols for the assessment of husbandry and animal welfare on farms both intensive and extensive.

In this chapter, I describe and discuss the principles, development, testing and implementation of practical protocols for the assessment of husbandry and welfare at the farm level. I shall begin with a brief critical review of the principles and essential elements of existing schemes, then describe in more detail the development of the Bristol Protocols for animal-based assessments of welfare outcomes, using as an example the protocol for dairy cattle.

4.1 Provisions and outcomes

Good husbandry includes the provision of appropriate resources of food and shelter, effective management and sympathetic stockmanship. It is the responsibility of farmers to provide these things in order to promote good welfare, and it is the responsibility of the assessors of any welfare-based QA scheme to ensure that farmers comply with the standards of husbandry as laid down by the scheme. However, compliance with husbandry standards does not guarantee good welfare for all of the animals all of the time and ultimately it is the welfare of the animal that matters. Quality control designed to provide QA as to standards of animal welfare needs to be based on assessment of the provision of resources and management and on assessment of outcomes, i.e. animal-based observations and records of welfare state. The Five Freedoms and Provisions (Table 1.2) offer a comprehensive framework on which to hang specific observations and records of both provision and outcome. The key elements of husbandry provision and welfare outcome are illustrated in Figure 4.1. The main categories of provision are described below in more detail and illustrated by example.

(1) Resources – physical resources necessary to ensure proper feeding, housing and hygiene:
   • well-constructed, properly replenished food stores;
   • accommodation that is hygienic, physically and thermally comfortable, and unlikely to cause injury;
   • facilities for routine preventative medicine and the care of individual sick animals.
(2) Records – strategic management designed to address the physiological, health and behavioural needs of the animals:
   • feeding, production, health and welfare plans devised and implemented with professional advice as appropriate;
   • comprehensive records relating to feeding, production, health and welfare.

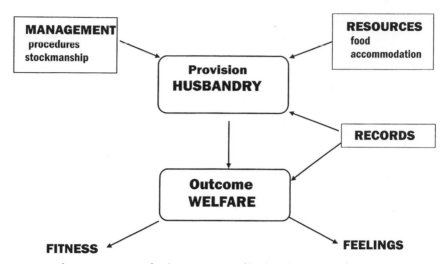

Figure 4.1 Elements necessary for the assessment of husbandry provision and its outcome, animal welfare.

(3) Management – competent 'stockmanship', sympathetic to the day-to-day physiological, health and behavioural needs of the animals:
- a skilled, sympathetic approach to animal handling;
- early recognition and attention to any signs of disease or injury;
- work practices that encourage good stock-keepers (and give them the time!) to develop empathy with the animals in their care.

Observations and records relating to welfare outcomes (and elements of provision directly related to welfare outcomes) can be categorised under the headings of fitness and feelings. These include the following.

(1) Fitness:
- good body condition, growth, fertility, etc. contingent upon good nutrition;
- good condition of the skin and coat, contingent upon comfortable, clean accommodation and absence of external parasites;
- good health, contingent upon good hygiene, preventative medicine and early recognition and attention to disease.
(2) Feelings:
- freedom from pain associated with lameness and injury;
- freedom from fear and stress induced by exposure to unsafe facilities, inconsiderate humans or other animals;
- freedom to exhibit most natural (socially acceptable) expressions of behaviour, in particular those associated with sensations of pleasure.

4.2 Tailoring QA schemes to individual needs

The examples of measurements and records presented above are by no means exhaustive and the list of things that could be included in a protocol for the assessment of husbandry and welfare can be extended almost indefinitely. Indeed, several existing protocols have, in my opinion, already carried the pursuit of things to record (or, more precisely, boxes to tick) far too far. Any QA scheme that relies on voluntary compliance will only succeed if those who subscribe to the scheme believe in it and are prepared to accept the cost of the scheme in terms of time, money and general disruption to the daily routine. Government schemes enforced by legislation are less subject to the constraint of market acceptability and more inclined to 'cover their backs' by appearing to account for anything that could possibly go wrong at any time, ever. Nevertheless, it is important therefore to avoid the bureaucratic obsession to include everything that might be of concern and rather to focus on what really matters. A good assessment protocol is therefore one that has been designed, refined and reduced to a form that most efficiently and parsimoniously meets the specific aims of the system it seeks to assess. As always, the aim should be to ensure that 'everything should be as simple as possible but no simpler'. Protocols for assessment of the welfare of animals in groups on farms, in the laboratory or in other commercial establishments may be directed towards one or more of the following aims.

- Research designed to improve husbandry systems through improved understanding of specific welfare issues (e.g. alternative husbandry systems for laying hens).
- Ensuring compliance with legislative requirements (e.g. minimal cage standards for laying hens or laboratory mice).
- Ensuring compliance with voluntary certification schemes (e.g. organic standards, 'Freedom Foods').
- Use as advisory/management tools for addressing general or specific problems of health and welfare on individual farms (e.g. lameness control schemes for dairy herds).

A good assessment protocol should meet the criteria of feasibility, validity, reliability, repeatability and objectivity. It is relatively easy to meet these criteria when assessment schemes are based on 'Yes or No' questions relating to provision of resources, records and management (e.g. housing design, participation in health schemes). They are less easy to meet when the assessment involves 'fuzzier', animal-based measurements of welfare outcomes. For this reason provision-based approaches are more likely to satisfy the requirements of legislation and certification schemes where the aim may simply be to establish compliance or non-compliance with the standards. For research, for advisory purposes, or to audit the effectiveness of provision-based QA schemes, more searching questions need to be addressed and here there is no option but to include animal-based measurements of welfare state.

If animal-based protocols for assessment of welfare outcomes are to meet the criteria of feasibility, validity, reliability, repeatability and objectivity, they clearly require expert, well-trained assessors. However, there is the danger that even the best and most objective of assessors may jump to the wrong conclusion on the basis of 'snap-shot' observations made at a single visit. This can be overcome in part by selecting observations (e.g. body condition, skin condition and evidence of injury) that reflect the quality of husbandry over a prolonged period. Moreover, observations made by the external assessor of animal fitness and behaviour on a single day should not be the sole source of evidence. They should be augmented by animal-based records and reports from the farmer/stock-keeper and interpreted in full recognition that these (especially the reports) may lack reliability and objectivity.

While animal-based measurements may be used most often to assess welfare outcomes, they can also be the most effective approach to assessing the effectiveness of key areas of provision. For example, the requirement for 'provision of an adequate diet' defines a resource but is best defined in terms of an outcome, since 'adequacy' is better assessed from the health and body condition of the animals than from (e.g.) records of the quantity of food provided. In this example, an animal-based measure (e.g. poor body condition) provides the evidence to indicate that the provision of food has been inadequate. Having identified a welfare problem in terms of a measure of outcome, it then becomes necessary to assess the provisions to discover where things have gone wrong. The corollary to this is that where there appears to be no welfare problem, there is no need to pry into every corner. Life is too short to worry about everything and 'if it ain't bust, don't fix it'. Thus it is neither efficient nor parsimonious to seek to observe and record everything that could possibly go wrong on every farm on every visit. It makes more sense to focus the initial assessment on identifying actual or incipient problems, then to expand the investigation of specific problems both backwards and forwards to identify, respectively, the sources of the problem and what should be done about it.

Any welfare-based QA scheme should start from the basis of an assessment protocol that incorporates elements of both provision and outcome. It is not, however, possible to give assurance as to animal welfare simply on the basis that it is being assessed. An assessor can only guarantee compliance with the provisions of the scheme if he/she incorporates procedures to ensure that effective action is taken to address any serious welfare problems that are identified during the assessment. He/she may, for example, identify a lameness problem in a herd of dairy cows. If this could clearly be attributed to a failure of provision (e.g. filthy floors and no attention to foot hygiene) then this would be cause for due warning and, if the faults were not remedied, dismissal from the scheme. However, an assessor may identify a lameness problem on a farm that appeared to be in compliance with all the standards of provision laid down by the scheme. This would not give sufficient cause for immediate dismissal. However, assessors cannot simply shut their eyes to the existence of a welfare problem on the grounds that they have been able to tick all the boxes necessary to demonstrate formal compliance with the elements of provision identified by the scheme. In this case the farmer would be directed to seek appropriate professional (e.g. veterinary) advice. Failure to seek and/or act upon this advice would be evidence of a failure of provision and thus due cause for dismissal.

4.3 Comparison of current schemes for assessing on-farm welfare

The development and animal welfare implications of existing Farm Assurance schemes have been reviewed by the Farm Animal Welfare Council (FAWC, 2001). They make the point that welfare is only one of many concerns for consumers, retailers and producers. Farm Assurance schemes must also incorporate elements relating to food safety, biosecurity, animal identification and traceability. The early development of Farm Quality Assurance schemes within the UK was centralised under government control until 1993. Since then the responsibility for developing QA schemes has been devolved to the farming and food industry. This has, inevitably, led to the creation of a multiplicity of schemes, which can be confusing to consumers, who do not know what they are getting, and exasperating to farmers, who find themselves under surveillance from all sides. However, there are national and international accreditation bodies to assess and accredit the competence and integrity of individual QA schemes. The United Kingdom Accreditation Service (UKAS) is the sole accreditation body for the UK and is a member of the European Co-operation for Accreditation. This body exists to 'provide the market with confidence in the impartiality and technical competence of its individual evaluators and to provide assurance that evaluators have sufficient resources and facilities'. This is linked to European Standards in relation to accreditation: EN45001 (Production Certification Standard) and EN 45004 (Inspection Standard). However, to quote FAWC (2001): 'It is worth noting that being accredited to EN45001 simply means that an organisation is competent to certify to a specific set of criteria as defined in a given standard. For example, this has allowed both British and Danish pig producers working to different technical standards which meet the needs of their respective stakeholders to be certified by EN 45011'. In other words, the EN 'standards' are not standards as such. They allow different nations to set their own different minimum standards for animal welfare and are satisfied so long as they abide by the standards they have set for themselves.

Farm Assurance schemes other than the organic (UKROFS) and high-welfare ('Freedom Food') schemes tend to be either system-based (e.g. the Assured Chicken Production Scheme, the National Dairy Farm Assurance Scheme) or regionally based (e.g. Scottish Food Quality Certification). I do not intend to compare and

Table 4.1 Summary, with examples, of the format of the DEFRA Revised Codes for the welfare of pigs and cattle (DEFRA, 2003).

General recommendations	Examples	
	Pigs	**Cattle**
Stockmanship	Health and welfare plan	Health and welfare plan
	Basic skills	Basic skills
	Health inspection	Health inspection
	Handling	Handling
Health	Biosecurity	Biosecurity
	Condition scoring	Condition scoring
	Lameness	Lameness
	Parasites	Parasites
	Sick and injured animals	Sick and injured animals
	Health records	Health records
Accommodation	Space allowances	Cubicles
	Floors	Cowsheds and straw yards
	Temperature and ventilation	
Food and water	Design of equipment	Access to roughage
	Trough space	Water requirements
Management	Farrowing sows and piglets	Pregnancy and calving
	Weaners and rearing pigs	Calf rearing
	Dry sows and gilts	Dairy cows
	Boars	Milking
	Outdoor husbandry systems	Management at pasture

contrast these schemes. Suffice it to say that they all set out in detail standards of husbandry provision designed to promote good welfare. They are all based on the DEFRA Codes of Recommendations for the Welfare of Livestock (www.defra.gov.uk), which 'aim to encourage all those who care for farm animals to adopt the highest standards of husbandry'. The Welfare Codes do not themselves constitute legislation, although they are supported by legislation and can be cited in evidence at a prosecution for abuse of farm animal welfare.

Table 4.1 summarises the approach used by DEFRA in the production of its two most recently revised Codes (at time of writing) for Cattle and Pigs (DEFRA, 2003). The Codes are prefaced by a statement of principle, namely the Five Freedoms and Provisions (Table 1.2) and reference to relevant legislation, e.g. the Welfare of Farmed Animals (England) Regulations (2000 with later amendments). They then proceed to consider the essentials of good husbandry: stockmanship, health care, accommodation, provision of food and water, and management specific to the needs of different classes and ages of animal. The elements of stock-manship are set out in detail, including the creation of a written health and welfare plan, acquisition of handling and husbandry skills (e.g. castration, tooth clipping) and the ability to recognise early signs of ill health. The sections on health dwell in some detail on important issues such as body condition scoring, lameness, control of parasites and the care of sick animals. The sections on accommodation, food and water and the specific recommendations for management also reflect in considerable detail the differing needs of the different species and classes of stock.

The revised Codes provide an excellent, authoritative (and refreshingly animal-orientated) introduction to the principles of good husbandry and are reinforced by suggestions for further reading. If we could guarantee that all farmers abided by all elements of the Welfare Codes then we could claim that all were doing their best to promote good welfare within the existing rules of engagement, e.g. legislation for minimum space allowances, cage sizes, etc. How these rules should evolve is, of course, a separate issue. My present theme is not to set down what should be done but to consider how best we can audit what is being done and effect action when action is necessary.

Inspection of the *Standards Manuals* drawn up by the various accreditation boards reveals, on first inspection, that they are very long, and, second, that they are based almost entirely upon elements of provision (e.g. see Assured British Pigs, 2001). The Assured British Pigs Certification Standard, for example, is based on self-assessment followed by inspection. The self-assessment requires the producer to tick 102 boxes, 100 of which deal with resources, records and management. Only two (condition score and injury) can be categorised as animal-based assessments of welfare. Self-assessment is followed by an inspection intended 'to check that you meet the requirements of the standard. We shall make a detailed inspection of the production facilities, your operational procedures and practices, together with relevant records'. Appendix 1 indicates in detail how the inspectors score 'Housekeeping'. The manual continues 'Inspection of livestock is integral to the scheme' but gives no specific indication of what the inspectors will be looking for, beyond the assessment of body condition which appears as Appendix 3.

The RSPCA Freedom Food Welfare Standards state that they are based on the Five Freedoms (as do the DEFRA Welfare Codes). One might expect therefore that they would be more animal-based. However, inspection of (for example) the Freedom Food standards for laying hens reveals 152 requirements (excluding those relating to transport and slaughter), 145 of which relate to provision and only seven of which may be defined as animal-based indicators of welfare. The magnificent seven do cover the most important welfare problems such as mortality, feather loss, pain and injury, parasitism and behavioural abnormalities, but this begs the question 'are the other 145 questions really necessary?' Another inefficiency of the Freedom Food scheme is that it does not include a mechanism that allows most of the items of provision to be established, in the first instance, by self-assessment. Thus the Freedom Food assessor is committed to spending a high proportion of the visit doing things other than assessing animal welfare.

It is fair to say that at the time of writing (2003) none of the current QA schemes for farm animals incorporates a significant element of animal-based welfare assessment. However, there is clear recognition among animal welfare scientists and others of the need for animal-based protocols, not necessarily to replace existing provisions-based schemes but to complement them. This was a central theme of the 2nd International Workshop on the Assessment of Animal Welfare at Farm and Group Level, held at Bristol in 2002 (Webster & Main, 2003).

4.4 Development of the Bristol protocol for animal-based welfare assessment

The 'Freedom Food' (FF) scheme, set up by the RSPCA in 1994, was the first farm assurance scheme to concentrate on animal welfare. The scheme has attracted international recognition and its principles have been adopted as the basis for similar schemes in many countries. The commitment of the RSPCA to the principles and practice of the FF scheme has undoubtedly been a powerful force for good whose impact has extended far beyond the strict confines of those farms currently registered within the scheme. However, the RSPCA Council, to their credit, recognised that they could not guarantee the FF standards of high welfare either to the customers or to the animals unless they were prepared to submit the scheme to an independent audit. The key questions are: (1) does compliance with the standards of the FF scheme ensure high welfare? and (2) does compliance with the standards of the FF scheme ensure *better* welfare than on non-FF farms?

These questions can only be answered on the basis of measurements of outcome, i.e. welfare state. To do this, one first has to develop animal-based protocols that meet the criteria of feasibility, validity, reliability, repeatability and objectivity. A team consisting of Becky Whay, David Main, Laura Green and myself was contracted by the RSPCA to develop the protocols, conduct the independent audit of FF and advise the RSPCA in the light of the results and their implications. In reference to the quotation that heads this chapter, we were invited to police the policemen. The sequence of steps involved in this process is outlined in Table 4.2.

Our initial contract has been to assess the welfare of dairy cows, growing pigs and laying hens on free-range units. The first step was to gather the opinions of animal welfare experts as to the most important welfare problems for these animals and the most appropriate animal-based measures for welfare assessment (Whay *et al.*, 2003a). This review of expert opinion was carried out using the Delphi technique. This involves the preparation of a structured (but non-leading) consultation document that is sent to a panel of experts who are asked to contribute, as individuals, their knowledge and opinions. The first round of replies is summarised and returned to the panel, who are then asked to comment on or rank the views of the other panel members. This two-stage approach leads progressively towards

Table 4.2 The sequence of steps necessary for the development, testing and implementation of animal-based protocols for assessing on-farm welfare.

(1) First review of expert opinion
(2) Relative importance of different welfare problems
(3) Approaches to measurement of welfare problems
(4) Development and testing of protocols for on-farm assessment of animal welfare
(5) Assessment of welfare on a statistically valid sample of farms
(6) Identification of strengths and weaknesses on individual farms
(7) Second review of expert opinion
(8) Needs for intervention to address specific welfare problems
(9) Development of action plan to address specific problems on individual farms

Table 4.3 The 'top-ten' measures for assessment of the welfare of dairy cattle, pigs and laying hens.

Rank	Cattle	Pigs	Laying hens
1	Observe lameness	Observe lameness	Observe feather appearance
2	Examine health records	Examine limb lesions (PM)	Examine mortality records
3	Observe disease	Examine mortality records	Examine health records
4	Observe mastitis	Examine medicine records	Feather pecking behaviour
5	Observe general demeanour	Examine lung pathology	Observe fear behaviour
6	Score body condition	Observe feeding behaviour	Observe pecking injuries
7	Observe stockmanship	Score body condition	Observe calmness
8	Observe lying behaviour	Observe limb lesions	Observe use of range
9	Examine production records	Response to novel object	Parasite treatment records
10	Observe skin lesions	Observe social behaviour	Observe perch use

PM Post mortem

a consensus of opinion and, because the experts never meet, one that is unlikely to be biased by the force of individual personalities.

Experts were asked to identify at least five welfare issues for each species, rank each according to its importance both to the individual animal and to the UK industry, and state their opinion as to the extent to which it could be avoided by good husbandry practice. Each question was ranked on a score of 0–5. They were then asked what measures could be used to assess each welfare issue, were they useful and were they practical? The 'top ten' measures for each species are listed in Table 4.3. Expert views as to the effectiveness of measures are given in Whay *et al.* (2003a) and will not be reproduced here. The essential point of this Delphi review was to ensure that our approach to assessing welfare on the farm truly reflected expert opinion and not simply our own prejudices. The experts who replied to our questionnaires included veterinarians, ethologists and animal production scientists. It is notable that criteria relating to both fitness and feelings were identified for all three species but that behavioural measures were given far more importance for the laying hen than for the other two species.

4.5 The dairy cow protocol

The first protocol to be developed, tested, implemented and published was that for dairy cattle (Whay *et al.*, 2003b). I present it here as an illustration of the process as it may be applied to assessing the welfare of any species or group of animals whether on farm, in the laboratory (etc.). I shall discuss its implications in more detail when I consider the welfare of dairy cows in Chapter 6. The protocol was based on direct indices of welfare derived from a combination of direct observations, recordings and farmers' estimates and used for a planned evaluation of welfare on 40 FF farms and 40 non-FF farms paired by farm type and location. All observations were made by Becky Whay. Unfortunately, the study was curtailed by the UK foot-and-mouth epidemic of 2001 after only 53 visits, but subsequent analysis revealed that this number was sufficient for our purposes. The results for all farms are summarised in Table 4.4. The observations and records have been grouped according to nutritional state, reproduction, disease, external appearance, environmental injury and behaviour. The incidence or prevalence of the various indices of welfare state are ranked as percentages and arranged 'from best to worst' into five quintiles A–E, so that 20% of herds are within each banding. Obviously, the allocation of a farm to a particular band is specific to each observation.

A complete analysis of the results is given in Whay *et al.* (2003b). Only a selection of the results is discussed here to illustrate major welfare concerns. Nutritional state was obtained from observations of body condition (thin or fat cows), state of the rumen, milk fever (periparturient hypocalcaemia) and other production-related diseases. Table 4.4 shows, for example, that for the specific observation 'thin cows' (condition score less than 2) prevalence in the 'best' 20% of herds (B and A) was 0–5.6%. In the 'worst' herds (band E) it ranged from 33 to 61%. Reported conception to first service was used as a simple index of infertility. This is not in itself a source of distress, but it is a key indicator of loss of fitness.

The recorded and estimated annual incidence of mastitis was in accord with other national surveys. There was a good association between farmer estimates of mastitis incidence and records of treatment. This reflects the policy of farmers to treat mastitis early and record each treatment. The prevalence of lameness, identified by our expert panel as the most important welfare problem for dairy cows, was approached in three ways. True prevalence (per cent) was assessed by observing the locomotion score of all cows as they left the milking parlour. The farmer's

Table 4.4 Results profile for indices of welfare on 53 dairy farms arranged in quintiles from 'best to worst'.

Measure	Type	Score categories (20% in each banding)				
		A	B	C	D	E
Nutritional state						
Thin cows (CS < 2)	Obs.	0–6	6.3–11	13–21	22–31	33–61
Fat cows (CS > 3.5)	Obs.	0	0	0	1–5	5–28
Bloated rumen (%)	Obs.	0	3–6	7–17	18–24	25–47
Hollow rumen (%)	Obs.	0–6	7–14	14–20	21–31	32–82
Milk fever (%/year)	Est.	0	0	0	1	1–31
Metabolic disease[1] (%/year)	Est.	0–3	3–4	5–7	7–9	10–19
Reproduction						
Conception to first service (%)	Est.	80–68	66–60	59–56	55–49	47–28
Assisted calving (%/year)	Est.	0	0	1	1–5	5–40
Disease		0				
Mastitis (%/year)	Rec.	0–9	11–21	21–34	41–46	47–120
Mastitis (%/year)	Est.	3–13	15–19	20–33	33–47	47–89
Lameness prevalence (%)	Obs.	0–14	14–18	19–23	24–30	30–50
Lameness incidence (%/year)	Rec.	0	0	2–4	4–11	11–42
Lameness prevalence (%/year)	Est.	3–9	9–14	15–21	21–34	35–54
Claw overgrowth (%)	Obs.	0–12	12–25	27–34	35–46	46–76
External appearance						
Dirty hind limbs (%)	Obs.	65–85	90–96	97–100	100	100
Dirty udder (%)	Obs.	0–8	10–18	18–23	24–33	36–70
Dirty flanks (%)	Obs.	0	2–7	8–11	14–23	26–78
Hair loss (%)	Obs.	0	4–7	8–13	15–31	33–88
Environmental injury						
Hock hair loss (%)	Obs.	0–8	10–22	22–45	47–71	74–92
Swollen hock (%)	Obs.	0–11	11–28	29–36	37–68	70–97
Ulcerated hock (%)	Obs.	0	3–4	5–12	12–25	29–50
Non-hock injuries (%)	Obs.	6–43	46–59	59–66	67–79	80–100
Behaviour						
Average flight distance[2] (m)	Obs.	0.6–1.1	1.2–1.5	1.5–1.7	1.7–1.9	2.1–3.4
'Idle' cows[3] (%)	Obs.	0–2.6	2.8–3.7	4.7–5.1	5.6–8.3	8.5–25
Rising restriction[4] (%)	Obs.	0–10	12–20	30	33–40	50–78

[1] Metabolic disease includes (e.g.) ketosis, hypomagnesaemia but not milk fever, mastitis or lameness
[2] Distance at which cows retreat from the observer
[3] Standing cows performing no activity
[4] Cows showing severe difficulty in rising, hitting fittings and 'dog-sitting'
CS = condition score; Obs. = observed; Est. = estimated by farmer; Rec. = recorded by farmer
Annual incidence is expressed as cases/100 cows per year (%/year)

perception of lameness was obtained from records of incidence (per cent per year) and their estimates of prevalence at the time of the visit. The proportion of cows recorded as moderately or severely lame from direct observation of locomotion score was 0–14% in band A, rising to 30–50% in band E. The overall lameness prevalence was 23% which compares closely with that recorded in the 1989 Liverpool study (Clarkson *et al.*, 1996). However, farmer estimates of lameness prevalence were, on average only about 20% of that observed during locomotion scoring. Moreover, there was no correspondence between farmer estimates of lameness prevalence and those identified by Whay as severely lame. This shows up a major welfare concern. When at any time 20% of animals are lame and a far greater proportion cannot be said to be walking truly sound, such behaviour can appear 'normal'. This is a powerful illustration of a general conclusion that one of the major tasks for those seeking to improve farm animal welfare is to improve farmer perception of the problem. There was also a significant correlation between the prevalence of true lameness and other environmental injuries, especially ulcerated hocks. Hock damage can serve as a simple and robust indicator of inadequate standards of comfort and injury for dairy cows.

The behavioural observations included in our protocol were average flight distance, rising restrictions and the percentage of cows observed to be standing 'idle' (not eating, ruminating, grooming, socialising, etc.). Flight distance is a good measure of whether cows are calm or nervous and this clearly reflects the social interaction between the cows and their stock-keepers. Rising restriction is a good index of physical discomfort, associated with a mismatch between the dimensions of cow and cubicle. Interpretation of the percentage of idle cows is rather too complex to discuss here, but I shall return to it in Chapter 6.

By allocating a score of 0 (best quintile) to 4 (worst quintile) for each individual welfare assessment, we could arrive at a cumulative 'Welfare Score' for each farm. Obviously some farms were worse than others, but, overall, there were no thoroughly good or thoroughly bad farms. All had some problems and these were specific to the farm. This implies that when you make a welfare assessment on a wide range of animal-based measurements it is, in most cases, impossible to reduce the results to the simplistic conclusion that welfare is 'good' or 'bad'. This may appear self-evident, but it begs the question 'How then can we conclude whether a farm is, or is not, in compliance with the welfare standards of a particular QA scheme?' I shall address this question in the next section.

Having obtained measures and records of the incidence and prevalence of these specific welfare issues, the next stage in the development of the protocol was to submit the information summarised in Table 4.4 to a second round of expert opinion. Veterinarians, ethologists and animal welfare scientists were asked to indicate the score category (quintile) at which they considered intervention would be necessary to remedy a welfare problem apparent at herd level. Arbitrarily, but I believe reasonably, we have identified a clear herd problem as one where the prevalence or incidence was such that 75% of experts recommended intervention.

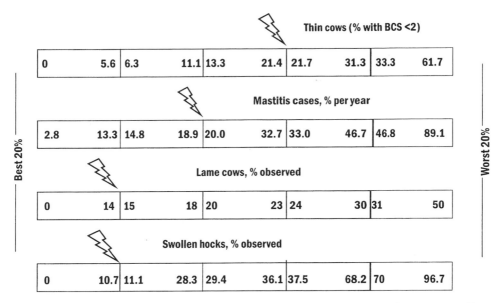

Figure 4.2 Examples of expert opinion as to the need for intervention in four major welfare problems for dairy cows.

Figure 4.2 presents four important examples of expert opinion as to the need for intervention (as illustrated by the jagged arrows). The prevalence ranges in each quintile are those given in Table 4.4. In the case of thin cows, 75% considered that intervention was necessary for farms in bands D and E (i.e. in 40% of the farms where prevalence was >21%). For mastitis, intervention was recommended at an annual incidence above 20% (60% of farms). For lameness and swollen hocks, intervention was recommended in bands B–E (when prevalence was greater than 13% and 11%, respectively). In other words, 75% of competent judges considered that lameness was a welfare problem that required attention at a herd level in 80% of the farms in our study!

The final step in development of the welfare assurance programme (Table 4.2) is to implement an action plan designed to address specific welfare problems. I repeat: farms did not perform consistently well or badly. Most were good at some aspects, poor at others. It follows from this that remedies for welfare problems need to be tailored according to the specific needs of specific farms. I should also point out at this stage that there was no difference in overall welfare score between FF and non-FF farms (for details see Main *et al.*, 2003). Thus, we were unable to conclude that membership of the FF scheme ensured better overall welfare than on non-participating farms. This may, at first sight, seem like bad news for the RSPCA. It does, however, highlight a very positive outcome to our study, namely that our animal-based protocol for assessment of welfare outcomes is able to identify specific problems on farms where the resources and management are in compliance with FF or any other welfare-based QA scheme. The Bristol protocol identified specific welfare problems (especially lameness) on some farms that were in compliance with the FF scheme. The RSPCA then, with our assistance, instituted action plans tailored towards specific problems on FF farms and implemented with the active collaboration of the farmers and their veterinary surgeons. Our independent audit of the FF scheme for dairy cows has not served to diminish the scheme but to strengthen it. It now includes a protocol that can identify specific welfare problems that may occur notwithstanding compliance with the standards of provision laid down by the scheme, and an action plan designed to resolve these specific problems.

4.6 Development of welfare-based quality control procedures

So where do we go from here? Let me recapitulate the key issues relating to the current state and future development of welfare-based quality assurance and quality control schemes for farm animals:

- Any comprehensive audit of animal welfare should incorporate a review of both provisions and outcome, i.e. husbandry and welfare.
- Current QA schemes are mostly based on long check lists of elements of provision (some produced by self-assessment).
- Assessment of welfare is only part of the QA requirement for Farm Assurance, which will also require assurances as to food safety, biosecurity, etc.
- Voluntary welfare-based QA schemes will only succeed if they are understood, trusted and seen to add value by all parties: consumers, retailers and farmers.

The current status of welfare-based QA schemes offered to or imposed upon farmers is far from satisfactory. Most involve a bureaucratic, time-consuming marathon of ticking boxes relating to items of provision. Even an obviously welfare-orientated scheme such as Freedom Foods can still fail to identify an important welfare problem such as lameness in dairy cows. Thus current schemes are both failing to measure the things they ought to have measured and measuring the things they ought not have measured. The aim for the future should be to develop protocols that can *both* highlight welfare problems *and* identify failures in provision that have contributed to these problems. My suggested approach is as follows:

- The QA scheme should lay down clear guidelines for husbandry, following a format similar to that of the DEFRA Codes of Recommendations for the Welfare of Livestock (Table 4.1) and modified, as necessary, to meet minimum standards for the scheme where these differ from the welfare codes (e.g. space allowances, enriched environments).

- The farmer should, in the first instance, be required to measure compliance with the standards by a process of self-assessment that would, in part, consist of ticking boxes relating to matters of fact but also require self-assessment of the quality of key areas of husbandry.
- The independent assessment of compliance with the provisions of the scheme should primarily involve animal-based observations and records of welfare outcomes. These would be conducted by trained assessors, who would also make a random selection of checks on some (not all) of the farmer's self-assessment of elements of provision.
- If the assessor identified no welfare problem serious enough to warrant attention (on a herd basis) and no deficiencies arising from spot checks on the self-assessment, then the farmer would pass the test of compliance with the standards of the scheme.
- If the assessor identified a welfare problem(s) serious enough to warrant attention, it would then be necessary to check specific items of provision (as defined in the standards) that may contribute to the specific welfare problem. These can be identified relatively easily (if slowly) within existing lists of standards. Computerising the process would make it both faster and more accurate.
- When specific welfare problems can be clearly linked to failures of provision, then the farmer would have to remedy these problems in order to remain in compliance with the standards of the scheme.
- If the assessor identified specific welfare problems but these could not be linked clearly to specific deficiencies of provision, then the farmer would be required to seek professional (e.g. veterinary) advice and prepare an action plan to resolve (or at least reduce) the problem. The assessor, in association with the farmer and his/her veterinarian, would review the situation after an appropriate interval to decide whether or not sufficient had been done to meet the standards of good husbandry required by the scheme (which does not necessarily imply elimination of the problem).

This approach addresses the objectives that I have set for identifying welfare problems, the causes of welfare problems and actions designed to remedy welfare problems. I have illustrated our approach by reference to the dairy cow protocol. Protocols for other groups of animals, on farm, in the laboratory, etc. will be discussed later. At this stage, however, it is important to emphasise the need for continued development and testing of the efficacy of practical protocols such as these against more searching indices of animal welfare established under experimental conditions with small numbers of animals. Ideally (for the animals) we should work towards achieving a satisfactory degree of international uniformity as to method and interpretation since welfare problems, as perceived by the animals, do not recognise national boundaries. This becomes especially important if minimum standards are to be set by legislation for both the provision of good husbandry and its outcome, good welfare.

Two further issues need to be considered in relation to the development of improved protocols for the assessment of husbandry and welfare. These are: (1) can we and should we attempt to integrate welfare indices? and (2) how may welfare assessment best be incorporated within the broader aims of sustainable economic agriculture? Some integration of individual indices is almost inevitable in any broad assessment of animal welfare. The Austrian 'Animal Needs Index' is one good example (Bartussek, 1999).

The level of integration may be partial, i.e. the integration of groups of associated measures to rank welfare status within a particular category, e.g. nutritional status or comfort. It may be deemed necessary to integrate all measures into a single overall value (a welfare 'score') or simple ranking (e.g. satisfactory or unsatisfactory). The necessity for integration and the nature and degree of integration should be determined by the aims of the assessment. Some degree of integration of individual measures to rank husbandry and welfare within defined, fairly broad categories (e.g. stockmanship, environment, nutrition, health) is both sensible and realistic. However, complete integration of these different categories in order to produce an overall welfare score raises the fundamental problem addressed in Chapter 1, namely that different groups will, for ethical or political reasons, give different weightings to different parameters (e.g. injury v. behavioural deprivation). The problem here is that one is trying to weight value judgements.

Some QA schemes may wish to rank overall welfare on individual farms to produce, for example, a 'league table' that would reward the champions and offer incentives to others to raise their standing within the league. This approach has some attractions and would, in my opinion, be relatively harmless if not taken too seriously. In other words, it could be used as an incentive for farms acting in compliance with the standards of the scheme to improve their husbandry and welfare and so progress up the league table. However, I believe that an overall integrated welfare score should never be used as the sole mark to determine whether a farm passed or failed the assessment. The great drawback of basing compliance on an overall score is that a farm that performed adequately according to most welfare categories might 'scrape a pass' despite severe deficiencies in a specific area, such as lameness. If this occurred, there would be no mechanism and no incentive to remedy specific problems. The protocol that I have outlined above is designed to promote general compliance with accepted standards of good husbandry, identify specific welfare problems as they occur and initiate actions designed to remedy these specific problems. Such a scheme does not require integration beyond that necessary to define categories of welfare from a range of observations and records. Participation in the scheme depends on compliance with agreed general standards of provision and effective action to address specific welfare problems as they occur.

The last question that I shall look at in relation to the development of animal-based protocols for assessing welfare in farm animals is 'How may welfare assessment best be incorporated within the broader aims of sustainable economic agriculture?' The first thing to say here is that animal welfare is important but not all-important. It has to be incorporated within a broader assessment of quality that takes proper account of the interests, views and demands of all parties, both those that have an active stake in the free market – consumers, retailers and producers – and those who do not – farm animals and the living environment. Thus animal welfare standards cannot be set in isolation and must inevitably involve compromise. There are, of course, exceptions. Beyond a certain level, defined by law as 'unnecessary suffering' caused by cruelty, abuse of animal welfare becomes unacceptable in any circumstances. However, the vast majority of welfare problems for the vast majority of farm animals are not caused by acts of cruelty or even negligence. They arise within systems that meet broad acceptance from the majority of society.

It is only too apparent that animal welfare is only one of many concerns in the minds of those who make it their business to check up on farmers. Hygiene, biosecurity, pollution, health and safety of employees, land allocations for 'set aside', all create large amounts of paperwork and impose controls on what a farmer can and cannot do on his/her own land. It is in the interests of everybody (save those who derive their living from making life difficult for others) to streamline these operations. This is not the place to discuss in any detail the co-ordination of all elements of Farm Assurance. I do suggest, however, that those whose prime concern is to ensure high standards of animal welfare through QA should seek to co-ordinate their procedures with other registration bodies. A farmer should not have to write the answer to the same question in six separate self-assessment forms, still less stand around while six separate assessors armed with clip boards read the questions out loud. The assessment protocol that I have described above calls for qualified assessors to evaluate welfare from animal-based observations and records. If these protocols, or developments of these protocols, were accepted as international standards of assessment (or even accepted across a broad range of voluntary QA systems) then the qualified assessors could be empowered to assess the outcomes of all or a wide range of QA schemes. This would be a giant leap forward towards the goals of feasibility, validity, repeatability and objectivity. It should also reassure both farmers and consumers that such schemes sought to be fair to all parties.

4.7 Implementation of welfare-based quality assurance and quality control

In a free-market society the ultimate success of any QA scheme will require recognition both by farmers and by consumers that it gives added value, where this concept includes a proper recognition of the intrinsic value of sentient animals. In this way all parties can benefit from the scheme. For the consumer, there will be more trust; for the farmer there will be more pride. As for the animals, they are more likely to be fit and feel good.

I have to conclude, with regret, that few of the voluntary schemes currently operating in Europe are making a significant contribution to added value for consumers, farmers or their animals. The success of free-range eggs is a conspicuous, if slightly contentious, exception to this rule (see Chapter 5). It is customary to market QA schemes to farmers on the basis that they will improve profitability by reducing costs. It is true that some improvements to animal welfare, implemented at the farm level, can be economically advantageous to the farmer. For example, sustaining the fitness of the dairy cow to prolong her working life from two to six lactations can improve her lifetime productive efficiency by 15–20% (see Chapter 6). However, many of the husbandry provisions necessary to improve welfare (better housing, improved veterinary care) can only be achieved at a cost to the farmer. It follows therefore that many farmers, currently doing the best they can within the current economic climate, will only improve standards of husbandry if they are paid a premium to do so.

Where improved welfare carries a significant cost to the farmer this can only be achieved through legislation, fairly imposed throughout the trading community (and this is much easier said than done). However, in Chapter 1 (Table 1.5) I showed that the cost to the consumer of achieving significant improvements in minimum welfare standards for farm animals in intensive 'factory farm' conditions could be significantly improved and could be imperceptibly small. A voluntary QA scheme is an instrument of competition. It follows from this that only the most successful schemes will survive. If a voluntary scheme is to succeed with the consumer, it has to promote the demand for higher-value animal products within a free market, where the measure of value incorporates an assessment of the 'non-product-related process and production methods'. This is the basis for QA schemes directed towards niche markets (e.g. organic, Freedom Foods). If it is to succeed with producers it must deliver, at best, a cash premium for their products. Failing this, it should be seen as an effective way to combat international competition for trade in animals as commodities by persuading the consumer to buy food produced according to the standards of a scheme that gives respect to the food animals as sentient beings.

Animals for Food: Industrialised Farming, Pigs and Poultry 5

Dogs look up to you, cats look down on you but a pig treats you as an equal.

Winston Churchill

The titles of this and the next four chapters begin with the words 'Animals for': animals for food, animals for science and biotechnology, animals for entertainment. The phrases are crude but accurate since they acknowledge that we breed and rear animals for food, for science or for field sports simply to serve our needs. Nobody (well, almost nobody*) breeds pigs simply out of respect for the intrinsic value of the species. Our motivation is self-interest. So far as we are concerned, the value of these animals is defined by their extrinsic value (to us). This chapter will consider the most extreme example of our treatment of animals as commodities, namely industrialised 'factory' farming, which has reached its apogee in the production of pigs and poultry.

5.1 The industrialisation of livestock farming

It is, at the outset, necessary to understand the forces that led to the industrialisation of livestock farming. Within traditional, family-scale farming systems, ruminants designed primarily for meat production (sheep and goats) were expected to forage for themselves, grazing land that the family did not own and consuming food that the family could not digest. The farmer and his family would, however, grow, cut, carry and conserve food for the house cow, since she could repay this investment through the production of milk and work. Her male calf would be killed to be eaten as veal on special occasions (e.g. return of prodigal son) and before it began to compete with its mother for food. Poultry and pigs (where culturally acceptable) acted as scavengers who ate food that would otherwise have

* Lord Emsworth perhaps?

gone to waste. Young pigs intended to provide food for the table or for preservation and sale as cured ham were kept in styes and fed on house and farm swill to ensure they fattened as quickly and as cost-effectively as possible. Breeding sows and chickens would usually be given the run of at least part of the farm, since this let them forage for some of their own food and reduced the cost and labour of housing, bedding and manure disposal. The traditional farmer who allowed his pigs and hens free range on his farm was not being inherently kinder than the manager of a modern poultry unit, he was simply adopting the strategy most appropriate to his own circumstances. The key to the success of the system was that, so far as possible, the animals harvested their own food and spread their own manure.

These simple principles formed the basis for livestock farming from the beginning of agriculture, almost to the present day. We can (with full bellies) commend the approach as demonstrably sustainable. However, it provided little more than subsistence for most of the farmers, most of the time and it certainly could not meet our modern expectations for a wide variety of good, safe, cheap food in all seasons. The industrial revolution in livestock farming really began only about 70 years ago, and only in the industrialised world. In undeveloped countries, it has hardly started. The single key that exposes all the differences between the modern industrialised livestock farm and traditional, sustainable but subsistence farming is that the output of the factory farm is no longer constrained by what can be produced off the land it occupies. Most or all of the inputs to the system – power, machinery (e.g. tractors) and other resources (e.g. food and fertilisers) – are bought in so that output is constrained only by the amount that the producer can afford to invest in capital and other resources and the capacity of the system to process them.

Figure 5.1 outlines the genealogy of the intensive livestock farm, as typified by modern intensively housed pig and poultry units. Some feed for pigs and poultry (e.g. cereals) may be grown within the farm enterprise, but this, along with purchased feed supplements to ensure a balanced diet, is trucked onto the unit and dispensed to animals in controlled environment houses by mechanical feeding systems. The capital required to set up such a unit is high. Mechanical and electrical power is used to control temperature and ventilation in the intensive housing units, to dispense feed and to remove and disperse the manure. Factory farming was born when it became cheaper, faster and more efficient to process feed through animals using machines than to let the animals do the work for themselves. Once the high set-up costs had been met, the input of cheap energy and other resources from off-farm was able to increase output and reduce running costs. In consequence, poultry meat from chickens and turkeys, once the food of family feasts, is now the cheapest meat on the market.

Potentially harmful outputs from intensive livestock systems (dashed lines in Figure 5.1) include increased pollution, infectious disease and abuse of animal welfare. I emphasise the word 'potential' to avoid succumbing to the simplistic

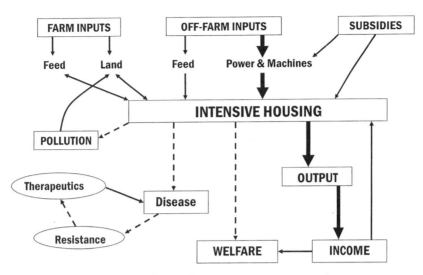

Figure 5.1 The genealogy of the factory farm.

mantra 'intensive bad, extensive good'. Most of the pollutants emerging from intensive livestock units are, in fact, organic fertilisers. The problem is not the material itself but too much of it in the wrong place, an inevitable consequence of divorcing the husbandry of livestock from the husbandry of the land. Bringing animals off the land and into close confinement inevitably increases the risks of infectious disease. To combat this increased risk it has been necessary to introduce strict new strategies to eliminate or at least reduce exposure to infection through improvements to biosecurity and hygiene. Where exposure to infection cannot be eliminated it is necessary to develop routine disease control measures through the use of vaccines, antibiotics and other therapeutic drugs. The key to biosecurity in an intensive pig unit is to preserve a minimal disease status in the herd by preventing any infection getting into the unit from outside. This requires strict controls on the movement of animals and stock-keepers who shower and don protective clothing before entering the unit. This will normally ensure the health of the animals (one essential element of welfare), but there are obvious limits to the expression of natural behaviour in a large isolation hospital. The key element of hygiene is to minimise contact between animals and their excreta. It is important to remind ourselves that one of the main reasons for putting laying hens into battery cages was to reduce the risks to the animals and to food safety of infectious diseases such as those carried by the *Salmonella* species of bacteria.

The other essential requisite for the control of infectious diseases in intensive livestock units has been the use of veterinary preparations, therapeutic agents such as vaccines, antibiotics and antiparasitic drugs. If access to cheap power had been all that was necessary for the success of intensive livestock farming, then this industrial revolution would have occurred in the 1920s. In fact it did not really take off until the 1950s when antibiotics effective against the major endemic bacterial diseases of housed livestock became cheap and freely available. Alternative, subtler approaches to disease control, such as the development of specific vaccines and strains of animals genetically resistant to specific diseases, have also contributed to the commercial success of intensive systems, especially in the case of poultry. However, it is fair to claim that industrialised farming of pigs and poultry has, for the last 40 years, been sustained by the routine use of antibiotics, coccidiostats and other chemotherapeutics to control endemic diseases. In some cases these diseases could be life-threatening. In most cases, however, chemotherapeutics have been used routinely to increase productivity by reducing the effects of chronic, low-grade infection.

However, the era when it was possible to rear pigs and poultry under blanket cover of prophylactic antibiotics is coming to an end, in Europe at least. EU legislation to impose a complete ban on the use of antibiotics as 'zootechnical additives' or 'growth promoters' is pending. The reason for this ban is increasing concern that the development of microbial resistance to antibiotics used as growth promoters will pose an increasing risk to the health of the animals and, especially, us the consumers. The scientific evidence in support of this legislation is not entirely convincing, mainly because the antibiotics currently licensed as growth promoters differ in character from those used therapeutically in veterinary and human medicine. Indeed, there is a real danger that this new prohibition will suffer a similar fate to previous worthy attempts at prohibition, and do more harm than good, partly through an increase in the black market, but more likely through a large increase in the 'legal' prescription of genuinely therapeutic antibiotics to farm animals. However, on balance, and in time, it has to be a good thing, both for the animals and ourselves, to restrict the routine use of antibiotics in livestock agriculture. It is an unequivocal insult to the principle of good husbandry to keep animals in conditions of such intensity, inappropriate feeding or squalor that their health can only be ensured by the routine administration of chemotherapeutics. It is also a breach of veterinary ethics to dispense therapeutic antibiotics on a routine basis to sustain the production of animals in an unacceptable environment. However, in limping towards this particular corner of Eden, a paradise of naturally healthy farm animals, it is necessary to tread carefully. The view from the Soil Association, the high moral ground of organic farming, is that antibiotics should only be used as a last resort to treat sick animals when prevention and other approaches, such as homeopathic preparations, have failed. The ultimate goal of this argument, a population of naturally healthy animals, is entirely laudable, and many of the routes to this goal are entirely sensible (though not the homeopathic one). Paradoxically, however, this policy is similar in its absolutist principles to UK government policy to ensure freedom from an epidemic disease such as foot-and-mouth virus through wholesale slaughter of infected animals and those in close contact. In both examples, the goal may be admirable, but a lot of animals are likely to suffer *en route*. Those who work with animals on a day-to-day basis, stock-keepers and veterinary surgeons, have a responsibility to ensure the welfare of those animals that are in their care, now. If, in their competent and caring judgement, this involves, from time to time, the use of prophylactic therapeutics not to 'promote growth', but to prevent or control a properly diagnosed outbreak of infectious disease, then so be it. They do not deserve to be condemned by those who proclaim principles that they will never be forced to put to the test.

Furthermore, it is simplistic to assume that intensification of livestock production is inherently detrimental to animal welfare. In the next section I shall consider welfare problems inherent to factory farming in some detail. At this stage I would simply state the obvious fact that in any system whereby hundreds of thousands of animals are contained within a single building it is impossible to care for animals as individuals. This is a potential welfare risk for the individual if things go wrong. Indeed any individual that falls behind the average by virtue of ill health, impaired development or reluctance to compete at the feed trough has little chance of being nursed back to normality through sympathetic stockmanship. Thus factory farming has imposed a neo-Darwinian variation on the principle of the survival of the fittest.

It is also a fact that the amount of care that farmers can give to the welfare of their animals is limited by what they can afford. If animals are to be housed in a building, then it is better for the animals that it should be a good building, and that usually means more expensive. In *Eden I*, I argued that the welfare of sheep has been greatly improved by housing ewes at lambing. This, in common with many other capital investments on farms, has been made possible by increasing income, partly through increased sales and partly through subsidy (Figure 5.1). There are many welfare problems inherent to intensive farming, but, I repeat, it is simplistic to assume that they can be automatically cured through extensification, i.e. a policy of lower inputs and lower outputs. Unless farmers are protected from further erosion of farm incomes, e.g. through appropriate redirection of subsidy, enforced extensification may do more harm than good for animal welfare.

5.2 Welfare problems inherent to factory farming

Table 5.1 outlines a series of welfare problems that are inherent to the factory farming of large numbers of animals in confinement systems. These are largely self-evident and well recognised by the designers and operators of large livestock units. Recognition of a problem is, however, only the beginning. In order to resolve a problem it is necessary to understand its origins. In this section I shall explore the nature and origins of the inherent welfare problems identified in Table 5.1 and identify pathways towards their resolution.

The central problem for animals in intensive livestock units is that they have little or no freedom of choice. In other words they are not in control of their own

Table 5.1   Welfare problems inherent to intensive livestock production.

Loss of choice
   Feed selection in sickness and in health
   Environmental selection: comfort, security, fresh air
Failures of stockmanship
   Inadequate time and access for individual contact
   Inadequate perception of the animals' physiological and behavioural needs
Failures of equipment
   Ventilation
   Feed and slurry handling
Increased transmission of infectious and parasitic diseases
   High stocking densities
   Accumulation of pathogens and pollutants
Inability to exhibit natural behaviour
   Insufficient space for normal movement
   Inability to establish normal social interactions
Problems of handling, transport and slaughter
   Difficulties with handling very large numbers
   Thermal and physical stresses during transportation
   Suffering at the place of slaughter

lives. Their physiological and behavioural needs are determined by the humans who run the enterprise (and their professional advisors) and dispensed, so far as possible, by machines. A vast amount of animal science and technology has been invested in determining (e.g.) the nutritional and environmental needs of farm animals, and this has been extremely successful in increasing the efficiency of livestock production. The nutrient requirements of farm animals have been documented in exquisite detail (e.g. in the publications of the National Research Council of the USA) down to a stated precision of milligrams/day of essential amino acids or trace elements. It would, however, be absurd to assume that these 'requirements' correspond exactly to what each individual animal would choose for itself at every stage of normal growth or lactation, and more absurd to assume that they would still apply to an animal when, for one reason or other, it felt less than entirely healthy. The word 'requirements' should properly be replaced by 'allowances', i.e. they are not a definition of what the animals need but what we think we should provide. While these allowances can achieve highly efficient production from most of the animals most of the time, they do not allow an individual animal to select a diet that makes it feel better when it is sick, nor one that allows it to 'catch up' during convalescence. There is an increasing body of scientific evidence to show that pigs, poultry and ruminants will, given the choice, select diets according to their specific physiological needs, e.g. during catch-up growth or when carrying a heavy parasite burden (Kyriazakis & Emmans, 1991). A number of enlightened producers of poultry meat have demonstrated advantages for both health and production from giving broiler chickens limited choice between two diets that permit them to balance the protein:carbohydrate ratio to meet their own perception of physiological needs. This is not the place to examine diet selection in detail (I have discussed it at greater length in *Eden I*, Chapter 3). I wish only to suggest that opportunities for diet selection should be considered in any plans for the installation, updating or day-to-day operation of any large livestock rearing enterprise.

It is equally simplistic to assume that all animals in a large group have exactly the same thermal and physical environmental requirements all the time. I have already described how pigs and poultry in environments containing ammonia at >10 ppm are motivated to seek fresh air, not all the time, but from time to time (Jones *et al.*, 1999). Pigs also choose to sleep in cooler environments during the night than the day and pass urine and faeces at sites remote from the areas where they feed and sleep. Hens that are not confined to the extremely barren environment of a battery cage will select favoured areas for egg laying and for security. Any livestock unit that gives animals no opportunity for action to modify how they feel (e.g. attend to their individual needs for comfort and security) is, by definition, an unsatisfactory environment.

Probably the biggest welfare problem inherent to intensive livestock units is that it renders impossible the practice of proper stockmanship. We have it on the highest authority that the good shepherd 'shall gather the lambs with his arm and carry them in his bosom' yet there is little more that the best-intentioned of stock-keepers in a broiler unit can do than cull the dying and carry out the dead. The system simply does not make it possible for the stock-keeper to observe each individual animal, let alone attend to their individual needs. I have written already that animals need stock-keepers in proportion to the extent to which they are denied the opportunity to attend to their own physiological and behavioural needs. The more intensive the unit, the greater the denial and therefore the greater the need for good stockmanship. In this regard machines that dispense feed and remove manure may be viewed as a blessing rather than a curse (so long as they are working properly) since they remove much of the drudgery from the job and, in theory, allow more time for inspection and care of animals. However, in practice, and in the current economic climate, such time is seldom made available. In Table 5.1 I cite 'inadequate perception of the animals' physiological and behavioural needs' as an inherent welfare problem in intensive systems. This is not intended as a criticism of stock-keepers as individuals. Many are extremely well-trained, conscientious and caring. My criticism is that it is simply not possible in the barren environment of an intensive livestock unit holding thousands of animals to recognise the needs of individuals, nor attend to them, nor (which is worse) give them the opportunity to act for themselves in a way that will help them to feel good.

Welfare problems due to failures of equipment are largely self-evident and potentially catastrophic. They are well recognised by the owners and operators of intensive units. Poultry units, for example, will have fail-safe mechanisms that operate in the event of a failure in mechanical ventilation to prevent birds dying from asphyxiation and hyperthermia. Nevertheless there have been cases where broilers have died in their thousands from hyperthermia, not because the artificial ventilation system failed, but because the 'environmental control' system simply did not have the capacity to maintain a tolerable air temperature within the building during periods of extreme hot weather.

I have already drawn attention to the inherent risks of infectious disease arising from keeping very large numbers of animals at high stocking density in a single air space and it is a subject that I have considered in detail elsewhere (Webster, 1990). At this stage I simply repeat that control through the blanket use of antibiotics and other chemotherapeutics will soon no longer be an option for many intensive producers. This will impose major and largely welcome changes on intensive production systems.

One of the most obvious insults to welfare in densely stocked intensive livestock units is that identified by the Brambell Committee (Brambell, 1965), namely the lack of freedom for the individual animal to 'stand up, sit down, turn round, groom itself and stretch its limbs'. The wish to rectify this denial of essential maintenance behaviour has been the prime motivator behind much of European legislation to improve minimum welfare standards for farm animals and has expressed itself (e.g.) as an increase in minimum space requirements for caged laying hens and a ban on the keeping of sows for prolonged periods in individual stalls. These are short, halting steps towards Eden; welcome insofar as they go, but they fall far short of the target of meeting behavioural needs. The other welfare problem inherent to units containing very large numbers of animals is that individuals are unable to establish normal social interactions. This arises partly because there are simply too many animals to establish a hierarchy, and partly because individuals that meet have neither the space nor the environmental resources (e.g. escape routes) to permit expression of those rituals of advance and retreat, aggression and appeasement, necessary to establish and maintain stable social relationships.

The final category of welfare problems inherent to industrialised livestock production are those relating to handling, transport and slaughter. Chapter 7 addresses these topics in detail and I shall do no more than highlight them at this stage. Suffice it to say that the bigger the unit, the more difficult it is to gather the animals for transport; the more animals in a vehicle, the more difficult it is to provide thermal and physical comfort. As units become bigger they become fewer and farther between, thus the further animals are made to travel *en route* to slaughter. The more animals 'processed' per day through an abattoir the more difficult it becomes to protect animals from the whole range of potential insults that may occur from the time the animal is disturbed in its home pen to the time that death brings to an end its capacity to suffer.

5.3 Breeding animals fit for purpose

Evolution through natural selection operates according to the principle of survival of the fittest. The animals whose genetic design is better adapted to a particular environment are those most likely to breed successfully and so pass their genetic superiority (in that environment) on to their offspring. Indeed, in the strictly Darwinian sense, the 'fitness' of an animal is defined by its success in passing its genes on to subsequent generations. By domesticating animals and controlling their breeding to suit our own needs we have redesigned the phenotype to produce what we want (e.g. food and clothing) within an environment that we control. The modern long, lean bacon pig bears little resemblance to the wild boar; the modern broiler chicken, bred to produce as much breast meat as possible in 6 weeks, bears even less resemblance to the jungle fowl. According to the most limited definition of Darwinian fitness, it can be claimed that the top five lines of broiler breeders represent an outstanding success since their offspring constitute over 80% of the world broiler population. Breeders of animals designed for intensive systems are able to claim that their strain of chicken, pig or dairy cow is 'superior' within the environment for which it is designed. It grows faster, gives more milk, converts food more efficiently, has a leaner carcass. Indeed, the breeders of modern intensively reared strains of pigs and poultry frequently congratulate themselves on the fact that they have achieved so much more progress than, for example, the breeders of sheep whose animals look much the same as they did 200 years ago.

The modern commercial genotypes of pigs and poultry that have, through international trade, achieved world dominance may, in a strictly limited Darwinian sense, be defined as the 'fittest'. However, for most people and for most purposes, fitness is better interpreted as a state of good health and vigour. This is certainly what I have in mind when I define good welfare as 'fit and feeling good'. When modern genotypes of farm animal bred for intensive systems are examined according to this definition, the breeders' claims to genetic superiority come apart at the seams. Broiler chickens that are crippled in large numbers or die from cardiac failure if reared beyond the conventional slaughter date of 42 days are clearly not fit. The food intake of adult broiler breeders has to be severely restricted to stop them eating themselves to death. Breeding sows so large, clumsy and/or lame that they have to be confined in farrowing stalls to prevent them from crushing their piglets as they crash uncontrollably to the ground are not fit. Dairy cows that have to be culled for reasons of infertility, mastitis or lameness after less than three lactations are not fit. In these examples the artificial selection of food animals for traits dominated by the quality and efficiency of food production *per se* has imposed a severe cost largely expressed as a loss of fitness in the breeding generation.

The most obvious reason why there has been so much apparent genetic 'improvement' (the word 'change' would be more accurate) in pigs and poultry and so little in sheep is that we have modified the environment for pigs and poultry

Table 5.2 Factors determining efficiency of meat production; allocation of feed energy to the breeding and slaughter generations in broiler chickens, pigs, sheep and suckler beef cattle.

Factors determining efficiency of meat production	Broilers	Pigs	Sheep	Beef cattle
Weight of breeding females (kg)	3.0	180	75	450
Carcass weight from meat animal (kg)	1.5	50	18	250
Ratio, wt carcass/wt dam	0.5	0.28	0.24	0.55
Progeny/year	240	22	1.6	0.9
Wt carcass per year/wt dam	120	6.2	0.38	0.5
Proportion of food energy/year				
To breeding generation	0.04	0.20	0.68	0.52
To slaughter generation	0.96	0.80	0.32	0.48

to the point where almost their only requisite for survival is to eat, whereas sheep and lambs out on the hill need to fend for themselves. There is another, more subtle reason illustrated by Table 5.2 which analyses the most important factors that determine the efficiency of meat production from broiler chickens, pigs, sheep and suckler beef cattle (i.e. production of beef from calves reared by their mothers). The first five lines provide the information necessary to estimate the mass of saleable carcass produced per annum from one breeding female. This is a function of the ratio of the carcass weight of the slaughtered animals to the live weight of their mothers multiplied by the number of progeny produced per year and reared to slaughter weight. Thus one breeding broiler hen producing 240 eggs/year can yield 120 times her own body weight per annum in terms of saleable meat (and bone). For the breeding sow producing 22 piglets per year, the ratio is 6.2. For the grazing ruminants sheep and beef cows producing respectively 1.6 and 0.9 off-spring per year the ratios are only 0.38 and 0.5 respectively. The apparent anomaly between the higher prolificacy of the sheep but lower ratio of carcass weight to mature weight is explained by the fact that most lambs grow fast and cheaply on grass and mother's milk and are slaughtered at a young age (approximately four months) and a relatively low proportion of mature body weight. Beef cattle tend to be grown more slowly and slaughtered at about two years of age at a higher degree of maturity.

The last two lines in Table 5.2 estimate the proportion of total food (energy) that is consumed by the breeding generation and by the offspring, or slaughter generation. In the extreme case of broiler chickens, 96% of all the chicken feed going into the system is eaten by the slaughter generation. In the case of pigs, it is 80%. At the other extreme is the sheep industry where 68% of all feed is con-sumed by the breeding generation of ewes (and a few rams). Moreover, in the case of sheep nearly all the expensive conserved or purchased feed is eaten by the breed-ing generation since they are the animals kept alive over winter. Thus on a sheep farm the cost of feeding the breeding generation will, in most cases, exceed 80% of total feed costs. When nearly all the feed is consumed by the slaughter generation, it is economically adroit to select animals for traits that improve efficiency in the slaughter generation. The most important of these are rapid growth, leanness and food conversion efficiency. Leanness and food conversion efficiency are closely correlated since it takes about eight times as much food energy to deposit one gram of fat as to deposit one gram of fat-free muscle. However, two of the facts of growth are that the bigger the animal the faster it grows and that as each animal approaches its mature weight it deposits progressively more fat and less lean. It follows therefore that selection for leanness and rapid growth to an optimal weight and 'finish' as determined by the butcher is strongly correlated with selection for slaughter at a progressively lower proportion of mature body weight. It follows from *this* that selection for leanness and rapid growth means a progressive increase in size of the breeding generation. Thus in the case of pigs we are producing larger and larger breeding females, increasingly prone to lameness, too big for existing farrowing crates, yet too clumsy to rear their piglets in the more humane environment of a pen of deep straw. In the case of broilers, we have produced breeding birds that must be kept on a severely restricted diet that prevents them from achieving their target mature *lean* weight to save them from the diseases of obesity, lameness and cardiac failure.

In strictly economic terms the intensive pig and poultry industries can carry the cost of reduced fitness in the breeding generation, because the impact on the overall enterprise is small (Table 5.2). In consequence they are prepared to accept an element of poor performance – *and even poorer welfare* – in the breeding generation as an acceptable tax on the system. However, the more extensive sheep and suckler beef (cow/calf in the USA) enterprises could not bear the economic cost of selection simply for 'superior' traits in the slaughter generation alone. If the sheep industry had elected to pursue genetic 'improvement' according to the same rules that operate in the pig and poultry industries, namely selection exclusively for commercial traits appropriate to the slaughter generation, it would now be operating with breeding ewes perhaps 50% heavier than the current average, each requiring 50% more food. Since the breeding ewes account for approximately 80% of total feed costs this policy would have led to a serious deterioration in the overall efficiency of the enterprise. I shall discuss the welfare of sheep and beef cattle in Chapter 6. At this stage it suffices to say that breeding ewes and suckler beef cows are, for the most part, phenotypically pretty well designed for survival for the good reason that their owners could not afford to have them otherwise.

There is, however, constant pressure on the beef and sheep industries from breeders and other advisors to breed for superiority in carcass traits. The most grotesque form of this trend is manifest in the 'double-muscled' Belgian Blue cattle, selected for such extreme muscle development, especially around the hindquarters, that the cows cannot give birth naturally and must be exposed to repeated Caesarian section; the calves born by Caesarian section are excessively prone to respiratory distress and risk of pneumonia. As a visibly obvious abuse of the normal principles of humanity, this far exceeds anything that has been achieved or even attempted through modern techniques in biotechnology and genetic engineering. I constantly assert that one of the guarantors of good animal welfare is pride in good husbandry. I cannot believe that anyone could honestly profess pride in rearing the double-muscled freaks that pass as Belgian Blue cattle.

The 'good husbandry' solution to reconciling the divergent needs of the butcher for good beef and lamb carcasses with the needs of the farmer for breeding stock that are fit and that last is through divergent selection and crossbreeding. Divergent selection implies selecting for different traits (and indeed different breeds) for the breeding males and breeding females. The relatively small numbers of bulls and rams can be selected for traits applicable to the slaughter generation. (In simple terms this means large and lean.) The much larger number of breeding females need to be selected for traits that minimise feed costs relative to the output of weaned offspring. (In simple terms this means small and fat.) This principle of divergent selection has achieved perhaps its most elegant expression in the extremely traditional, sustainable, stratified system of rearing sheep in the British Isles. Breeds of small hardy ewes such as the Scottish Blackface or the Welsh Mountain (with the potential to get fat if they ever saw enough food) live out at little cost in the harsh, very extensive environment of the high hills and are expected to produce one small lamb per year. About half of these hardy hill ewes are crossbred with 'Improver' rams (e.g. Blue-faced Leicester) to produce a larger half-bred ewe for sale to more productive lowland farms where she will be expected to produce two larger lambs per year. This 'improved' half-bred ewe will then be mated with a ram from a breed selected primarily for the slaughter generation traits of growth rate and carcass composition (e.g. Suffolk, Texel). The offspring of this second generation of crossbreeding are then sent for slaughter as high-quality meat lambs. This traditional, elegant strategy ensures the most efficient marriage between breeds differing widely in phenotype within systems that make efficient and sustainable use of a wide range of grassland environments. Unfortunately it does not make a lot of money, mainly because it is still heavily reliant on inputs from the land rather than the purchase of cheap but ultimately unsustainable inputs of feed and power that currently drive intensive farming (see Figure 5.1). It also requires sheep to spend quite a lot of time in lorries.

In the case of milk production from dairy cows and eggs from laying hens, it is the breeding females who are the major source of income for the enterprise. In this case one would expect genetic selection pressure to favour traits associated with sustained fitness in the adults. Unfortunately this is not the case. The hen at point of lay and the dairy heifer due to calve for the first time will normally give every appearance of excellent health and vigour. Nevertheless, in a short time, both laying hens and dairy cows are simply worn out. In the case of hens it is seldom economically viable to keep them in lay for more than one year so it matters little to the producer that they are said to be 'spent' by this time. As I shall explain later,

Table 5.3 Genetic and phenotypic correlations between selection for increased milk yield and infertility (increased calving interval), mastitis and lameness in dairy cattle (Pryce *et al.*, 1998).

| | Correlations with milk yield | |
	Genetic	Phenotypic
Calving interval (days)	+0.39	+0.20
Mastitis incidence	+0.26	−0.01
Lameness incidence	+0.17	+0.04

it does impose an economic cost on the dairy farmer if his or her cows fail to thrive for at least five lactations. However, in many modern intensive dairy herds average life expectancy is falling below three lactations, cows having to be culled for infertility, mastitis and lameness. In both cases the animals have been selected to maximise output of saleable product relative to input of animal feed, *in the short term*. Each individual is being made to work harder and harder and in consequence they are increasingly likely to break down. The first great truth of animal breeding is that you get what you select for. The second is that you never get only what you select for; you also get correlated responses that may often be deleterious. In the case of dairy cattle there is clear evidence that selection for increased milk yield is associated with a genetic deterioration in fertility, mastitis and lameness (Pryce *et al.*, 1998). The overall phenotypic expression of mastitis and lameness in dairy cows is remaining relatively constant (Table 5.3). In the case of these two production diseases, farmers are, through harder work and better husbandry, just managing to hold the line against animals that are increasingly unfit for purpose. In the case of infertility, the battle is already being lost.

In this section I have asked the question 'Are the welfare problems of farm animals attributable in part to the fact that farmers are compelled to work with animals that are increasingly unfit for purpose?' The depressing answer to this question is 'Yes'. Breeding pigs and meat birds are faced with welfare problems arising from the fact that they are not designed for sustained fitness and, in strictly economic terms, this does not matter. Laying hens and dairy cows are designed to be fit at the start of their adult working life but burn out quickly. In the case of the laying hen, the breeders have not presented the producers with an economic problem. For dairy producers, the breeders have claimed to offer quick solutions to the economic problems of the dairy industry but are increasingly becoming a major part of the problem itself. In all these examples, improper animal design has led to an impaired ability to sustain fitness as an adult. This is, by definition, always an insult to welfare and frequently a source of suffering.

Having marshalled convincing evidence in support of the case that the selective breeding of farm animals is creating strains increasingly unfit for purpose, it is necessary to quote paragraph 29 of the Welfare of Farmed Animals (England) Regulations (2000), which states:

No animals shall be kept for farming purposes unless it can reasonably be expected, on the basis of their genotype or phenotype, that they can be kept without detrimental effect on their health or welfare.

This is a worthy aspiration but a nonsense regulation. It can reasonably be expected, on the basis of their genotype and phenotype, that the majority of broiler chickens, breeding sows and dairy cows cannot be kept under commercial conditions without detrimental effect on their health or welfare.

5.4 Problems and progress in animal welfare: analysis of systems

It is now time to consider specific animal welfare problems in specific farming systems; where we have made progress in addressing these problems; and where much remains to be done. In the remainder of this chapter I shall deal with some welfare problems of pigs and poultry. Many whole books and conference proceedings have addressed the welfare of each species (e.g. pigs, poultry). Moreover, the recently revised UK Codes of Recommendations for the Welfare of Livestock, Pigs, Laying Hens and Poultry Reared for Meat provide excellent, comprehensive but concise descriptions of routes to good welfare through attention to stockmanship, accommodation, management, health and hygiene. These are accompanied by reference to relevant welfare legislation contained (mostly) in the Protection of Animals Acts (1911–2000) and the Welfare of Farmed Animals (England) Regulations (2000–2003). This frees me from the need to attempt yet another comprehensive review of all aspects of husbandry and welfare in each species. Instead I shall examine just some of the more important features of current and developing production systems and, for each, pose the following questions:

- How well (or badly) does the system appear to meet the physiological and behavioural needs of the animals?
- How can we assess the quality of alternative husbandry systems from animal-based measurements of animal welfare?
- What changes in husbandry have occurred in the last ten years, either through legislation or natural development, and what impact have they had on animal welfare as assessed from animal-based measurements?
- What are the unsolved problems and how may these be resolved?

5.5 The welfare of pigs

5.5.1 Physiological and behavioural needs

I made it clear in Chapter 1 that I do not consider it essential to the welfare of any animal that it is offered the full range of resources and experiences that it might encounter in a natural environment. However, in planning the environment for any domestic animal (in this case the pig) it is necessary to give due attention to their physiological and behavioural needs. To this end, it is highly instructive to observe how pigs attend to their own needs in a natural (or near-natural) environment and consider how this behaviour is directed (instinctively) towards their genetic fitness and (sentiently) towards their wish to feel good. In a forest or 'pig park' (Newberry & Wood-Gush, 1986), breeding sows will normally form relatively small groups in which each establishes a reasonably hassle-free position in the social hierarchy through a series of encounters more or less ritualised to minimise the risk of aggression getting out of hand. However, the domestic sow, like the wild pig, is not a particularly gregarious animal because it has no need to be. Unlike the relatively defenceless chicken or sheep, group living is not particularly important to its success as a species. Thus pigs in company tend to be more competitive than cooperative. During the day pigs will forage for several hours, turning up the ground with their snouts in search of buried food. When a sow senses that she is about to give birth, she gathers materials to build a deep, warm nest in which to deliver and feed her litter of piglets. Feeding (in ideal circumstances) is prefaced by interactive behaviour between sow and litter. She grunts and kneels down on her front legs. The piglets gather to one side. She then drops to a fully lying position with her teats facing the gathered piglets who proceed to their chosen teat and begin to feed. Piglets will begin to leave the nest and seek other sources of food at about ten days of age and weaning is effectively complete by about 16 weeks of age.

A typical commercial breeding sow will be mated for the first time at approximately 220 days of age. She will then be confined in the company of large numbers of other dry (non-lactating) pregnant sows in specialised accommodation until, after 114 days, she is ready to give birth to her first litter of about 10 piglets. In advance of parturition she will be moved to a farrowing crate where she will be held in extreme confinement for about one month until her piglets are removed and weaned. She may successfully rear nine of these piglets. She will return to oestrus and be remated about five to ten days later to repeat the process at intervals of approximately 140 days, thereby producing 23 weaned piglets per year. This cycle will continue until her productivity falters, whereupon she will be culled. For most sows, this will occur sometime between her second and eighth litters. Piglets weaned from their mothers at 28 days of age will be moved to accommodation (probably a succession of buildings) designed to ensure optimal growth rate and food conversion efficiency up to the point of slaughter at four to six months of age.

These two life styles are very different. Following the sequence of the Five Freedoms I list a number of potential problems arising through failure to meet physiological and behavioural needs within the environment of a commercial pig unit. This list is by no means inclusive.

(1) Nutrition and oral satisfaction
   • Inadequate opportunity for foraging possibly leading to oral stereotypies
   • Unphysiologically early weaning leading to digestive disorders and predisposition to infection

(2) Thermal and physical comfort
- Chronic cold and discomfort in sows and growing pigs confined to concrete floors

(3) Pain, injury and disease
- Skin lesions arising from chronic contact with hard lying surfaces
- Osteoporosis and arthritis in penned sows arising from chronic inactivity
- Ascending urinary infections in sows 'dog sitting' in dirty, cramped cubicles

(4) Fear and stress
- Fighting between pigs in unstable social groups (both adult sows and growing pigs)
- Tail biting in growing pigs

(5) Constraints on natural behaviour
- Denial of normal maternal behaviour in farrowing crates
- Denial of normal maintenance behaviour in pregnancy stalls and farrowing crates.

Most of these welfare problems are inherent to the production system, in particular the design of accommodation for pregnant sows, lactating sows and piglets, and growing pigs. Confinement of sows during pregnancy, especially in individual stalls or on tethers, can be cold, uncomfortable and injurious, and imposes severe restrictions on natural behaviour. Confinement during farrowing and lactation in crates designed to minimise the deaths of piglets from crushing practically eliminates any possibility of movement or normal maternal behaviour. Confinement of early weaned growing pigs on concrete floors in barren environments predisposes to injury, either from contact with the hardware or through abnormal behaviour, fighting and tail biting.

There are those who would seek to justify the farrowing crate and pregnant sow stall on welfare grounds. The farrowing crate is justified on the basis that the benefits accruing from a reduction in piglet deaths more than compensate for the costs to the sow. The case that sow stalls are good for welfare is that they protect sows from injuries incurred through fighting. Both cases rest on the premise that it is acceptable to prevent an undesirable pattern of behaviour by restricting all forms of behaviour. It would be as valid to claim that prisons would be so much more manageable if all the inmates were kept permanently in solitary confinement. In Europe, though not in the USA and most other industrialised countries, there are now regulations to prohibit the confinement of pregnant sows in individual stalls. The UK Welfare of Farmed Animals Regulations (2003) state:

36. Sows and gilts shall be kept in groups except during the period between seven days before the predicted date of farrowing and the day on which the weaning of piglets . . . is complete.

* This does not apply to farm units with less than ten sows provided the individual pens meet minimum space requirements.

42. All dry sows and gilts must be given a sufficient quantity of bulky or high fibre food, as well as high energy food, to satisfy their hunger and need to chew.

The UK authorities have reviewed the scientific evidence and made the value judgement that the needs of sows for the social satisfaction of living in groups and the oral satisfaction provided by bulky feed are sufficiently important to be enforced by regulation. In effect, this compels farmers to run pregnant sows in yards or out of doors. In (e.g.) the USA and Australia, the authorities remain satisfied that conventional intensive systems, namely sow stalls with no access to straw, are acceptable on welfare grounds. As I pointed out in Chapter 1, European and USA legislators reviewed the same scientific evidence. They came to different conclusions by applying different value judgements, in relation not only to the relative importance of different physiological and behavioural needs to the welfare of the sows but also to the aspirations of the citizens whom they had been elected to represent. Issues in animal welfare are always political.

5.5.2 Animal-based welfare assessment

I return now to the central theme ('the big tune') that recurs throughout this book. What can we do now to improve the welfare of pigs in practice? There is a fairly general consensus as to the nature of the major potential welfare problems faced by pigs. All would agree with the need to minimise ill health and injury. There is more argument about the significance of behavioural needs, not least because we still do not fully understand the emotional and cognitive motivation that drives abnormal behaviour patterns such as stereotypic bar chewing by sows or tail biting by growing piglets. Nevertheless, we accept that abnormal behaviour tends to reflect life in an unsatisfactory environment.

The general principles of our approach to developing animal-based measures for the assessment of welfare state in farm animals were outlined in Chapter 4. Experts were asked to identify the important welfare problems for individual pigs and for the pig industry, suggest observations and records that could be used as on-farm indicators of these problems, and comment on the extent to which these problems could, or could not, be resolved by attention to husbandry within different, currently acceptable systems of production (Whay *et al.*, 2003a). Table 5.4 summarises their responses within four categories – injury, disease, poor nutrition and abnormal behaviour – and lists the observations and records deemed most suitable for their assessment.

Based on this we have developed a protocol for the animal-based assessment of welfare state in growing pigs. Table 5.5 summarises the key elements of the protocol and presents some results from a preliminary study of pigs all reared in straw-bedded pens, i.e. relatively 'high-welfare' accommodation. Table 5.5 is intended only to indicate our approach to the evaluation of welfare state. We are not yet in a position to compare welfare in different rearing systems, nor have we yet devel-

Table 5.4　Summary of expert opinion as to the major categories of welfare problems for pigs and animal-based measures that may be used to assess them.

Welfare problem	Assessment measures
Injury	Record lameness
	Record limb lesions *in vivo* and *post mortem*
	Record injuries from fighting and tail biting
Disease	Examine records of mortality and use of medicines
	Examine lung records *post mortem*
Poor nutrition	Observe feeding behaviour
	Score body condition
Abnormal behaviour	Observe response to novel object
	Observe social behaviour (e.g. fighting, play, bunting, tail biting)

Table 5.5　Animal-based assessment of welfare state in growing pigs.

	Measures	Median	Lower quartile	Upper quartile
Attitude	Response to observer (% retreat)	62	26	90
	Response to novel object (% interested)	28	9	34
Oral behaviour (% active)	Manipulating object	26	23	32
	Manipulating pig	13	10	15
Social behaviour*	Pushing	10.4	3.1	19.5
	Aggression	9.7	7.4	23.6
	Sexual behaviour	6.2	3.2	8.4
	Play	4.9	3.0	12.0
	Biting	4.1	0.6	8.8
	Abnormal respiration	5.7	3.6	13.1
Condition (% affected)	Limb lesions	30	15	40
	Ear lesions	25	15	34
	Flank lesions	22	15	30
	Lameness	15	11	20
	Tail lesions	5	0	10

*Social behaviours expressed as the number of events observed in ten minutes in a pen of 100 pigs

oped a protocol for the study of pregnant sows, although the approach would be essentially the same. Our first step on entering the pig house is to assess the general attitude (or mood) of the pigs from their approach to the observer and to a novel object. This permits us to rank the mood of the group on a two-dimensional scale of passive–active and anxious–confident, an approach that has been developed further by Wemelsfelder *et al.* (2001). Oral behaviour (an important behavioural need for pigs) is assessed on the basis of numbers orally manipulating substrates (e.g. straw, toys) or other pigs. Elements of social behaviour (pushing, aggression, sexual behaviour, play, biting) are recorded as events occurring within a ten-minute period of observation and standardised to 100 pigs in a pen. Behaviour is examined first with as little interference as possible. The observers then enter the pens to examine the physical condition of the pigs. In this study with growing pigs the most prevalent physical problems were limb lesions (e.g. abraded and swollen hocks) presumably induced by contact with injurious surfaces, and flank and tail lesions caused by fighting and tail biting. Had the observations been made on pregnant sows, other elements such as body condition score would probably have assumed greater importance.

I do not intend to draw any firm conclusions from the preliminary results listed in Table 5.5. The intention at this stage is to outline our approach to on-farm assessment of welfare state. Such observations can be used to provide direct comparisons of (e.g.) leg injuries to pigs on concrete v. straw, or tail biting in pigs reared in barren v. enriched environments. It is also possible to explore relationships between behaviour, environment and attitude. For example, are anxious pigs more inclined to injure one another? (Probably.) Do growing pigs show more confidence and less anxiety in an enriched environment, or is their attitude influenced more by the quality of the stockmanship? (Don't know.) I simply restate the case made in Chapter 4, namely the need to develop and standardise protocols for the animal-based assessment of welfare state. These can be used to inform the political debate as to the relative merits and acceptability of alternative rearing systems for legislative or quality assurance purposes. They will also become a valuable diagnostic tool for farmers and veterinarians to identify welfare problems and solutions specific to the animals in their care.

5.5.3 Developments in husbandry
Dry sows
The UK Welfare of Farmed Animals Regulations (2003) ban the prolonged confinement of dry, pregnant sows in individual stalls and require them to have access to high-fibre feed. This Act has compelled our pig farmers to develop alternative systems of husbandry that can compete economically in a buyers' market. For practical purposes this has meant group-housing sows in straw yards or running them in outdoor units that give them free range to forage in groups but access to individual covered arks in which they may obtain comfort, shelter and security. This is, of course, a welcome return to proper husbandry since the only farms now suitable for pig production are those that grow their own cereals and straw and/or have access to light, well-drained land on which sows may over-winter without drowning in a sea of mud. It is no longer realistic to set up a factory pig farm in which the animals are permanently housed on concrete, all feed is bought in and the land used merely as a repository for slurry.

There have been problems associated with the development of group housing for sows in straw yards. The most serious have been those involving aggression at the time of feeding. The ration of high-energy food offered to pregnant sows is far less than they would choose to eat. Consequently there is a lot of excitement, aggression and frustration around the time of eating. This can lead to sows getting hurt and/or not getting their fair share of food. Several solutions to this problem have been tried, tested and shown to work. Computer-controlled feeding stalls that recognise and admit sows wearing transponders have the obvious merit that each sow can be fed to meet individual requirements (unless another sow steals its transponder – this can happen!). Some of the early systems led to some dreadful injuries as sows queued for, or even worse, sought to back out from the feeding stalls. Designs have improved greatly to ensure one-way movement through the feeding stations and minimise aggressive interactions at the points of entry. However, the only real advantage of the expensive computerised feeding stall is to minimise feeding costs by ensuring that each sow gets no more than her allowance. I believe that dump-feed systems that scatter sow pellets over a relatively wide area of deep straw are, by most measures, superior to computerised feeding stalls. This approach minimises aggression and allows the sows to forage happily for hours. It may not be ideal for sows that have become especially thin at the end of lacta-tion, but such individuals merit special care anyway. However, by mid-pregnancy all healthy sows appear to thrive in the comfortable and relaxed environment of a straw barn with scatter feeding.

Outdoor units with well-designed, well-maintained arks fully meet the essential physiological and behavioural needs of sows most of the time. The set-up costs are relatively low on the right farms with low rainfall and well-drained land. However, caring for outdoor pigs in all weathers is hard work and frequently uncomfortable. Carting feed and bedding to arks when the ground is saturated with rain can be an expensive nightmare. Application of the ethical matrix would reveal a major concern for the welfare of the stock-keepers. Provided that food and bedding continue to arrive, adult sows, adapted to the outdoor environment, are able to achieve reasonable thermal and physical comfort nearly all the time. Moreover, unlike the sow in the confinement stall, they are able to meet the most vital of all behavioural needs, namely the need to take positive action designed to make them feel good (or better, at least).

I shall not consider the welfare of the sow in the confinement stall in any detail since in Europe we have limped, or are about to limp, out of that unhappy state. Suffice it to recapitulate the essentials. Sows on concrete in confinement stalls suffer abuse according to all the Five Freedoms:

- lack of oral satisfaction;
- lack of thermal and physical comfort;
- pain and lameness from injuries, muscle weakness and osteoporosis;
- stress-related oral stereotypies;
- almost complete denial of normal maintenance behaviour (e.g. grooming, limb stretching).

Those nations that still permit the confinement stall have either not yet reviewed the evidence or chosen to discard those elements of welfare abuse that I list above. This is, of course, not a scientific decision but a political one. When there is sufficient pressure of public opinion to persuade them that it is unjust then they will change their minds, because that is what politicians do.

Farrowing and nursery accommodation

No one could possibly deny that farrowing crates are rotten for the sow. She is constricted to the point where she can do no more than struggle to her feet and fall over. She is moreover denied any expression of her powerful motivational needs, to create a satisfactory environment for her piglets, to feed them in due order and to educate them in the ways of pigs. Nevertheless, in law, and even in many welfare-based quality assurance schemes, farrowing crates are tolerated on the basis that piglet survival is paramount. This is primarily an economic argument. One may advance a welfare argument on a strictly utilitarian basis that the survival of perhaps two piglets justifies four to five weeks of abuse to the sow (I would not). However, any ethical analysis that includes the principle of autonomy, or respect for the individual, should rule the farrowing crate out of court.

This begs the question 'Is the farrowing crate really as essential as we deem it to be and, if so, why?' Halverson (2002) has reviewed factors relating to piglet mortality in different systems. Data from the USA indicate an 8.3% increase in piglet mortality over the last ten years in pig breeding units using farrowing crates. There is no reason to suppose that the design of the crates has deteriorated during this time. Indeed, one would have expected some overall improvement. This strongly suggests that accommodation design is failing to keep pace with deterioration in the genotype of the sow. The most obvious manifestation of this is sows that are too big for the crates. Even when crate sizes have increased, mortality appears to be rising, not least because larger sows are clumsier sows. In farrowing/nursing units where sows have freedom of movement and piglets are protected more or less adequately by straw bedding and anti-crush rails, piglet mortality owing to crushing or hypothermia is, on average, one to two pigs per litter greater than when farrowing crates are used. However, this average disguises a large amount of variation, much of it amenable to control. Honeyman *et al.* (1998) analysed piglet crushing mortality by hut type in outdoor farrowing units. In this study mortality rates ranged from 3% to 30% and most of the difference could be accounted for in terms of hut design. The best unit (one death per three litters) used the UK-designed 'Pig Saver' hut with steep-angled walls, well-designed anti-crush rails and the door in a corner so the sow could lie diagonally across the pen.

It is well recognised within the pig industry that the strain of hybrid sow best suited to outdoor units is inherently fitter than that selected for confinement in farrowing crates. She is smaller and potentially fatter, but more agile and has better mothering ability. However, as I explained earlier, traits best suited to the breeding generation tend to be negatively correlated with economically important traits (leanness and rapid growth) in the slaughter generation. Since, in pig rearing systems, the slaughter generation eats 80% of the food (Table 5.2), breeders weight their selection indices overwhelmingly in favour of traits that are best expressed in the slaughter generation. However, the evidence reviewed by Halverson (2002) suggests that, despite the farrowing crate, intensive sow producers are failing to hold the line against the genotypic deterioration in breeding sows that are becoming increasingly unfit for purpose. The best way forward from this unhappy position is not yet clear and will require some good, practical, multidisciplinary research involving breeders, agricultural engineers and ethologists. Nevertheless we already have quite enough evidence to indicate that the farrowing crate is not the only solution to the problem of piglet mortality.

In this regard it is pertinent to remind ourselves that piglet deaths from crushing and hypothermia occur almost entirely in the first 48 hours of life. The sow may enter the crate four days before she farrows and leave it 28 days after she farrows. Thus for 30/32 days the whole complicated, expensive, abusive machinery of the farrowing crate is completely unnecessary. It is used simply because it is deemed too expensive to provide breeding sows and piglets with separate farrowing and nursery accommodation. This practice developed when the policy in the most intensive units was to wean piglets at as early an age as possible (21 days or less). The UK Welfare of Farmed Animals Regulations (2003) now make it an offence to wean piglets at less than 28 days. One reason for this is to ensure that piglets are sufficiently mature at weaning to enter a naturally ventilated, straw-bedded building rather than the artificially heated and ventilated barren 'flat-deck' cages deemed necessary for piglets weaned at three weeks of age. This enforced extension of the nursing period increases the economic viability of a rearing system that separates farrowing accommodation from nursing accommodation. In the most intensive of systems, and with sow phenotypes unable to avoid crashing down and crushing their neonates, the duration of time spent in a crate in the expensive farrowing accommodation could be reduced to a maximum of about six days. Nursing accommodation would become much cheaper and, in these circumstances, it could prove economic to delay weaning until piglets are six to eight weeks of age. Once again this proposed development in husbandry will need to be tested in practice using all disciplines necessary to evaluate health, behaviour and production economics.

Growing pigs

The Welfare of Farmed Animals (England) Regulations 2000–2003 state (*inter alia*):

- Accommodation used for pigs shall be constructed in such a way as to:
  - have a clean, comfortable and adequately drained place in which it [the pig] can rest;
  - have enough space to allow all the animals to lie down at the same time.

- Floors should not cause injury or suffering to pigs standing or lying on them.
- Feeding and watering equipment shall be designed so that harmful effects of competition between animals are minimised.
- Pigs shall be placed in groups as soon as possible after weaning. They shall be kept in stable groups with as little mixing as possible.

These regulations have done much to improve minimum standards within the UK pig industry and deserve to be copied throughout the world. They are especially wise because they tend to be worded in terms of welfare outcomes rather than husbandry provisions. Thus they do not impose a regulation to house growing pigs on straw but state that floors 'should not cause injury'. They do not require all pigs to be fed at the same time but require feeding equipment and practice to be designed to minimise 'harmful effects of competition'. I repeat, I do not want to make too much of the results of our relatively small study of the welfare of growing pigs (128 pens on 20 units, Table 5.5). However, it is necessary to point out that in all these units the pigs were on straw yet the prevalence of lameness and leg injuries was in many cases higher than we would have wished. Provision of straw is a good thing, but it is not a panacea. This, once again, reinforces my central argument that welfare needs to be assessed from animal-based measures to identify specific problems and specific solutions on individual farms. Simple compliance with husbandry standards, whether set by law or by a QA scheme, is no guarantee of satisfactory welfare.

The most outstanding welfare problem for growing pigs is 'post-weaning scours', a generic expression that describes a range of digestive disorders and infections occurring shortly after weaning. These must be categorised unequivocally as production diseases since the major risk factor is the abrupt removal of sow's milk and introduction of a formulated rearing diet. At 21–28 days of age the digestive tract of the piglet is insufficiently mature, and has neither the enzymes nor the immune mechanisms nor the appropriate balance of intestinal microorganisms to cope satisfactorily with this abrupt change of diet. Poorly digested food, allergic responses to food and the absence of beneficial (probiotic) microorganisms all conspire to damage the lining of the gut wall and predispose to infection. Nutritionists and feed manufacturers are constantly striving to minimise these risks by improving the quality of the weaning diet. However, it remains a fact that in most intensive units weaning piglets at 28 days or less, post-weaning scours and related syndromes are only being kept under control by the routine prophylactic use of antibiotics. Legislation to ban this routine administration of antibiotics to weaner pigs will, in the short term, cause an increase in the incidence of post-weaning scours and thus a deterioration in pig welfare. It will, if properly enforced, also cause a significant deterioration in the productivity of the unit unless the farmer radically revises his/her whole weaning strategy. In the long term therefore, a ban on the routine prophylactic use of antibiotics in livestock farming (properly enforced) will have a beneficial effect on the welfare of growing pigs since it will force farmers to adopt weaning strategies that do not ravage their piglets' guts.

5.6 The welfare of laying hens

In the UK, the conventional, unenriched cage for battery hens currently affording 550 cm² floor space per bird is, to adopt a phrase well understood by the poultry industry, 'spent'. The Welfare of Farmed Animals (England) (Amendment) Regulations 2002, that give effect to the European Council Directive 99/74/EC, state that 'from 1st January 2003 no person shall build or bring into service' a conventional unenriched cage for laying hens and that from 1st January 2012 'no person shall keep any laying hen' in such a cage. So as to waste neither your time nor mine, I shall start from the premise that the unenriched battery cage simply does not meet the physiological and behavioural requirements of the laying hen, which makes any quibbling about minimum requirements for floor space superfluous. The debate can then proceed quickly to the question 'What are the satisfactory alternatives to the battery cage and why?' The two broad options that remain open under European law are the enriched cage and non-cage systems for accommodating large colonies of hens in barns or on free-range units.

The 1992 Regulations state that laying hens in enriched cages must have (*inter alia*) 'at least 750 cm² of cage area per hen, 600 cm² of which shall be usable, a nest, litter such that pecking and scratching are possible, appropriate perches allowing at least 15 cm per hen and suitable claw-shortening devices'. In *Eden I* (Webster, 1994), I recommended a nest, a perch and 900 cm² of 'usable' space additional to that occupied by the nest boxes. The regulations have added litter and claw-shortening devices but cut back on space allowance. My recommendation for 900 cm² of 'usable' space was based on evidence that hens are powerfully motivated to work for space when confined at less than 900 cm². The evidence at that time concerning the motivation of hens to work for litter was equivocal and, I believe, still is. Nevertheless I am entirely satisfied with the decision to insist on the provision of litter. Hens may or may not be stressed by its absence, but there is no doubt that they enjoy it when it is there. I am not satisfied by the decision to restrict usable space allowance to 600 cm² of usable space.

Minimum standards for colony systems require at least one nest for every seven hens or, if group nests are used, 1 m² of nest space for a maximum of 120 hens; no more than four levels of perches providing at least 15 cm per hen; and at least 250 cm² littered area per hen. On free-range units where hens have access to open runs there must be sufficient pop holes extending along the entire length of the building and giving a total opening of 2 m per group of 1000 hens. Open runs 'must be of an area appropriate to the stocking density and to the nature of the ground in order to prevent any contamination, and equipped with shelter from inclement weather and predators'. The revised DEFRA Code of Welfare for Laying

Table 5.6 The ethical matrix: alternative husbandry systems for laying hens.

	Barren cage	**Enriched cage**	**Free range**
Hens	Severe restriction of behaviour	Meets most important behavioural needs	Full expression of behaviour
			Some injury, pain, fear, stress
	Chronic injury and pain	Low fear and stress	Increased mortality
	– Unacceptable	– Acceptable	– Acceptable
Consumers	Cheap and wholesome	Unacceptable to welfarists	Preferred choice of many
Producers	Commodity with no added value	No added value?	Added value
			Pride in production

Hens includes the essential elements of all relevant regulations and provides an excellent, succinct summary of the housing and management necessary to promote (though not ensure) hen welfare to a standard deemed acceptable within current legislation. This frees me from the need to provide a comprehensive list of all husbandry provisions deemed necessary for good welfare. I shall therefore proceed at once to the main contentious issue, namely 'Which is preferable, free range, or the enriched cage?', expressed more forcibly by welfare charities such as Compassion in World Farming as 'Free range for all'.

In *Eden I*, I argued the relative merits of free range v. the enriched cage simply in terms of welfare as perceived by the hens themselves on the basis of information drawn mostly from motivational studies conducted on small groups of birds under laboratory conditions. I now acknowledge the limitations of building any animal welfare argument on science alone. Values form an inescapable part of the equation, whether these values be ethical or driven by the marketplace. Table 5.6 briefly identifies the major pros and cons of alternative husbandry systems for laying hens as perceived by consumers, producers and the hens themselves. I include the unenriched cage in this comparison because, in many parts of the world, it remains legitimate and is the most common system.

The main criticism of the unenriched cage, dating back to the Brambell report (Brambell, 1965), is that it imposes an unacceptably severe restriction on the hens' ability to meet their behavioural needs for grooming, stretching, wing-flapping, nest building and litter bathing. Extreme confinement in barren wire cages also predisposes to external injuries to feet and feathers, and exacerbates the development of osteoporosis, leading to bone fractures and chronic pain. The main argument in favour of the enriched cage has been that it meets the most powerful motivational needs of the hen to seek a nest in which to lay her eggs and achieves a significant improvement in comfort and satisfaction through the provision of a perch and litter. The minimum space allowance has been set more by economics than a primary concern for hen welfare. The argument has been advanced that given a space allowance in excess of $600\,cm^2$ hens are more inclined to injure one another through feather pecking. My personal belief is that the benefits to the hen of at least $900\,cm^2$ floor space outweigh the harm done through beak trimming to restrict feather pecking when this is done with professional competence and according to regulation at less than 10 days of age. Thus the enriched cage meets many but not all the behavioural needs of the laying hen. It should also ensure the low mortality rates achieved in conventional cage systems.

In colony systems hens are kept in barns. Normally each barn houses more than 4000 birds. If the birds are confined permanently within the barn without access to open runs, the eggs are sold as 'barn eggs'. When they have access to a suitable and sufficient outdoor run, the eggs may be sold as 'free range'. In theory, all birds are provided with the space and the opportunity to express their full range of natural behaviour; nesting, perching, grooming, litter bathing, ground pecking, exploration and, of course, feather pecking or, at worst, cannibalism. In practice, it is not always easy for a hen to exhibit its full behavioural repertoire in the close company of thousands of other birds who may present a threat or simply get in the way when it feels the need to enter a nest or pop out through a pop hole. There is good evidence that in many commercial 'free-range' units a high proportion of the birds never leave the house at all. Thus the large commercial colony unit provides no guarantee of full behavioural expression. The prevalence of injuries due to feather pecking and mortality rates in colony units are very variable but consistently higher than in cages. Clearly both enriched cages and colony systems go much further towards meeting the behavioural needs of laying hens than the conventional unenriched cage. However, both have their limitations and, strictly on the basis of available scientific evidence as to the physiological and behavioural needs of the laying hen, it is not possible to claim that either system is clearly superior. Thus the European Commission has deemed both systems to be acceptable.

Unfortunately the most important criterion for the success of any 'high-welfare' system of food production from animals is not whether it makes the animals feel better but whether it makes us feel better. If the enriched cage is not perceived as free enough by those prepared to pay good money to buy freedom for the hens, then it will not attract the money that these people are prepared to pay. On the world market, hens in unenriched cages will continue to provide nutritionally wholesome eggs at the cheapest possible commodity price set by producers unconstrained by welfare regulations (or even concerns). Free-range eggs will sell well when there is consumer demand and this demand is likely to increase. Where I live, the market for free-range eggs is over 30% and rising*. Local farmers producing free-range eggs are benefiting from a premium that is keeping them solvent. Moreover, in talking with them, I have sensed a healthy return of pride and enthusiasm for chicken farming. The producer currently operating with conventional cages and contemplating conversion to the enriched cage is facing the prospect of

---

* Excluding eggs used for processing.

a substantial capital outlay and an increase of about 30% in running costs*. He is, moreover, faced by the problem that the consumer is unlikely to view eggs from hens in enriched cages as a high-welfare, value-added product since, in the EC at least, these will become the minimum standard. The producer will therefore still face international competition to produce a staple commodity according to economic rules defined by the lowest common denominator. Moreover, as the cost of producing standard eggs increases, the 'mark-up' on free-range eggs should decline and this should increase their market share. All this sounds extremely attractive, but it begs the question 'Is the welfare of hens generally satisfactory on large, commercial free-range units?' At present we do not have a good answer to this question, since we have not yet gathered sufficient evidence from robust, animal-based measures of the welfare of hens kept in large colonies under a wide range of conditions of accommodation and management.

5.6.1 Animal-based assessment of the welfare of hens in colony systems

Table 5.7 briefly illustrates the protocol we have developed at Bristol for assessment of the welfare of hens in free-range units. As with pigs and cattle, the welfare priorities and best measures were established through expert consultation (Whay et al., 2003a). The procedures begin, as always, with those observations of attitude and behaviour that can be made with minimal disturbance to the animals' normal routine. These include observations intended to assess the overall attitude (or mood) of each colony of birds within a two-dimensional space defined by the axes 'passive–aroused' and 'anxious–confident'. There are strong suggestions that the overall 'group personality' of colonies of hens may, over time, develop in very different ways, even in colonies of hens living on the same farm, or succeeding one another in the same building. A colony may be anxious and aggressive. This mood may increase the incidence of feather pecking and this may ratchet up the anxiety and set up a vicious cycle of increasing injury and mortality. Another colony may be calm and non-competitive at the outset. This may set up a virtuous cycle as the birds acquire an increasing sense of security; and both production and welfare will remain good throughout the life of the colony. The question we cannot yet answer is how far these trends can be controlled by the producer or whether they are an uncontrollable risk arising as an inevitable consequence of bringing thousands of birds together and leaving them to their own devices.

The protocol gives much attention to feather pecking, both the action and its consequences. The problem of feather pecking in laying hens continues to attract a great deal of scientific research (recent studies include El-Lethy et al., 2000; Jones et al., 2002; and Albentosa et al., 2003). The only conclusion one can draw from all this work is that there is no simple explanation. Feather pecking, and its more serious associations, vent pecking and cannibalism, may be an expression of aggression, frustration in the absence of a suitable pecking substrate, redirected

* Including costs of amortisation on capital developments.

Table 5.7 Protocol for assessment of the welfare of hens in free-range units. Each step in the procedure should be carried out in three areas: the slatted floor/perching area, the littered area and outdoors on range.

Flock examination	
Overall calmness/arousal	Score
Flight distance (m)	Record for ten hens in each area
Response to novel object	Overall behaviour: fearful – avoidance – disinterest – interest
Vocalisation	Quiet – steady murmur – loud chatter
Behavioural indices of health	Head shaking (respiratory challenge)
	Hunched, reluctant to move, head tucked under wing
	Poor perching and crash landing on perches and fittings
Aggression between hens	Encounters in 10 minutes: none – mild – medium – severe
Feather pecking: events	Encounters in 10 minutes: none – picking – pecking – pulling
Feather pecking: prevalence	Estimate percentage involved in activity
Feather loss: prevalence	Estimate overall percentage of birds with significant feather loss
Feather loss: location	Indicate sites of feather loss on hen profiles
Feather loss: overall severity	None – mild – medium – severe
Comb colour (%)	Pink – dark pink – red
Panting	None – mild – medium – severe (evidence of heat stress)
Individual assessment	20 birds (four from perches, two from nests, 14 from floor)
Body weight (kg)	
State of beak	None – tipped – trimmed – severe trim
State of plumage	Score soiling and loss of feathers
State of limbs	Examine feet and hocks for injury, mutilation, scalding, etc.
Evidence of external injury	Feather loss, vent pecking, skin injuries, etc.
Evidence of fractures	Breast bone, clavicles, wings and legs
Evidence of red mites	Observe under wings
Comb colour	Pink – dark pink – red
Overall health and demeanour	E.g. alert, well hydrated, bright eyed, etc.
Resistance to handling	Score

ground pecking (not involving frustration), an instinctive, genetically predetermined response to specific cues, or simply mindless. In our protocol, aggression and feather pecking are first assessed on a flock basis both as activities and consequences. Comb colour is scored on a scale of pink – dark pink – red. A red comb indicates a bird that spends a lot of time out on free range; birds with pale pink combs are those that hardly if ever venture out of doors. Preliminary results suggest that in many so-called free-range units, more than half the birds have pink combs, i.e. have elected to stay permanently within the building. This may be because they tried going outside and found it alarming, or were faced by aggression at the pop holes, or were preconditioned to stay indoors because the pop holes were closed when they were introduced to the house.

The protocol also calls for detailed inspection of 20 birds, four taken from perches, two from nests and 14 from the floor. In order to minimise any disturbance, we ask the stock-keeper to pick up the birds within the house and make no attempt to catch birds out of doors. The individual inspections provide evidence of body condition, external injuries and parasitism (red mites), and bone fractures, especially to the breastbone (sternum) clavicles, wings and legs. One of the main criticisms of the conventional battery cage has been that enforced inactivity has induced osteoporosis and this has increased the incidence of bone fractures, both in the cages and during handling and transport prior to slaughter (Gregory & Wilkins, 1989). Hens in colony systems with perches have stronger bones but more scope for injuries, e.g. fractures to the sternum incurred when crash landing on perches. It should be possible to reduce the incidence of fractures through improvements to building design both in the laying house and during the rearing period. The hens at point of lay should be fully adapted to all the activities necessary to ensure their comfort and security in the laying house. They should know how and where to fly to find a perch. They should know what a pop hole is and what attractions await out of doors. Most especially they should have acquired the confidence to exploit these resources.

In general, I am delighted to witness the trend towards free-range egg production, but a lot more development of these systems is required before they can truly be said to meet the expectations of both the hens and the purchaser of high-welfare eggs. Animal-based protocols for assessment of welfare outcomes (e.g. Table 5.7) will play a vital role in the development of these systems. I must stress, however, that current deficiencies in free-range systems cannot be used as a defence of the unenriched battery cage. Although free-range egg production, like outdoor rearing of pigs or group rearing of veal calves, appears at first sight to represent a return to traditional farming systems, these systems are almost entirely new and untried at the scale necessary for commercial survival. It is unreasonable to expect them to operate at once at the same efficiency expressed in terms of (e.g.) production and mortality as conventional intensive, machine-driven systems that have been in operation for many years. At the same time, we cannot simply assume that because hens (or pigs) are given access to free range, all will be well. The price of good animal welfare will always be constant vigilance.

5.7 The welfare of poultry reared for meat

At the time of *Eden I* (Webster, 1994) I wrote 'The modern commercial broiler is reared in large flocks (5000 to 50000 birds per flock) on litter and with near continuous lighting (23 hours on: 1 hour off) to reach a slaughter weight of 1.8 to 3.0 kg at an age of 42 days. This spectacular rate of production has been achieved in part by advances in nutrition and building design but mainly by intense genetic selection for absolute growth rate in muscle (especially the more attractive breast muscle) to the virtual exclusion of all other traits that may affect fitness. Similarly the turkey has been intensively selected to produce very large breasted birds that will typically be slaughtered at ages from 16 to 24 weeks and weights from 8 to 20 kg'. I went on to say that selection for rapid growth and gross hypertrophy of the breast muscle has created serious problems of 'leg weakness'. This is a euphemism for a range of pathological conditions of bones (e.g. tibial dyschondroplasia), joints (e.g. septic arthritis), tendons (e.g. perosis) and skin (e.g. hock burn). Kestin *et al.* (1992) reported that the incidence of leg weakness sufficient to cause moderate or severe lameness approached 25% in the most common heavy strains of broiler chicken as they approached their slaughter age of 42 days. Kestin *et al.* used a gait scoring system that has been widely adopted as a method for assessing lameness. Birds with a score of zero are said to be sound. Scores of 1–3 indicate progressive abnormality in locomotion. A bird with a score of 4 can move but with extreme difficulty and reluctance. At a score of 5, it is immobile.

> On the basis of this evidence I concluded that: . . . *approximately one third of the heavy strains of broiler chicken and turkey are in chronic pain for approximately one third of their lives. Given that poultry meat consumption in the UK exceeds one million tonnes per annum this must constitute, in both magnitude and severity, the single most severe, systematic example of man's inhumanity to another sentient animal.*

These were strong words. However, they expressed a widespread concern that was endorsed by the UK Farm Animal Welfare Council Report on the Welfare of Broiler Chickens (1992). It is necessary now to explore how far the industry has gone to address this concern. Although the aetiology of leg disorders in broiler chickens is complex (Butterworth, 1999), the incidence is very low in slow-growing strains (e.g. birds bred to be egg layers). The predominant predisposing factor for leg weakness has always been birds that outgrow their strength.

The UK Code for the Welfare of Meat Chickens (2002) states the following:

- Management measures should be taken to prevent lameness. The strain and source of chicks, stocking density, lighting patterns, feed composition, and feeding routines should all be considered.
- It is important to bird welfare to provide them with a period of darkness (not less than 30 minutes) in each 24-hour cycle. This helps to prevent panic in the event of a power failure.
- The maximum stocking density for chickens kept to produce meat for the table should be 34 kg/m^2 which should not be exceeded at any time during the growing period.

The regulation regarding stocking density means that birds weighing on average 2.5 kg on the day before slaughter will have a (shared) space allocation of 735 cm^2

per bird. The legal minimum space allowance for smaller laying hens confined on the ground in colony systems is $833\,cm^2$. The regulation concerning lighting is designed only to avoid panic and does not address the more serious issue that the object of near-continuous lighting is to encourage the birds to eat for as long as possible, and so outgrow their strength.

The expression 'Management measures should be taken to prevent lameness' carries no clout. However, some enlightened commercial companies have developed systems for broiler production that have achieved significant reductions in lameness incidence without compromising profitability through intelligent control of lighting, feed composition and feed selection. In essence they seek to restrict food energy intake in the early stage of development and permit 'catch-up' later on. This is yet another example of a modification to husbandry imposed by the need to compensate for phenotypic faults arising from the selection of birds that are not fit for purpose.

The evidence from Kestin et al. that 25% of broiler fowl were in pain for one third of their lives prompted a call from FAWC (1992) to remedy the situation within 5 years. There has, through selection, been a significant reduction in some problems such as tibial dyschondroplasia. Indeed most cases of severe lameness (gait score 4–5; Kestin et al., 1992) are now associated with cases of infectious arthritis (Butterworth, 1999). This would appear to suggest that most severe lameness can now be attributed to problems of hygiene in the hatchery, in transit or during early rearing. However, the direct evidence for this is unconvincing and the fact remains that it is not a problem in lighter, slower-growing birds, reared for laying. Kestin et al. (2001) reported a further study of the relationship between growth rate, liveweight and lameness in broiler chickens made almost 10 years after his original exposure of the problems of lameness in heavy strains of broiler birds. In this new study he imposed a rather more severe test, by recording lameness at 54 and 81 days of age in light and heavy strains of birds grown at different rates. There were, as expected, differences in lameness attributable to strain and feeding regimen. However, when the data were analysed to remove the effects of differences in liveweight by including it as a covariable, almost all of the differences attributable to strain, feeding regimen, etc. disappeared. Almost all the differences in lameness between treatment groups could be attributed to weight for age (i.e. relative growth rate). This provides unequivocal evidence that the predominant cause of lameness in broiler chickens is still the selection of genotypes that outgrow their strength.

Nevertheless, in the last ten years there has been some progress in reducing some causes of lameness in broilers. Some of this (not enough) has been achieved through selection (e.g. a reduction in tibial dyschrondroplasia); more has been achieved through improvements to husbandry (feeding and lighting). Recent lameness surveys carried out by DEFRA indicate that the prevalence of moderate to severe lameness (gait scores 3–5) is well below 10% in most commercial units, as against the prevalence of over 20% reported by Kestin et al. (1992). This does represent progress. It does not, however, mean that the problem is *en route* to solution. The problem is pain and this problem is worse than we thought. Danbury *et al.* (1999) carried out a classic study in which broiler birds were allowed to select food that did, or did not, contain the anti-inflammatory, analgesic drug carprofen. Those birds whose locomotion was normal preferentially selected the food without carprofen, perhaps because they were slightly averse to the taste. However, at all gait scores above zero (scores 1–4) the birds adjusted their food selection to increase their intake of the analgesic drug. My analysis of the original data reveals that carprofen intake was significantly greater at gait scores 1–4 than at gait score zero, but that there was no significant difference in intake between scores 1–4. This implies that birds sensed that they were in pain at all gait scores above zero, but their motivation to relieve pain did not increase in proportion to the abnormality of their locomotion. This suggests very strongly that we should not arbitrarily set a gait score of 4 (or 3) as the threshold of unacceptability. All lameness hurts.

5.7.1 Animal-based assessment of the welfare of chickens in broiler units

It is clear that some commercial, 'conventional' broiler units are achieving better welfare than others, as assessed by criteria such as mortality and lameness. Moreover, there is a trend, as yet small, towards free-range and other more sympathetic husbandry systems for broiler chickens and especially turkeys intended for the specialist Christmas market. As always it will only be possible to evaluate the relative merits of alternative systems and the standards of welfare on individual units within systems on the basis of robust animal-based measurements of welfare outcomes. The most widespread (and the worst) approach is the European Poultry Efficiency Factor (EPEF) where:

$$\text{EPEF} = \frac{\text{Liveability (\%)} \times \text{Mean slaughter weight (kg)}}{\text{Age at slaughter (days)} \times \text{Food conversion ratio (kg feed:kg gain)}}$$

This cannot be considered a welfare index since, with the exception of liveability, all measurements simply reflect production efficiency. Animal-based traits that may be used as robust measures of welfare include the following:

- mortality: obtained from farm records;
- contact dermatitis (hock burn, foot burn): from observation of a representative sample of birds;
- lameness: leg weakness assessed by gait scoring 100 birds at random;
- feather loss and skin damage;
- weight distribution at slaughter.

Haslam (2003) has developed a systematic approach to scoring these traits and weighting them, together with measures of provision such as stocking density and environmental enrichment, into a single Unified Welfare Index (UWI). As indicated in Chapter 4, I believe that overall welfare scores are of limited value. They can be used to define the overall pass mark necessary to meet the standards laid down by a QA scheme such as the RSPCA Freedom Food scheme. However, in practice, different units have different problems. It is necessary to identify these specific problems and propose specific solutions. Nevertheless the study of Haslam (2003) does identify the most important welfare problems and propose practical and robust measures for their assessment.

Haslam proposes an overall Equivalent Leg Weakness Score (ELWS) based on observation of 100 birds and records of numbers N_D, N_E and N_F at gait scores 3, 4 and 5 respectively. Then:

$$ELWS = N_D + 2N_E + 3N_F$$

Thus ten birds at score 3 plus three at 4 and one at 5 would yield an ELWS of 19. Haslam suggests, from consultation of expert opinion that the threshold of unacceptability should be above 20. The two main risk factors for contact dermatitis (foot burn and hock burn) are wet litter and birds that are extremely reluctant to stand because of leg pain. There is a strong negative correlation between gait score and the time a broiler will willingly remain on its feet. Most birds at scores of 3–4 will lie down within a few seconds of being made to stand. Evidence of feather pecking is included in the protocol. This has not proved a problem in intensive units, but it is a remote possibility in free-range systems.

Weight distribution at slaughter is included as an animal-based assessment of the potential failure of the system to allow all birds to meet their physiological and behavioural needs. The variation in body weights just prior to slaughter is described as the number of weight bands with a band width of 150g, and excluding the upper and lower extremes. In the Haslam study the lowest weight distribution score was 7 (i.e. a weight range of 1050g), the highest 13 (weight range 1950g). A weight range of 1.9kg at an average slaughter weight of 2.5kg is a pretty convincing indicator of bad husbandry.

Animals for Food: Cattle and Other Ruminants

The cow, crunching with depressed head surpasses any statue.... They are so placid and self-contained. I stand and look at them long and long.

Walt Whitman

Cattle, sheep and goats are ruminant species that have evolved to graze and browse the grasses, herbs and leaves of the bush and the open plains. The special characteristic of these animals is the rumen itself, a fermentation chamber wherein an enormous population of micro-organisms works to digest cellulose and other plant fibres to yield nutrients (energy, protein, etc.) to support the maintenance of life and the productive functions of growth and lactation in the host animal. Downstream of the rumen, the processes of digestion and metabolism in a ruminant cow or sheep are very similar to those in a simple-stomached pig or human. The owner of cattle, sheep or goats in a primitive pastoral society was able to derive food, clothing, work and fuel from animals that thrived on plants that he was unable to digest, and on land that he did not own. The main contribution of sheep and male goats was a meal of meat large enough to feast an extended family. Their value was limited by the fact that they could make this contribution only once, so they were largely left to fend for themselves and corralled only as necessary. Cattle, however, were of much greater individual value and more value alive than dead. All adult animals could be made to work at the plough. Their dung fertilised the ploughed soil and fed the fires. Some cultures, such as the Masai, would repeatedly bleed their animals to provide a sustainable source of food. For many nomadic cultures, the number of cattle in the possession of a family or tribe was a direct measure of their wealth. The idea that large numbers of apparently unproductive cattle could be viewed as a source of wealth is difficult to capture through modern Western eyes. However, all animals that can extract value for their owners from plants they need not grow and on land they do not own are a source of wealth when times are good and a capital reserve when times are bad.

For all cultures that have developed in close association with cattle as chattels for their personal use (the two words have the same root), the most valuable individual has been the lactating cow. She is a daily provider of food in the form of milk that may be consumed at once or conserved as butter, cheese, ghee or yoghurt. Not only is this highly nutritious food for the family, it is also available for sale on a daily basis and thus a regular source of income. The farmer and his family invested time and labour to grow, cut, carry and conserve food for the house cow, and the cow more than repaid this investment through the production of milk for home consumption and for sale. Thus dairy production became the first expression of high input/high output animal production as a source of disposable income; a currency that could lift farmers from subsistence agriculture towards some freedom of choice in the marketplace. The value of the dairy cow as a source of both food and income finds expression in the phrase *milch cow*, defined in *Chambers Dictionary* as 'a cow yielding milk, or kept for milking; a ready source of gain or money'.

It is important to recognise that dairy production is the only facet of cattle farming that is sufficiently productive of food as a commodity to justify substantial expenditure of capital and labour. Before the age of refrigeration, it seldom made sense to rear male calves to produce mature beef as we now understand it. This would have been a clear case of cutting off more than one (or even the village) could chew! The calf born to the milking house cow was fed on some of its mother's milk and slaughtered at a young age for white veal before it began to compete with its mother for food. Refrigeration and transport has made it economic to rear beef animals to slaughter weights in excess of 500 kg. However, in Europe about 50% of beef is still produced as a by-product of the dairy industry. 'Natural' beef from calves reared by their mothers, the suckler cows, is a luxury item highly valued in societies where some of the people have more money and some of the people have more land than they really need. Modern production of white veal is an efficient mechanism for 'using up' by-products: surplus male calves born to dairy cows and skim milk and whey surplus to the production of butter and cheese. I have severely criticised the welfare abuses associated with the production of white veal (Webster, 1984) and shall do so again. However, here, as always, it can be dangerous to destroy something until you have something better (or potentially better) to put in its place. At present, millions of male calves born to dairy cows are being slaughtered at birth because they have no value. It is entirely valid to claim that these calves will not have to experience three to four months of suffering in an intensive veal unit. Nevertheless it is a terrible waste of lives.

This chapter on the welfare of cattle and other ruminants introduces problems associated with the full spectrum of husbandry, from highly intensive, highly mechanised dairy production, to highly extensive ranching of scarcely domesticated animals on marginal land. At one end of the spectrum, high-yielding dairy cows are fed and housed but may be worked to exhaustion. At the other, sheep on open range may be left to die because they are not worth the cost of feed, nor even a bullet to put them out of their misery.

6.1 The welfare of the dairy cow

Good welfare is defined, as always, as staying fit and feeling good. Provision of good welfare requires attention to the Five Freedoms. In Chapter 1, I illustrated how a scan through the Five Freedoms can be used to identify systematic welfare problems for farm animals. Applying these rules to the dairy cow:

- She may both suffer and fail to sustain fitness through hunger, malnutrition or metabolic disease if she is unable to consume or digest sufficient nutrients to support her genetic and physiological potential to produce milk.
- She may suffer chronic discomfort if housing design, especially the design of her lying area, is inappropriate to her size and shape. Problems of poor cubicle design and inadequate bedding may become worse if she loses condition through malnutrition.
- She may suffer pain through lameness or mastitis.
- She may show an increased susceptibility to infectious disease as a consequence of metabolic stress.
- She may be bullied or denied proper rest by other cows.
- She may experience metabolic or physical exhaustion caused by the stress of prolonged high production.

These potential sources of poor health and welfare can be interdependent and additive. For example, the high-genetic-merit dairy cow, housed in cubicles and fed a diet based on wet grass silage and concentrate in the parlour, may suffer from both hunger and chronic discomfort, partly because the quality of the feed has failed to meet her nutrient requirements for lactation and she has lost condition, partly because the wet silage has contributed to poor hygiene and predisposed to foot lameness, and partly because genetic selection has created a cow too big for the cubicles. Note please that these are problems arising in systems of feeding and housing inappropriate for the high-yielding cow. They are not a criticism of high genetic merit *per se*. However, it is an undeniable fact that genetic selection of cows for greatly increased milk yield has made it progressively harder for the farmer to meet their needs, whether for optimal productivity, health or welfare.

6.1.1 The work of lactation

Lactation is hard work. Table 6.1 examines the physiological costs of producing milk in different mammals. Daily milk yield is first expressed in litres, kJ milk energy and grams of milk protein. However, in order to compare inputs and outputs, such as rates of milk yield, food consumption and metabolic rate in the different species, I have scaled all measurements according to the function of body

Table 6.1 Comparison of the milk yield, food energy intake (MJ ME) and work rate (MJ heat production) of different mammals scaled for comparison according to metabolic body size (kg $W^{0.75}$/day).

	Dairy cow (Holstein)	Beef cow (one calf)	Sow (10 piglets)	Bitch (8 pups)	Woman (one baby)
Body weight (kg)	700	450	200	26	60
Metabolic size	136	97	53	11.50	21.50
Milk yield (l/day)	40	10	7.5	1.3	1.2
Milk energy (kJ/day)	124032	31040	40810	8222	3397
Milk protein (g/day)	1319	330	445	108	15
Milk yield/kg $W^{0.75}$/day					
Milk energy (kJ)	912	320	770	715	158
Milk protein (g)	9.7	3.4	8.4	9.4	0.72
Food intake (MJ ME/kg $W^{0.75}$/day)	2.06	1.06	1.76	1.64	0.75
Work rate (MJ heat/kg $W^{0.75}$/day)	1.15	0.75	1.00	0.93	0.60

weight kg$W^{0.75}$. This is a standard convention, usually defined as *metabolic body size*, used to confer proportionality on rate measurements in homeothermic animals. In simple terms, it accounts for differences directly attributable to body size and so permits comparisons between cattle and sheep, mice and elephants*. The examples in Table 6.1 include a typical (although not extreme) high-genetic-merit Holstein cow, weighing 700 kg and yielding 40 l milk/day; a suckler beef cow producing 10 l/day to feed one calf; a sow and a bitch, two species that give birth to litters (a sow with ten piglets and a Labrador bitch with eight puppies); and finally a human mother with a single baby. When body size has been taken into account, by dividing all measures of input and output by kg$W^{0.75}$ the daily yield of milk energy (912 kJ/kg$W^{0.75}$/day) and protein (9.7 g/kg$W^{0.75}$/day) from the Holstein is larger, but not conspicuously larger, than that of the lactating sow (770 and 8.4 respectively) or bitch (715 and 9.4 respectively). Thus the high-yielding dairy cow is not as genetically extreme, in terms of maximum yield, as might be imagined. Other species that give birth to litters (and indeed the highly selected dairy goat) achieve almost as high a daily rate of production. The big difference is, of course, that the sow or bitch is unlikely to produce milk at this rate for more than about eight weeks. Anyone who has cared for a bitch during an eight-week

* For a more detailed explanation see Webster (1992).

lactation knows that she can end up emaciated, even when given highly digestible food rich in energy and protein. Commercial dairy cows and goats are expected to produce milk at a high rate for ten months of the year on diets that are less digestible. The dairy cow carries the further cost of producing one calf per year, mainly to ensure a near-continuous supply of milk. Most of the welfare problems (the 'production diseases') of the dairy cow arise from the fact that she has to work so hard for so long. The dairy goat has the capacity to sustain a productive level of lactation for several years following a single parturition. This is to the advantage of the producer for whom milk is the main source of income and kids a liability. It is also to her own advantage, since most health and welfare problems occur in early lactation.

The suckler cow, feeding one calf, produces about 10 l milk/day, compared with 40 l/day from the typical Holstein and over 70 l/day from the most productive animals. She can achieve this 'natural' rate of milk production at approximately half the food intake of the dairy cow [measured as megajoules (MJ) of metabolisable energy (ME)], i.e. 1.06 v. 2.06 MJ ME/kg $W^{0.75}$/day. Her work rate measured as MJ of heat production (H) is 65% that of the dairy cow, i.e. 0.75 v. 1.15 MJ H/kg $W^{0.75}$/day. The work rate of a human male in a sedentary job is about 0.45 MJ H/kg $W^{0.75}$/day, that of a grazing, non-productive adult beef cow about 0.5 MJ H/kg $W^{0.75}$/day. The amount of ME required to maintain body weight in non-productive animals such as sedentary humans and idling ruminants is equal to their energy expenditure as heat (i.e. 0.45 and 0.5 MJ ME/kg $W^{0.75}$/day). In order to sustain milk production at 40 l/day the Holstein cow must therefore eat more than four times as much food (2.06 v. 0.5 MJ ME/kg $W^{0.75}$/day) and work more than twice as hard (1.15 v. 0.5 MJ H/kg $W^{0.75}$/day) as the non-productive cow at pasture. I have described the dairy cow as the apotheosis of the overworked mother. This may sound like a fanciful claim, but the evidence is beyond cavil.

6.1.2 Sustaining fitness

In Chapter 5, I considered the implications for both productivity and welfare of genetic selection exclusively on the basis of productivity traits while neglecting correlated traits that contribute to a loss of fitness. In the case of dairy cattle, selection for increased milk yield in first lactation has contributed to a loss of fitness through increased predisposition to infertility, mastitis and lameness (Table 5.3). In the poultry industry, this loss of fitness has not really hurt the producers (although it has hurt the chickens) since broilers are not expected to survive more than six weeks of rapid growth, nor hens more than one year in lay. However, in the dairy industry everyone has been hurt by the drive to increased production at all costs. Strong selection pressure for milk yield has achieved a rate of genetic improvement of 2% per year in first lactation. Moreover the response is still linear; there is as yet no sign that response is levelling off. All other things being equal therefore, a 2% improvement per annum will, by compound interest, over ten years increase output by 19.5%. This sounds like an offer that the dairy farmer cannot refuse. However, all else is not equal.

Figure 6.1 illustrates the effect of increasing longevity on lifetime efficiency, expressed as total litres of milk produced in relation to lifetime food intake (gigajoules, GJ ME). The two graphs refer respectively to cows with lactation yields of 12 000 and 4000 l in the third to fifth lactations. In each case the overall efficiency of the enterprise is calculated in two situations: assuming no genetic improvement (G = 0%) and assuming five years of genetic improvement at 2% per annum (GE = 2%). In both examples, optimal lifetime efficiency is reached after five to six lactations although there is little net improvement after four. For cows yielding 4000 l/year on a typical low input/low output system sustained mainly from fresh and conserved grass, a life expectancy of only three lactations reduces lifetime efficiency by 7%; a life expectancy of two lactations reduces it by 12%. For 12 000-l cows the effect is slightly less in relative terms – 5 and 10% for three and two lactations respectively. Figure 6.1 shows that a culling policy based on selection for increased milk yield that replaces cows after four lactations, will, after five years just match the consequences of keeping cows fit for six lactations and practising no selection at all. Thereafter, of course, the lifetime performance of the genetically superior herd will start to forge ahead. Herds that are culled, for whatever reason, after less than four lactations are still less efficient than those averaging six lactations despite five years of genetic progress at 2% per annum. In many high-genetic-merit dairy herds in both the UK and USA average longevity is below three lactations. Moreover the majority of the cows are being culled not as a planned instrument of selection for improved performance but as the unplanned consequence of a breakdown in fitness through mastitis, lameness and, especially, infertility.

Fortunately for all, dairy farmers are becoming increasingly aware that they were for many years being conned by the breeders and increasingly vocal in their demands for a better cow. It is now generally accepted that dairy cattle should be selected on the basis of an index that gives proper weight to traits consistent with satisfactory lifetime performance. One good example of this is the new USA Department of Agriculture Index of Lifetime Net Merit. This weights different selection traits as follows.

Milk fat and protein yield	62%
Somatic cell score	−9%
Udder conformation	7%
Productive life	14%
Feet and legs	4%
Body size	−4%

This selection index quite properly puts the highest weighting (62%) on yield of the two most valuable constituents of milk, namely protein and fat. However, it also acknowledges the need to improve productive life achieved directly through

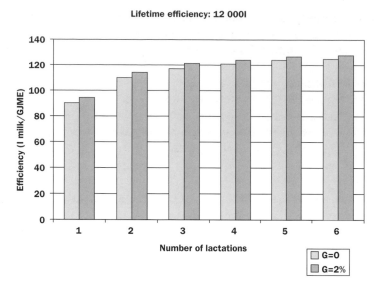

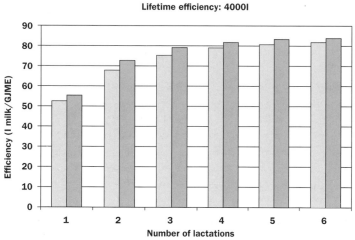

Figure 6.1 Effects of increasing longevity and genetic selection on lifetime efficiency in dairy cows. Efficiency is measured as lifetime milk production (litres)/lifetime food intake (gigajoules metabolisable energy). The groups G = 0% and G = 2% refer, respectively, to efficiencies in cows with no genetic improvement and after five years of genetic improvement at 2% per annum.

a reduction in infertility and also through an improvement in genetic fitness with regard to mastitis (udder conformation and reduced somatic cell score) and lameness (feet and legs). The inclusion of a negative weighting term for body size is subtle. The low weighting is not likely to result in a reduction in size of the modern Holstein cow. However, it should halt the trend towards selection for heavier and heavier cows because it seeks to break the correlation between increasing yield of milk and increasing size of cow. This is important because heavier cows are more prone to chronic discomfort, lameness and injury in most confinement barns.

The decision to incorporate traits relating directly to productive life and the main production diseases, infertility, mastitis and lameness, is a real positive step towards improved welfare, or, at least, redressing some of the errors of the past. However, it is no more than a partial solution since the heritability of the trait 'productive life' is low (8.5%). In the short term, the most effective way to achieve sustained fitness, and thereby the welfare of the dairy cow, is through a system of management (feeding, housing, hygiene, etc.) appropriate to the phenotype. Table 5.3 (from Pryce et al., 1998) shows that, at present, dairy farmers are just holding the line against loss of genetic fitness with regard to mastitis and lameness, but losing the battle against infertility. Genetic improvement to the phenotype (or, at least, a halt in the rate of genetic decline) will be a help, but most of the improvements will have to be made by the farmer on the farm with the animals he or she has got.

6.1.3 Disorders of digestion and metabolism

One of the great truths concerning the high-genetic-merit dairy cow is that the capacity of her mammary gland to produce milk far exceeds the capacity of the cow upstream to supply the nutrients necessary for milk synthesis. The first constraint to the productivity of the dairy cow is her capacity to consume and digest sufficient food to meet her nutrient requirement for milk synthesis. Table 6.2 estimates the food intake (expressed as dry matter, DM) that high-genetic-merit Holstein cows may reasonably be expected to achieve at pasture, when fed silage plus concentrates twice daily or when fed a well-balanced 'total mixed ration' (TMR). It then relates this to the level of milk production (litres/day) that this amount of food can sustain. A cow at pasture is restricted to an intake of about 16 kg DM/day simply because she has neither the time nor the machinery to harvest more. The housed cow with continuous access to grass silage but given concentrate feeds only during milking may eat 20 kg DM and this can sustain 36 l milk/day. However, a hungry, healthy cow producing 55 l milk/day may manage to eat 26 kg DM/day or more if a balanced diet is constantly available and in suitable physical and chemical form to promote rapid, safe fermentation of food energy and digestion of protein in the rumen. The formulation of balanced TMRs

Table 6.2 Milk yields and dry matter intakes of Holstein/Friesian cows in different circumstances.

	DM intake (kg/day)	Sustained yield (l/day)
Pasture	16	25
Grass silage + concentrates (×2/day)	20	36
Total mixed ration	26	55

has been the main vehicle that has permitted dairy cows to express their physiological potential to produce milk at rates of 50–70 l/day. This is two to three times greater than that which can be sustained by the same cow when grazing at pasture, partly because the food is more freely available, partly because the ration is of higher nutritive value, and partly because it should promote rapid but stable digestion in the rumen. It follows, however, that cows can only sustain yields over 50 l/day if they are kept almost permanently off grass. This provokes three questions of welfare.

(1)   Is it more stressful to a dairy cow to produce 55 l milk/day than 25 l/day?
(2)   Is it stressful to a restrict a cow with the genetic potential to produce 55 l/day to a diet that can only sustain 25 l/day?
(3)   Is it stressful to restrict a cow to a zero-grazing system for most or all of her adult life?

In addressing these questions it is helpful to remember that what motivates cows to eat is not the need to produce milk *per se* but the need to feel good. In short, they regulate food intake to ensure maximum comfort (or, more precisely, to minimise discomfort). The physiological demand for nutrients to support lactation creates a condition of 'metabolic hunger'. The cow senses not only the continuous uptake of nutrients by the mammary gland, but also the cumulative effect of loss of her body reserves of energy and protein. Clear evidence for this is provided by the responses of cows to injections of recombinant bovine growth hormone (rBGH or rBST). Milk yield typically increases by 15% within 24 hours. Food intake does not rise immediately so the cow loses condition as she draws on her body reserves. After an interval of about 14 days, this loss of condition becomes severe enough to trigger an increase in metabolic hunger and the cow will eat more, if she can. For most lactating cows, most of the time, the primary stimulus to eat is metabolic hunger. At the same time she is presented with powerful stimuli to *stop* eating. At pasture, food intake is limited by the rate at which she can harvest the grass. When housed and given *ad libitum* access to conserved forage but concentrates only in the milking parlour then her intake is constrained physically by gut fill and physiologically by the rate of absorption of certain end products of rumen digestion. Fibre that ferments slowly fills up the rumen and restricts food intake since the rate at which new food can enter the rumen is constrained by the rate at which partially digested material can be moved out. Asynchrony between the digestion of crude protein and carbohydrate in the rumen can increase the absorption of ammonia, giving rise to an increased concentration of urea in blood and this can impair appetite. The aim of the TMR is to promote rapid, stable fermentation, and so reduce the constraints presented by both rumen fill and high blood urea concentrations.

To summarise this physiology in terms of how it feels to the high-yielding cow: she is motivated to eat by metabolic hunger (a function of both milk yield and body condition); she is motivated to *stop* eating by sensations (conscious or uncon-

Table 6.3 Relative importance of different constraints on the food intake of dairy cows.

	Pasture	Silage + cake	TMR
Need to rest	+++	+	+
Gut fill		+++	
Unbalanced digestion	+	++ to +++	

scious) associated with gut fill, unbalanced absorption of certain end products of rumen digestion (especially ammonia), and the conflicting desire to do something other than eat, such as rest. Table 6.3 illustrates the relative importance of these constraints on food intake. At pasture, the first constraint on food intake is the rate at which the cow can physically consume the grass. Thus the motivation for the cow to stop eating is more likely to arise from the desire to rest than from the sensation of gut fill. On very high nitrogen pastures food intake may be constrained by ammonia absorption. A high-yielding cow offered poorly made, high ammonia grass silage, plus concentrate in parlour only, faces an impossible compromise between metabolic hunger, gut fill, chemically induced inappetence and the need to rest. According to the model of McFarland's Egg (Figure 3.2) she is moved towards a state of suffering because the stress is too complex and too prolonged. Her feelings may be defined, with brutal accuracy, as simultaneously hungry, tired, full up and feeling sick. Food intake in a barn-fed cow yielding over 50 l milk/day and offered a well-balanced TMR should be constrained to a far lesser extent by feelings of gut fill or sickness. However, consumption of 26 kg DM/day (possibly 100 kg fresh material/day) is hard work, even for a hungry cow, and she will face the conflicting motivation to stop eating and lie down. The observations of cow behaviour listed in Table 4.4 included numbers (%) standing idle. This was included as a measure of the amount of time available for the cow simply to 'stand and stare', having attended to her maintenance needs. As milk yields increased, so time spent standing idle decreased. It would appear that very-high-yielding dairy cows have practically no spare time at all.

Is it stressful therefore to expect a dairy cow to produce 55 l milk/day? It is certainly possible to formulate reasonably healthy feeds and feeding systems that will sustain milk yields of over 50 l/day *and* body condition on a day-to-day basis in cows but only if they are kept off pasture. However, they are operating at their limits of activity, both physiological and behavioural. They may yearn for green fields, but they have neither the time nor probably the energy to display much behavioural evidence of either good or bad welfare (e.g. play or frustration respectively). More serious welfare problems are likely to arise in cows that are unable to consume and digest enough food to meet the metabolic demands of lactation. It is normal for cows to 'milk off their backs' in early lactation, i.e. to draw on body reserves. Problems, especially the problem of infertility, arise when the loss of body condition in early lactation is too severe, or too prolonged. Failure to maintain body condition is undoubtedly the most useful long-term indicator of failure to achieve the first of the Five Freedoms, freedom from hunger.

It has been argued that selecting a cow with the capacity to produce 60 l/day, then feeding her at a rate sufficient for 25 l/day is comparable to buying a car capable of 140 m.p.h. then cruising at 60. This argument does not stand close inspection. This is a complex problem (see Webster, 1993), but I shall try to explain it in a few words. The capacity of the mammary gland to produce milk is limited by the supply of nutrients in the blood. The first limiting nutrients are usually amino acids from dietary protein. The greater the supply of amino acids, the greater the milk yield. However, the greater the milk yield the greater the overall requirement of the cow for food energy to support both maintenance and lactation. Most dairy farmers feed diets with a high protein concentration because they maximise milk production *in the short term*. This increases the probability that cows will be in energy deficit and so lose body condition. If cows are fed diets in which protein is the first limiting nutrient, milk yield is restricted by the low supply of amino acids. This reduces energy demand. Thus the cow produces less milk but sustains body condition and general fitness. It is therefore possible to devise diets that will enable a high-genetic-merit Holstein cow to sustain a yield of 25 l/day on a low protein ration in metabolic comfort, in the same way that a Porsche can cruise comfortably at 50 m.p.h. However, farmers competing in the milk race do not formulate rations to reduce milk production. They select cows with a high genetic potential for milk production and feed them high protein feeds in an effort to realise that potential. This can impose the following stresses:

- behavioural conflict between the motivation to eat and that to rest;
- abnormalities of rumen fermentation and digestion leading (e.g.) to inappetence, acidosis, bloat, displaced abomasum or lameness induced by laminitis;
- acute abnormalities of metabolism of energy, protein and minerals leading (e.g.) to ketosis, fatty liver syndrome or hypomagnesaemia;
- chronic consequences of a deficiency of dietary energy leading to loss of body condition, infertility or increased susceptibility to infection and injury.

Observations and records of body condition and the prevalence of production diseases provide good indicators of the extent to which the welfare of a herd of dairy cows may be compromised by disorders of digestion and metabolism. Thus, if a herd of barn-fed Holstein cows that achieve a peak daily yield of 60 l/day can sustain this yield, *and* sustain body condition and fertility, and have a very low incidence of disorders of digestion and metabolism, then, by these criteria, their welfare will be satisfactory. (This is a long series of 'ifs'.) Indeed their welfare is likely to be better than a herd of cows of similar genotype put into a pastoral system and expected to produce 20 l/day of milk from grass. The New Zealand dairy industry, for example, has aimed to produce 'clean and green' dairy products from cows kept at pasture throughout the year. There are many attractions of this system, not least its sustainability measured in terms of land use. It is not, however, a sustainable system for the dairy cows, who are likely to be culled for infertility after a lifetime of less than three lactations. The New Zealanders are discovering to their cost that the high-genetic-merit Holstein is not for them. She has been designed to live and feed in a barn.

6.1.4 Lameness

The importance of a welfare problem may be defined by its incidence, its duration and its severity. By these criteria, lameness is indisputably the major welfare problem for the dairy cow. Most surveys of lameness in dairy cattle in Europe and the USA report an annual incidence of about 50% and prevalence of over 20% (Clarkson et al., 1996; Whay et al., 2003b). In simple words this means half the cows go lame in any one year and 20% are lame at any one time. In 1990 the majority of cases in the UK could be attributed to claw horn disruption (CHD), haemorrhages into the sole and white line arising from mechanical damage within the internal suspensory apparatus of the foot. In more recent years infectious causes of lameness, especially digital dermatitis (DD), have become more common on both sides of the Atlantic.

This is not the place for detailed exposition of all the factors that can cause a cow to become lame. For further reading see Vermunt & Greenough (1996). It is necessary, however, to examine the risk factors for lameness and identify the extent to which they may or may not be controlled through attention to good husbandry. Table 6.4 lists the most important risk factors for the most common categories of

Table 6.4 Risk factors for hoof lameness in dairy cattle.

Category	Examples	Mechanisms
Claw horn disease		
Environmental	Concrete floors	High external load
	Quality of bedding area	Prolonged standing time
Nutritional	Nutritionally induced laminitis	Disruption of foot suspension
	Wet forage	Wet acid slurry
Managemental	Hoof trimming (good)	'Normalises' weight bearing
	Hoof trimming (bad)	Inadequate soles and heels
Cow-based	Size, conformation (CHD)	Uneven weight bearing
	Parturition and early lactation (CHD)	Increased laxity in foot suspension
Infections		
Environmental	Deep slurry in houses and yards (DD)	Anaerobic bacteria
	Damaging paths and gateways ('foul')	Infected injuries
Managemental	Buying in cows (DD)	Introduces new pathogens
	Poor attention to hygiene	Anaerobic bacteria

CHD, Claw horn disruption (sole and white line haemorrhages); DD, Digital dermatitis lameness, CHD and DD, and outlines the mechanisms involved. DD is caused by a number of anaerobic bacteria. If the specific bacteria are not present on the farm then DD will not occur; thus the first onset of DD usually follows the purchase of infected animals. DD can be treated with appropriate antibiotics, but once it has become endemic it is very difficult to eradicate. However, because the DD organisms are anaerobes, they can be controlled to a great extent by ensuring that the cows' feet are kept reasonably clean and, at the very least, they are not forced to stand with their feet immersed in slurry.

Approximately 75% of clinical cases of lameness due to sole ulcers and severe white line disease (two types of CHD) occur in the outer claws of the hind feet and most of these become apparent within the first ten weeks after calving. In most circumstances farmers only elect to treat the most severe cases of CHD, e.g. the sole ulcer, when there has been complete penetration of the sole, inducing deep pain from standing on concrete and scalding pain through exposure of the sensitive underlying tissues to acid slurry. However, these severe cases are only the tip of the iceberg. In my experience, nearly all newly calved cows and heifers kept in typical UK cubicle houses show some degree of sole haemorrhage in early lactation (Webster, 2002). The haemorrhage results from internal pressure from the pedal bone progressively eroding the sole from within (Ossent & Lischer, 1998). This is caused by a failure to accommodate the strength and duration of the forces acting on the foot. External forces become excessive if cows are compelled to walk excessive distances or stand for prolonged periods, especially on concrete. In cubicle houses this may occur when cows (and especially heifers) are denied access to cubicles by other cows, or simply through an absolute shortage of cubicles. It may also occur when they are reluctant to lie in cubicles, either because the bed is uncomfortable or because the design of the cubicle makes it difficult for them to stand up and lie down. Cow-based factors contributing to excessive load on the suspension apparatus of the foot include body weight and conformation. The fact that most sole ulcers occur in the lateral claw of the hind feet can be attributed to uneven weight bearing, due in large part to the developing presence of the large udder between the hind legs. This can be overcome to some extent by selection for good leg conformation and controlled to some extent by proper foot trimming to ensure even weight bearing. However, over-zealous foot trimming can do more harm than good by reducing both the thickness of the sole and especially the heels, which in cattle (unlike horses) play a major role in cushioning the forces acting on the foot.

The high incidence of lameness (and almost ubiquitous development of sole haemorrhages) in early lactation has traditionally been attributed to changes in feeding, housing and management as cows come into milk. This problem can be especially severe in heifers who may be crippled by sole ulcers within ten weeks of commencing their productive life. Undoubtedly heifers entering the dairy herd for the first time are presented with many new challenges: access to large quantities of high starch, high protein concentrates, prolonged standing on concrete in collecting yards and competition with adult cows for access to cubicles wherein they may rest their feet. Many of these problems can be overcome through good management. Nevertheless, there is increasing evidence that normal physiological changes accompanying parturition and the onset of lactation may weaken the suspension apparatus within the feet, thereby rendering cows especially liable to damage from mechanical forces in the early weeks of lactation. It follows from this that cows and heifers may be protected from developing CHD by reducing their exposure to mechanical forces during the critical weeks around calving and the onset of lactation. In a study at Bristol, heifers were either introduced to a cubicle house as they calved (a typical commercial situation) or kept in a straw yard until the eighth week of lactation. All animals showed some evidence of sole haemorrhage four weeks after calving, but this only progressed to the point of inducing clinical lameness in those heifers housed in cubicles from the outset. Those that started out in a straw yard had effectively overcome the slight initial problem by the time they entered the cubicle house and did not relapse (Webster, 2002).

6.1.5 The problem of pain

The main reason that lameness is a welfare problem is because it hurts! Although the number of limping cows in a typical dairy herd is likely to exceed 20%, the number of cows actually culled for lameness is only about 5%. This is consistent with our observation that most farmers fail to recognise more than 25% of their lame cows (Whay et al., 2003b). These numbers mean that a very large number of cows are being left to suffer. The important question to ask then is how much does it hurt and how much do they suffer? Pain is a subjective experience. When I am in pain, I know how much it hurts. But when you are in pain, I not only do not know how badly you are hurting, I also do not know whether the fuss you are making is justified by the pain you are feeling. How much more difficult it is when the animal in question is a cow. There is a widespread belief that cows are relatively insensitive to pain. This belief is based on the observation that cows often do not seem to display the signs of distress that we would expect (e.g. bellowing, immobility, loss of appetite) when one or more feet are showing signs of severe damage. It is important, however, to remember that, in nature, cows and other ruminants are prey animals who go around in herds to reduce their individual risk of attack from predators. In these circumstances, the animal that limps becomes the target. Thus it pays not to limp. Cows are natural stoics, but because they are not showing signs of distress it does not mean that it does not hurt. In fact, pain thresholds in cows are similar to those in man. Moreover, pain thresholds are significantly reduced in cows that are already in chronic pain from CHD or digital dermatitis (Whay et al., 1998). In cows as in man, chronic pain gets worse with time. The mechanism involves a 'wind-up' or amplification of pain sensation at nerve junctions within the spinal cord. Although we cannot claim that cows experience pain in the same subjective way as we do, we can say with confidence that the intensity of the sensation is as bad for them as it is for us.

Foot lameness in dairy cows is not just a problem of getting about; it is an expression of distress. Awareness of this imposes a responsibility to do what we can to prevent, treat and relieve the condition. I have already considered how to reduce the incidence and severity of lameness through husbandry designed to address the major risk factors (Table 6.4). It is also necessary to address the problem of pain in the cow that has become lame. Infectious conditions such as DD are very painful indeed but respond quickly to treatment. The problem of CHD is that the pain is chronic. Fixing a block to the 'unaffected' claw of a cow with a solar ulcer obviously relieves the pain on the affected claw. However, it is common to see haemorrhage on both claws, attributable to internal pressure from the pedal bone. This means that the claw with the block is likely to be painful too. Thus a block is not enough; cows need a comfortable bed as well. Wherever possible, individual cows with severe CHD (e.g. solar ulcers) should be removed from the cubicle house and kept in well-bedded pens or yards where they can lie down as much as possible. Ideally they should be given at least six weeks to recover.

Reduced to its simplest terms, the problem of lameness in dairy cows can be attributed to:

- the prevalence and severity of the condition (over 20% of cows in pain);
- the complexity of the risk factors (only some of which are amenable to control on a typical farm);
- the failure of farmers to recognise and treat the condition.

The last factor is not intended as a condemnation of dairy farmers. Many dairy farmers are as exhausted as their cows and have neither the time nor the money necessary to embark on a major strategic problem of lameness control. The herdsperson who daily follows his or her cows as they pick their tender-footed or painful way to pasture not only tends towards compassion fatigue but also comes to perceive their locomotion as normal. Moreover, it is a fact that many lame cows will continue to milk satisfactorily. Thus the economic cost of lameness to the farmer is usually less than the costs of infertility or mastitis. Chronically lame cows are often expected to struggle on until they are culled when they have completed their lactation. The stated reason for culling may be infertility, although loss of condition resulting from chronic lameness may have been the cause of infertility in the first place. The economic cost of lameness in the UK dairy herd has been estimated as at least 1 p/l of milk (5% of income). We should never forget that the cost to the cow is much greater.

6.1.6 Assessment and control of welfare on dairy farms

In Chapter 4 I outlined our protocol for assessing the welfare state of dairy cows as an example of our general approach to the evaluation of the welfare of groups

of animals on farms and in other commercial establishments. The protocol is summarised in Table 4.4 and need not be recapitulated here in any detail. One key
conclusion is, however, worth restating (several times). All-embracing audits of
husbandry provisions and welfare outcomes may be necessary to ensure compliance with the standards of QA schemes. They also provide a useful check that
none of the Five Freedoms is being neglected. It was, however, clear from our study
that we could not simply rank farms as good, satisfactory or bad. All farms had
one or more problems, some but not all serious enough to warrant immediate
attention. Most of the serious problems could be placed within the three broad
categories of metabolic stress, chronic discomfort and lameness. However, each of
these categories of poor welfare can involve a multiplicity of risk factors, the relative importance of which will differ from farm to farm. It follows therefore that
any approach to improving the welfare status of cows in a dairy herd should not
be based on the award (or not) of a simple badge of approval but on a systematic
professional farm-specific herd 'good husbandry' plan that will:

- prioritise those welfare concerns requiring immediate action;
- identify the main risk factors for the prior concerns and the critical control
  points for these risks;
- identify changes in the provision of nutrition, comfort, hygiene and stockmanship appropriate to the specified risks and implement those that can be put
  into effect immediately;
- identify and prioritise longer-term needs for improvements in resources and
  management that will require capital investment and establish a strategic plan
  to work towards meeting these needs;
- implement (and stick with!) a programme for the regular recording of welfare
  indices, e.g. involuntary culling rates, body condition, infertility, mastitis,
  lameness, skin abrasions and injuries, behaviour in cubicles (lying and chang-
  ing position);
- review and modify the husbandry plan in the light of changes (or not) in welfare
  outcomes.

6.2 The welfare of dairy calves

In a herd of wild cattle, or suckler beef cows, it is normal for the cow to feed her
calf for at least six months from birth. It is also normal for a cow on open range
to separate from the herd at the time of calving and 'hide' its young calf in isolation and away from the main herd. This evolutionary strategy has succeeded by
enhancing the calf's chances of survival. Thus it is consistent with both the physiological and behavioural needs of the calf that it should spend much of the time
apart from its mother. In the stable, semi-wild environment of a herd of beef cows
on range, it is normal for calves to lie in isolation for long periods in the first weeks

of life, then develop social 'play groups' with other calves of the same age, returning to their mothers for three to five good milk meals in every 24 hours. This contrasts strongly with the behaviour of some other grazing species, such as the horse. The young foal usually spends most of the time with its mother and feeds at hourly intervals.

In a typical dairy herd, calves are removed from their mothers very early in life, primarily to ensure that as much milk as possible is available for sale. All farmers know that it is essential that the calf receives an adequate supply of colostrum, the first milk from the cow which contains the antibodies necessary to give the calf immediate passive immunity to infection. Many dairy farmers separate the cow and calf in the first day of life, milk the cow and feed the colostrum from a bucket. At first glance this may appear to be both unnecessarily severe and unnecessarily laborious. However, it is not necessarily in the calf's best interests to do the 'natural' thing and leave mother and calf together for the first few days. One practical problem is that the calf may not manage to drink successfully because the udder of the dairy cow is abnormally pendulous so that the teats are not in the place where the neonatal calf has been programmed to look. The biggest welfare problem is that the longer the cow and calf are left together the stronger becomes the bond that develops between the two. Cows may briefly display signs of distress when their calves are removed in the first days of life. If calves are left with their mothers for two to three weeks they get a very good start in life. However, if they are then separated on a permanent basis, the distress shown by both mother and calf is loud and prolonged. I speak from experience since I live in earshot of such practice. Early weaning (the French word *sevrage* is more honest) is undoubtedly a source of distress. However, I am inclined to agree with Macbeth: 'When 'tis done, then 'twere well it were done quickly'.

Some farmers may permit their dairy cows to suckle their calves for at least two months, on the grounds of compassion and/or to meet the requirements of a QA scheme with exacting welfare standards. In these circumstances it is entirely consistent with normal behavioural development to run the calves in a group and only give them access to their mothers for twice-daily feeds. Other enlightened farmers (e.g. my neighbours) turn groups of calves out to pasture with an old nurse cow, retired (if only temporarily) from the production line. She provides the calves with a little milk, a lot of security and (probably) something of an education in conduct at pasture.

There is no doubt that the calf is well equipped to survive an artificial rearing strategy that simply does not work for most other farmed species such as the foal, lamb or piglet. When I first published *Calf Husbandry, Health and Welfare* (Webster, 1984) the cash value of male calves born to dairy cows ranged from about £150 for a pure dairy type to over £250 for a calf sired by a prime beef breed such as the Limousin or Charolais. At that time calf mortality rates (excluding deaths in the first day of life) were typically less than 3% simply because they were too valuable to lose. In areas such as the major centres of dairy production in the USA where male dairy-type calves carried little or no potential value as meat animals, they were either killed at birth or committed to rearing systems for the production of white veal or low-cost intensive beef, wherein mortality rates were typically about 20%. The high cash value of male dairy-type calves born in the UK in the early 1980s was sustained in large part by the export of calves for the white veal trade in continental Europe. This trade was destroyed by bovine spongiform encephalopathy (BSE or 'mad cow disease'). Male dairy-type calves are now spared the ordeal of exportation into veal crates but increasingly likely to be killed at birth or reared in low-cost intensive beef systems with high mortality rates simply because it is not financially worthwhile to strive to keep them alive.

I have repeatedly attacked traditional intensive systems of white veal production for systematic abuse of all Five Freedoms (Webster, 1984, 1994). I shall not replay this argument here since it has not changed either in principle or in detail. Legislation currently in force in the UK and pending in Europe has banned the worst excesses, namely rearing systems that commit veal calves for life to physical isolation in individual pens and a liquid diet that lacks sufficient roughage to permit rumen development. This is a beginning, but it remains a pretty dreadful system, one that will always fail the 'Pride' test. I simply cannot imagine a conventional producer of white veal inviting members of the public to 'Come and see my animals. They will be going off for slaughter next week and don't they look magnificent!'

The general awfulness of conventional white veal production raises two important, related questions, one ethical, one practical. The ethical question asks 'Is it more acceptable to kill dairy calves at birth than to condemn them to a life in a production system that will almost certainly seriously compromise both their health and their welfare?' I incline to the former view. Nevertheless, it is a terrible waste of life. The practical question asks 'How can we realise the potential value of the male dairy calf in a way that is consistent with our duty of care to a sentient life?' The intrinsic problem for the male calf is that genetic selection for milk production (especially but not exclusively in the Holstein breed) has created a phenotype with a conformation (e.g. muscle/bone ratio) that can be used for veal production at less than six months of age but is highly unsuitable for the production of mature prime beef. One solution to this problem for farmers aiming for sustainable, high-welfare production of added-value products for niche markets is to change the phenotype of the cow towards that of a dual-purpose animal. Absolute milk production will fall, but a greater proportion of the milk will be generated by nutrients from fresh and conserved grass. Moreover, all calves will be able to contribute to the capacity of the farm to create value from the resources of its own land. An affluent society that places a high value on sustainable agriculture, quality of the countryside *and prime beef*, but finds itself awash with liquid milk, can surely summon the will to encourage this development.

An alternative and complementary value judgement is to recognise that many people pay high prices to eat veal in restaurants and more would undoubtedly do the same if they were not dissuaded by concerns as to the method of production. I have demonstrated that it is perfectly possible to produce high-quality veal from calves reared in groups in deep straw, with sufficient dietary iron to avoid anaemia and sufficient roughage to permit normal rumen development and ensure reasonable freedom from the digestive disorders that plague calves reared on all-liquid diets (Webster, 1984). Such calves can be healthy, comfortable and free to engage in social behaviour. They are also spared the mutilations of dehorning and castration. Their life may be brief (14–16 weeks), but they should not suffer. I believe that a well-run high-welfare veal unit can pass the 'Pride' test with flying colours. Although 'high-welfare veal' sounds like an oxymoron, it is a concept recognised by the RSPCA Freedom Food scheme. On the basis of pure reason, it should be possible to develop a niche market for veal among those who value their meat on the grounds of not only taste but also animal welfare. However, as I wrote in Chapter 3, we are all sentient animals. We will not eat veal until we feel good about it and that will not happen until we can go on to veal units and see healthy, happy calves with our own eyes.

To return to the main theme: Table 6.5 (from Whay *et al.*, 2003c) summarises our approach to the animal-based assessment of welfare state as applied to calves from dairy herds, early weaned and artificially reared, whether for beef or as replacement heifers. The approach involves the usual combination of observations

Table 6.5 Animal-based indices of health and welfare in artificially reared calves (from Whay *et al.*, 2003c).

Category	Observations	Records
Hunger and thirst	Body condition	Electrolyte therapy
	Rumen (bloated, hollow, impacted)	
	Coat (dull, staring)	
	Hollow eyes, 'tenting' skin	
Discomfort	Skin abrasions and injuries	Treatments for external parasites
	External parasites	
	Excessive self-grooming	
Digestive disorders	Body posture	Treatments per 100 calves/year
	Diarrhoea	
Respiratory disorders	Coughing	Treatments per 100 calves/year
	Dyspnoea (laboured respiration)	
Dirtiness	Dirt (flanks, limbs, perineum)	
Behaviour	General demeanour (active–apathetic)	
	Oral behaviours (cross sucking, tongue rolling)	
	Social grooming	
	Play	

and records but gives special attention to health and welfare problems known to affect young calves. Thus under the general heading of nutrition and hydration our observations are directed towards gathering evidence as to abnormalities of early rumen development (e.g. bloat, impacted rumen) or dehydration (hollow eyes, skin that feels tight and 'tents' when pinched). Physical injuries in young calves reared on adequate bedding are rare, but external parasites are common. The most conspicuous problem is ringworm. However, lice infestation appears to be much more distressing to the calves. They may show bare patches especially around the shoulders and tail head. They will also spend so much time grooming themselves that no assessor should fail to recognise the problem during a visit lasting more than a few minutes.

Diarrhoea ('scours') resulting from enteric infections is probably the major cause of death and disease in young calves. Death usually results from toxaemia and dehydration. Many cases of diarrhoea in calves (as in babies) can be controlled by electrolyte replacement therapy, given as a drink or by stomach tube. Thus many calves can be kept alive at little cost. However, calves that have had an enteric infection are three times more likely to succumb to subsequent infections, typically pneumonia. The calf that has had severe bouts of both scours and pneumonia in early life may fail to thrive thereafter and become a 'poor doer' throughout its life.

Healthy young calves, unlike tired old dairy cows, have both the energy and inclination to indulge in social behaviour and play. This is a clear indication of positive welfare. On the other hand, the display of compulsive oral stereotypies such as bar sucking and tongue rolling is likely to indicate either a lack of oral satisfaction or abdominal discomfort, or both. Such stereotypies are very common in veal calves on all-liquid diets and relatively common in calves intensively reared for beef on diets high in starchy cereals but low in roughage.

6.3 The welfare of beef cattle and sheep

The production of meat from herds of suckler beef cattle and flocks of sheep at pasture or on open range is clearly the most 'natural' of all forms of animal production since the animals are, for the most part, kept in a habitat similar to that of wild ruminants and left to fend for themselves. If freedom to express natural behaviour were the whole of welfare then such systems would be beyond reproach. However, it is not. Table 6.6 compares the Five Freedoms for beef cows and their calves with sheep and lambs on open range. Clearly one of the biggest problems for grazing animals in extensive conditions is obtaining adequate nutrition, especially during the winter in the high latitudes and the dry season in the tropics. This is not simply a matter of finding something to eat. During the non-growing season dormant grasses are very fibrous and indigestible. Thus animals with a high nutrient requirement for pregnancy, lactation or growth may be faced by the same

Table 6.6 A comparison of the main potential welfare issues for beef cattle and sheep on open range.

Category	Beef cattle	Sheep
Hunger and thirst	Cows: poor body condition ++	Ewes: poor body condition +++
	Calves: dehydration +	Lambs: starvation +++
Discomfort	Cows: mud, cold, wet, filth ++	Ewes: thermal discomfort rare
	Calves: hypothermia +	Lambs: hypothermia +++
	External parasites +	External parasites ++
Disease	Cows: few endemic problems	Infectious foot rot +++
	Calves: diarrhoea	Ketosis +
Injury	Lameness +	Ewes: lameness +++
		Lambs: predators ++
Mutilations	Castration	Castration
	Dehorning	Tail docking
Behaviour	Sunbathing +	Sunbathing
		Lambs at play
Fear and stress	Little problem	Predation (perception and fact)

dilemma as the dairy cow: a metabolic hunger for nutrients but a rumen full of undigested roughage. The consequence of prolonged undernutrition is, of course, loss of body condition. This is clearly visible in a cow, but may pass unnoticed in sheep in full winter fleece. Body condition should properly be assessed by palpation of lumbar muscle and fat in both species. Sheep are also more susceptible than beef cattle to metabolic complications of undernutrition during pregnancy. Ketosis or 'twin lamb disease' is a potentially fatal metabolic disease of sheep carrying two or more lambs partly because the developing lambs have a high demand for glucose and partly because they occupy so much space within the abdomen that they leave too little room for the rumen. Pregnancy ketosis is seldom a problem for beef cows, partly because they normally carry only one calf and partly because larger animals have more space for the rumen relative to their nutrient requirements.

The newborn lamb is very susceptible to hypothermia. The lamb that becomes chilled within the first hours of life becomes too weak to suck, so the effects of hypothermia become exacerbated by hypoglycaemia. The progressively moribund lamb then becomes an easy target for predators such as foxes or crows, which may peck out its eyes while it is still alive. When outdoor lambing coincides with chilling conditions of cold, wind, rain or snow on extensive sheep ranges in (e.g.) Scotland or New Zealand, losses of newborn lambs may exceed 20%. The natural environment of the hillsides can be a pretty terrible place for the young lamb and its mother. It is an undeniable fact that the practice of housing ewes at lambing – a significant intensification of the sheep industry – has greatly improved both the productivity and the welfare of sheep. The newborn calf is considerably more cold tolerant than the lamb and, on commercial beef ranches, at much less risk from predators. Death (and even discomfort) from hypothermia is rare.

Calves and lambs, like all young animals, are particularly vulnerable to enteric infections leading to diarrhoea and dehydration and the risk is much greater when the animals are housed in close proximity to one another. Sheep are housed at lambing primarily to minimise losses of lambs from hypothermia, hypoglycaemia, predation and obstetric problems. However, whenever possible they are turned out to pasture within about two days of birth to minimise the risks of enteric infection. Lambs that are turned out of doors in late winter (e.g. February in the UK) when they are more than 48 hours old, have bonded to their mothers and begun to drink with vigour will frequently be stressed by cold but seldom killed by it. It is becoming increasingly common practice to house beef cattle during the UK winter, not primarily for their comfort and security but because the feet of these heavy animals can destroy ('poach') the pastures during the wet winter months. Adult cattle kept out over a wet UK winter are more likely to suffer discomfort than sheep because they are more likely to be found standing up to their oxters in mud. For the same reason, beef cows that are brought indoors to calve during the winter are unlikely to be turned out to grass within 48 hours of the birth of their calves. Thus sucklers' calves kept indoors are at greater risk of enteric disease than lambs turned out to grass. The standard treatment for artificially reared, bucket-fed calves with diarrhoea is to restrict milk intake and substitute electrolytes. This is less easy to accomplish when the dehydrated and thirsty calf continues to drink milk from its mother. Enteric disease is therefore a high welfare risk for beef calves kept in confinement during early life.

Problems of disease and injury, fear and stress are rare for adult beef cows on open range. Indeed these animals are remarkably easy to manage since they can do most things for themselves and, in my opinion, have a pretty good life. Adult sheep, on the other hand, are faced with a range of potential sources of pain, fear and stress. They are at real risk of injury from marauding dogs. Moreover their perception of the risk of injury and death from predation must be more intense than that of beef cows. Lameness due to foot rot is *the* major welfare problem for sheep grazing in the UK. The expression 'foot rot' oversimplifies a complex series of conditions. Feet softened by wet conditions and allowed to overgrow through lack of regular foot trimming are highly susceptible to physical injury. However, many cases of simple foot damage become infected, the severity of the infection varying according to the organisms involved. Infectious foot rot can be controlled by appropriate attention to hygiene and pasture management. In regions of Australia it has been eliminated through rigorous culling and control of sheep movements. Sheep farmers have a responsibility to recognise lameness as a very painful condition and a duty to do what they can to keep the problem under control. A sheep farmer that fails to fulfil this duty may be deemed guilty of causing unnecessary suffering through neglect. However, no sheep farmer, with the best will in the world, can hope to keep on top of lameness all the time. It is an inescapable fact that sheep require an enormous amount of care and then still discover unfore-seen ways of getting themselves killed or maimed. When, as a naïve young grad-uate, I went to work in western Canada, I landed a contract to write monthly articles for an agriculture journal. I recall with particular embarrassment one article entitled 'Why so few sheep?'. In it I argued on perfectly sound scientific grounds that sheep were physiologically extremely well adapted to the grasses and the dry, cold climate of the prairies and castigated the local ranchers for their unthinking devotion to beef cattle. What I totally failed to realise was that when your spread extends to several square miles you need animals that can look after themselves. Beef cows find it easy. Sheep do not.

Table 6.6 identifies mutilations as a welfare problem for both calves and lambs. Most calves will be dehorned and most lambs tail-docked 'for their own good', to reduce the risk of injury in cattle and infestation with maggots following 'blow fly strike' in lambs. The reasons given for castration are to prevent indiscriminate breeding, to control temperament and to encourage early fattening. Recent research on pain in association with castration in lambs reveals that it is severely painful at any age (i.e. castration in the first days of life does not reduce the suf-fering). Moreover the animal will show some degree of pain for several days after the procedure. The least painful method is probably to administer a local anal-gesic, crush the spermatic cords with a bloodless castrator (Burdizzo) and then apply a rubber ring to the crushed area (Moloney *et al.*, 1993, 1995). This requires three separate steps: first the analgesic, then a wait for it to take effect, then the double procedure of crushing followed by application of the rubber ring. There is at present no regulation compelling sheep farmers to conform with this recom-mended procedure. The most attractive option for all parties is to avoid castration altogether. However, as with beak trimming in poultry, the more extensive the system the greater the need for mutilations. Calves and lambs that are taken off grass and put in feedlots to grow and fatten quickly can achieve optimal carcass quality without the need for castration. Moreover they can be confined in single-sex groups to avoid the problems of indiscriminate breeding. Most calves intended for finishing at grass at about two years of age will need to be castrated both to ensure good carcass quality and because entire bulls can become dangerous at this age. Lambs that cannot be finished at grass by about three months of age will need to be castrated both to ensure carcass quality and to prevent indiscriminate breed-ing. The aim should be to avoid castration whenever possible, but often, especially in the most extensive and 'natural' husbandry systems, it becomes an unavoidable mutilation; a source of suffering that is necessary but should be minimised by all reasonable means.

6.3.1 Intensive fattening

In most systems of lamb production and beef production from suckler cows, most of the animals spend most of their time at pasture or on open range. In the UK, the aim is to produce lambs that can achieve slaughter weight at three to four months of age on a diet simply consisting of grass and mother's milk. A minority of lambs that cannot be finished at grass will be confined in yards and fed a mixture of conserved forage and cereals for the last few weeks of their lives. The environment experienced by these lambs is broadly similar to that experienced by their mothers when housed over winter. Lambs finished in yards are prone to the diseases of confinement, especially pneumonia. This is a potential welfare problem and one that can be difficult to control, especially if animals are held at a high stocking density. In consequence, space allowances for finishing lambs are usually relatively generous in comparison with broilers or growing pigs. I have no major concerns regarding the welfare of lambs being finished for slaughter in confinement systems.

When considering the intensive fattening of beef cattle, it is necessary to distinguish between beef produced from artificially reared calves born to dairy cows and that produced from calves reared by their mothers in a suckler herd. The most extreme (and most criticised) example of the latter is presented by the typical North American feedlot holding tens of thousands of calves taken off range, confined in close proximity, injected with anabolic steroids and fed high starch diets to maximise food energy intake and liveweight gain. Using, as always, the Five Freedoms as a check-list, one can identify the following problems as inherent to the system:

- disorders of digestion and metabolism caused by diets that compromise normal rumen digestion;
- thermal stress (especially heat stress) in animals closely confined with inadequate access to shelter;
- severe respiratory diseases, e.g. the 'Shipping Fever' complex;
- chronic lameness and pain from laminitis consequent to ruminal acidosis;
- stress resulting from social competition and aggressive sexual behaviour.

Most finishing diets for feedlot cattle are formulated to contain a high ratio of starch to roughage and this predisposes the animals to ruminal acidosis. This can be a direct source of discomfort. It can also lead to serious secondary complications including liver abscesses and, especially, laminitis, probably the most painful of all forms of foot lameness. Finishing cattle confined in many feedlots may be exposed to severe heat stress when compelled to stand in direct sunlight. It is, however, possible to construct sunshades. Where these are present, finishing cattle can be more comfortable in feedlots than on open range. Behavioural problems can also be severe. Oral stereotypies such as tongue rolling and bar sucking can be attributed to a lack of oral satisfaction and/or abdominal discomfort on the high starch diets. Many male calves destined for feedlots are not castrated. When pubertal male and female cattle are confined in large numbers (albeit separately) there is a great deal of sexually inspired riding and jostling and this can create a lot of disturbance. Even castrated steers are not spared the unwelcome attention of others if they have been 'treated' with synthetic sex hormones since these will increase libido.

There is much to criticise in large-scale feedlot production; less, I would argue, than in broiler production and not enough, I believe, to warrant new legislation*. However, there are enough undesirables within this system designed for the mass production of a commodity, whether viewed through the eyes of the cattle, the consumer or the producer, to encourage those who seek to do things better. Beef is a luxury item and it makes sense to market it as a product that has been produced with care. One of the few positive outcomes of the generally disastrous, self-inflicted epidemic of BSE in the British cattle herd has been the public demand for assurance as to farm of origin and method of production. Some proud and perceptive producers have seen this as an opportunity to market added-value beef, sold as organic, or finished at grass and advertised often with an invitation to visit the farm and see the animals at pasture.

Any criticism of the intensive feedlot system for finishing calves born to suckler cows on open range (e.g. in the USA) needs to be qualified by the observation that the period on feedlot typically lasts only about 150 days. Thus the calves spend most of their lives on open range and the cows spend all of their lives on open range. Even the perennial criticism (e.g. Rifkin, 1993) that North American feedlot cattle are not eating grass, as nature intended, but cereals and soya that could be used to feed the poor (if they could afford them), does not withstand close inspection. By far the greatest input of food to the overall system comes from the open range. Only about 35% of energy and 16% of protein comes from food that could be used directly for human consumption (Webster, 1993).

The intensive production of beef in Britain and the EU presents similar welfare problems to those I have outlined for the US feedlots, if not on such a large scale. However, in Britain and northern Europe, more than 50% of beef comes from artificially reared beef × dairy calves housed, in many cases, from birth to slaughter without ever having enjoyed life at pasture. Northern European diets tend to contain more (wet) forage and less corn starch than USA diets, so are less likely to cause problems associated with ruminal acidosis. However, wet diets (and higher rainfall) encourage producers to house their animals in very close confinement on concrete slats. The slats are physically uncomfortable and predispose to limb abrasions and injuries. High stocking densities are necessary to ensure that dung is trodden through the slats but impose a greater restriction on normal behaviour than on a typical feedlot.

Beef production in Britain does, however, provide a good example of the constructive use of subsidy as an incentive both to improved welfare and more sustainable agriculture. The simple decision to pay the beef subsidy in two tranches at 10 and 20 months of age rather than as a single payment made at 10 months

---

* The use of hormones as growth promoters for beef cattle is currently prohibited within the EU.

provided a strong financial incentive to production systems wherein beef cattle are finished for slaughter after two summers at pasture. It is easy, and usually valid, to criticise agricultural subsidies on the grounds that they confer unfair advantages to local producers at the expense of the consumer and international trade. However, a subsidy that promotes improved animal welfare, respects the desire of the consumer for improved standards of production and redirects farmers towards more environmentally friendly production systems shows respect for all parties identified within the ethical matrix.

6.3.2 Rendering unto Caesars: the Belgian Blue problem

Finally in this section on beef cattle I wish to raise the 'Belgian Blue' issue; namely the production of beef from animals selectively bred to a produce a degree of muscle hypertrophy that makes elective Caesarian section a 'necessary breeding technique'. The problem is not unique to the Belgian Blue (BWB), but in certain strains of this breed 90% of calves are routinely and repeatedly delivered in this fashion (Uysteprust *et al.*, 2002). It is, by definition, an unnatural procedure and unlikely to feature in any campaign to persuade people to eat more beef. Nevertheless it is legal and public opinion has not stopped it so far. It is, however, valid to pose two questions: (1) Does the practice (both the breeding and the consequences) impair the welfare of the cow and/or her calf, i.e. their capacity to sustain fitness and avoid suffering? (2) Should the practice be banned? In current British law, this focuses on the question: 'Does it deliberately invoke a significant degree of unnecessary suffering?' (Protection of Animals Act 1911).

It may be argued that the breeding of BWB cattle with extreme muscle hypertrophy is no worse than many production methods known to have systematically imposed an element of suffering, e.g. the creation of 'leg weakness' in broilers. However, 'leg weakness' was not imposed deliberately but was an unforeseen consequence of selecting and feeding birds for rapid weight gain. This is not intended as an excuse for the broiler breeders. Nonetheless, all parties (breeders and welfarists) agree in principle that leg weakness should be avoided if possible, whether or not they seek to put this principle into practice. The traditional and broadly accepted husbandry practice of castration deliberately imposes a degree of suffering, at least in part for the benefit of the producer, not the animal. Moreover, one of the main objectives of castration, namely control of carcass composition, is similar to that involved in breeding for double-muscling. In both cases this imposes the responsibility to acknowledge that suffering occurs and to seek to minimise it. There is, however, one big difference. As I have indicated earlier, cattle, pig and sheep producers increasingly tend to avoid castration whenever possible, which implies that when it *is* done it is considered a necessary mutilation. Although elective Caesarian section (ECS) may be defined as a 'necessary breeding technique' for double-muscled cows, the breeding of double-muscled cows is not *necessary* to beef production, whether defined by quality or efficiency. Thus, by definition, any significant imposition of suffering may be deemed unnecessary and so constitute cruelty under the 1911 Protection of Animals Act.

It is important therefore to consider carefully what elements of the overall practice of breeding and rearing BWB and other double-muscled cattle may impair welfare, or, at worst, induce a significant degree of distress. These elements include: (1) effects of ECS on the breeding cow; (2) effects of ECS on the calf; and (3) effects of double-muscling on the capacity of the cattle to sustain fitness and avoid suffering. The most obvious question is could ECS, when performed repeatedly, impose significantly greater pain and distress than natural delivery? Clearly ECS, when performed under effective anaesthesia, should reduce pain at the time of delivery. The critical question is 'What proportion of cows experience chronic pain as a consequence of post-operative complications such as intra-abdominal adhesions?' I am unaware of any attempts to answer this question, but it is amenable to study, e.g. by seeking evidence of chronic hyperalgesia as described by Whay *et al.* (1998). Double-muscled calves delivered by ECS are at high risk of respiratory disorders, in particular the acute respiratory distress syndrome. This is linked to anatomical abnormalities of the pharynx and upper respiratory tract.

Most of the economic benefits of the double-muscled BWB phenotype are conferred in the F1 hybrid generation following BWB insemination of a 'normal' cow. A calf born from a Holstein cow inseminated by a BWB bull presents no special problems of dystocia and does produce a beef carcass that fetches a high price. Nevertheless, the fact remains that the whole system depends absolutely on the deliberate production of a population of fundamentally unfit breeding animals, lethal recessives in fact, which can only be sustained by ECS. This abuses the first criterion for welfare, namely sustained fitness. We cannot yet prove that these abnormalities, and the consequent need for ECS, induce a significant degree of suffering in the cow (e.g. through chronic pain accompanied by hyperalgesia), but it is a question that should be addressed with some urgency.

This cautious, scientific analysis as to whether the production of double-muscled animals by repeated ECS does or does not constitute unnecessary suffering is necessary for legal purposes, but it is also a vivid illustration of the limitations of the scientific argument in matters of animal welfare. Anyone with a sense of respect for *telos*, the intrinsic 'cowness' of the cow, should reject this practice out of hand. Even producers motivated only by self-interest should recognise that consumers are increasingly turning against meat produced by methods they find repellent. Whereas much of the most extreme criticism of animal production methods may be unfair, I cannot believe that any farmers could truly claim to be proud of breeding animals that they know are unfit to survive without recourse to elective surgery. It is in nobody's interests to try to defend the indefensible.

Animals for Food: Handling, Transport and Slaughter

Though I walk through the valley of the shadow of death, I shall fear no evil.

Psalm 23

The aims of good husbandry on the farm are to ensure that the animals are well-fed, comfortable, fit and feeling good. This may, or may not involve direct contact. For artificially reared calves, the arrival of the stock-keeper with a bucket of milk will be the high spot of the day. For ewes with their lambs at spring grass, the presence of a shepherd with his dog will be viewed with some anxiety as a potential threat. For beef cows with their calves on open range, the arrival of a cowboy on a horse is likely to be treated with supreme indifference provided they do not get too close. In all three examples the welfare of the animals is satisfactory because they have access to the provisions they require, they are in a comfortable, familiar environment and, so long as they are undisturbed, they are unlikely to feel threatened. I have already argued that farm animals only need a stock-keeper in proportion to the extent that the stock-keeper has removed the resources they need to look after themselves. The responsibility of the stock-keeper is to do what is necessary to ensure that the animals are fit and feeling good. In some circumstances, it may be appropriate (and fun) for keepers to establish a stable, unthreatening, even friendly, social interaction with their stock, but it would be a foolish conceit to imagine that we should somehow strive to make our farm animals love us.

Inevitably, however, the time will come when the life of even the most comfortable and serene farm animal will be shattered and it will be exposed to a range of novel and physically unpleasant experiences: during handling on the farm for routine veterinary procedures, in transport and, finally, at the point of slaughter. It may seem outrageous to many to preface this chapter with a quotation from Psalm 23, but it is strictly accurate. All who choose to eat meat give tacit approval to those who carry out a number of unpleasant procedures on our animals, more often than not for our own benefit, and to those who kill them. The

157

aim of the good shepherd, charged with these duties, should be to see that the animals fear no evil in anticipation of the procedures and do not suffer when they occur.

This is easier said than done. Since most farm animals are accustomed to an almost unchanging daily routine, any sudden departure from that routine is likely to constitute a threat. During transport and at the place of slaughter some degree of discomfort and fear is inevitable. Two recent pieces of UK legislation, the Welfare of Animals (Transport) Order 1997 and the Welfare of Animals (Slaughter or Killing) Regulations 1995, have been drafted in response to European Council Regulations that, in effect, accept that these processes are inherently stressful and seek to minimise suffering. This legislation, which I shall discuss later in more detail, does represent a significant achievement in improving welfare standards. Another 'consolation' for animals transported to the point of slaughter is that stresses incurred at this time may also damage or otherwise reduce the quality of the meat, either as a direct result of injury or owing to changes in the chemical composition of the meat resulting from fear, dehydration or exhaustion. Thus the imposition of substantial pre-slaughter stresses carries both legal and commercial penalties.

Without apology, but at risk of becoming boring, I offer once again the Five Freedoms as a framework for preliminary but comprehensive analysis of potential welfare problems associated with the handling, transport and slaughter of farm animals. Table 7.1 presents a rather hard-hearted list of the most severe welfare problems likely to be experienced by poultry, pigs, cattle and sheep in transport and at the point of slaughter. There are circumstances where each of these species may suffer from abuse of each or all of the Five Freedoms. In practice, however, the different species are faced by different risks for reasons that are determined to a large extent by the special features of their anatomy and physiology.

Table 7.1 Application of the Five Freedoms test to identify the most severe welfare problems for farm animals in transport and at the point of slaughter.

	Poultry	Pigs	Cattle	Sheep
Hunger and thirst			Thirst (esp. calves)	Thirst
Physical discomfort	Overcrowding +++ Shackling ++	Overcrowding +	Exhaustion	Exhaustion
Thermal discomfort	Heat stress ++ Cold stress +	Heat stress +++	Tolerable	Rarely intolerable
Pain and injury Infection	Layers: fractures Day-old chicks?		Bruising (cows) + Young calves ++	Smothering
Inhibition of behaviour	Severe	Moderate	Severe	Severe
Fear and stress	High risk	Motion sickness Fighting	Fighting	Neophobia

Poultry and pigs have a very limited ability to regulate heat loss by evaporation. Most obviously, they do not sweat. Cattle and sheep are much better equipped in this regard; cattle through a combination of sweating and thermal panting (rapid ventilation of the heat exchangers in the nose), sheep almost entirely through thermal panting. Thus poultry and pigs are at much greater risk of death from heat stress during transportation in hot lorries than cattle and sheep. This is now well understood by the trade. Abattoir records in the 1980s revealed that the number of pigs discovered dead on arrival (in the UK) increased progressively as ambient temperature rose above 8°C! At the time of that report most pigs were carried in lorries without refrigeration or adequate ventilation and most were heat stressed most of the time. Our own work (Webster *et al.*, 1993) has shown that there are practically no circumstances where 5000 chickens crammed into a conventional, naturally ventilated lorry and producing 60 kW of body heat will not experience either heat stress while the vehicle is stationary or cold stress while it is in motion. Livestock hauliers now clearly recognise the need to prevent intolerable thermal stress for poultry and pigs whether through vehicle design, air conditioning, control of stocking density, travelling at night, or simply ensuring that the journeys are as short as possible.

Cattle and sheep, on the other hand, are much better able to dissipate heat by evaporation so are unlikely to be killed by acute heat stress. In consequence therefore they can be subjected to much longer journeys. The longer the journey, the greater the risk of suffering from physical exhaustion, dehydration and thirst. Although it is normal to withhold food from animals for some hours prior to transport primarily to reduce faeces production and so ensure that they arrive reasonably clean at the point of slaughter, hunger is unlikely to be a major welfare problem. This assumes, of course, that animals are transported according to EU regulations that set maximum journey times and times between feeding and watering. Dehydration and thirst are problems for cattle and sheep transported long distances, and these problems are exacerbated in hot conditions that compel them to increase heat and water loss by evaporation.

The problem of exhaustion is greatest for mature cattle. Young calves and pigs can and do lie down in relative comfort and security while vehicles are in motion. Cows and beef cattle at slaughter weight remain standing for the very good reason that any animal that lies down puts itself at severe risk of injury from the other animals. At the recommended stocking density of about 0.25–0.3 m²/animal, sheep are able to lie down without incurring injury, but many hauliers prefer to minimise the risk of injury or smothering by seeking to keep them on their feet (Knowles, 1998).

Most injuries are incurred during handling or as a result of fighting. Laying hens with osteoporosis are highly susceptible to bone fractures when pulled out of cages in the battery house or clamped onto shackles in the abattoir. Pigs and beef cattle (especially bulls) are at risk of injury from fighting in lairage, especially when unfamiliar animals are mixed. Carcasses from cull cows may show a high incidence of bruising as a result of beating by drovers (McNally & Warriss, 1996). This is a particularly distressing statistic. Old dairy cows should require the least goading to drive them through passages since this is something they do every day. They may be beaten simply because they are slow. They may be slow because it hurts to walk. The drover may not be restrained from inflicting bruises because the carcass is worth little or, as a consequence of the UK BSE epidemic, nothing.

All farm animals will experience some degree of fear when taken from their familiar surroundings, driven or manhandled into lorries, transported, driven again into lairage, mixed with unfamiliar, equally stressed individuals, then finally marshalled to the point of slaughter. A great deal can be done to reduce the intensity of stress through intelligent design of the facilities and a sympathetic approach to human–animal contact. However, it is important at this preliminary stage to recognise that the most ubiquitous source of fear and stress associated with handling and transport is neophobia, or fear of the unknown. Beef cattle, sheep or deer that have spent almost their entire lives out of contact with humans and on open range are most likely to be stressed by the procedures involved in getting them onto a lorry or to the killing point in the abattoir. Once on the lorry, pigs that have spent most of their lives crammed together on concrete may, on the other hand, find the environment all too (depressingly) familiar. There is good evidence to show that the stress responses to transport in sheep and cattle (e.g. plasma cortisol concentration) are normally greatest on the first journey. Good hauliers also report that sheep and cattle become progressively easier to load with successive journeys. This implies that transportation, done properly, is not aversive *per se*. The greatest fear is the fear of the unknown. It follows therefore that the prime aim of any strategy for handling animals whether on the farm, in transit or at the point of slaughter should be to minimise the element of unfamiliarity. The environment, as perceived by the animals, should be one in which they remain in the close, reassuring presence of familiar members of their flock or herd and are, as far as possible, unaware of what else is going on around them. Temple Grandin (1993) has been *the* good shepherd in regard to this approach and I shall make reference to her work as I come to discuss specifics.

7.1 Stockmanship and the human–animal bond

The good shepherd is one who cares for his/her sheep. Nevertheless, we should never forget that farm animals need us in proportion to the extent to which we have taken away the resources they need to look after themselves. For much of the time it may be that the best thing we can do for most farm animals is simply to keep out of the way and let them get on with their lives. However, there are times when close contact is inevitable. Moreover, even when we are acting in the best interests of the animal (e.g. treating a painful condition such as mastitis or lameness) these are the times that it is most likely to be stressed. We have a responsibility therefore to ensure that the animals' perception of their contact with us is, at least, non-aversive and, wherever possible, a feel-good experience. It is self-evident that a good stock-keeper should be someone who *likes* animals, recognises them as sentient creatures capable of suffering and pleasure, and respects their intrinsic value. However, it is not sufficient simply to like animals. We must understand them as well. In particular we need to understand how they regard us and interpret our actions.

The first key to successful interactions with other animals is to identify specific cues that they can interpret as signs of aggression, invitation or simply as useful information. For example, sheep will interpret the appearance of a man with a sack of grain as an invitation to feed but a man with a dog as a potential threat. However, if both man and dog position themselves at the right distance and the right angle, the sheep will receive a clear signal, either to stand still or to move out of harm's way. The potential threat presented by man and dog will be interpreted not as a source of stress but simply as information. The response of the sheep may be compared with that of the zebra at the waterhole who sees the lion, maintains a sensible distance but sees no need to panic. It may equally be compared with the human pedestrian who recognises the motor car as a potentially lethal weapon but one that can be avoided by staying on the pavement. The skill in driving animals, especially herding animals unused to human contact, is to convey the information necessary to move them quietly in the desired direction. Once man or dog encroaches within the flight distance of the driven animal, fear kicks in and their behaviour becomes less predictable. For animals that are more accustomed to associate human contact with good experiences, such as the arrival of food, then it frequently makes more sense to direct animals by invitation, e.g. rattling a bucket.

The generic question 'How do domesticated farm animals such as cows and pigs regard humans?' is more difficult to answer. Most species of wild animal such as the badger and fox are born with an innate fear of humans in the same way that humans and other primates are born with an innate fear of snakes (Figure 3.3). Innate fear is genetically inherited, but like all acquired traits it has evolved over time as an adaptation to environments where man has been the great predator. Thus species such as penguins which have not evolved in dangerous proximity to man appear not to have evolved this innate fear. In species that have 'allowed themselves' to be domesticated, the genetic basis of the human–animal bond, as perceived by the animal, has evolved towards one that ranges from wary acceptance in the sheep to unqualified adoration in the dog. However, for all animals, their innate perception of man on a scale ranging from predatory killer to loving provider can be greatly modified by experience, in particular, experience in the early, formative stages of life. Thus the lamb reared by its mother on the hillside will flee at the appearance of man. The orphan lamb reared on a bottle in the kitchen is likely to be quite fearless (and a thorough nuisance).

Boivin *et al.* (2003) have perceptively reviewed evidence relating to the question 'How do farm animals regard us and why?' A key common feature of the species that have allowed themselves to be domesticated for food production is that they are social animals accustomed to life in stable, hierarchic groups. The stability of the hierarchy is reinforced by more or less subtle anatomical, physiological and behavioural signals designed to establish the place of each individual within the pecking order and reward individual behaviour that is consistent with the lasting fitness and general peace of mind of the group*. It would be interesting, though not perhaps very important, to know the extent to which animals such as dogs, horses and cows may regard humans as conspecifics, i.e. one of their social circle, differing only in terms of the threat we may present or the rewards we may bring. There are quite good reasons for concluding that dogs reared from weaning at eight weeks as part of a human family act as if they were one of the family and are sensitive to emotional interactions not only between dog and human but also between human and human. The Monty Roberts (1998) approach to taming (rather than breaking in) horses is based on presenting stimuli permitting responses that are part of the horse's repertoire for normal social interactions within the herd. The young horse to be gentled into submission to its rider is committed to a social interaction with an apparently dominant individual within an environment where evasion is not an easy option. The horse gives out submissive signals to reduce the risk of the encounter turning dangerous and is rewarded for this submission by discovery that the experience turns out to be much less stressful than it feared. It does not really matter whether or not the horse views its trainer (and, by association, other humans) as a dominant member of its own herd. What *is* important is that both horse and trainer are able to understand both the signals and responses. They are communicating in the same language. Moreover the actions of both parties are appropriate to the environment and designed to avoid stress.

The vocabulary of signals necessary for communication with most farm animals is small relative to that which may be achieved between human and dog, human and horse. (Cow dressage has a very limited appeal!) Most close interactions between keepers and their stock occur when it is necessary to move animals, usually into a place of confinement and restraint. Nevertheless the principles remain the same. The signals should be informative, unambiguous and in a language that the animal can understand. The design of the facilities should be such that the natural response of the animal allows it to move without anxiety through the facilities in a manner that is consistent with the aims of the drover.

---

* This does not imply that the individual is acting for the benefit of the group; simply that the actions it performs out of self-interest are consistent with the overall fitness of the group.

7.2 Humane handling

Cattle

The principles and practice of cattle handling on the farm, in transit and especially at the abattoir have been described in detail by Grandin (1993, 1998). It is only necessary here to identify the key features since these can be applied in almost all circumstances. These are:

- Cattle are gregarious animals who feel secure within the herd and are stressed by isolation.
- Cattle are particularly responsive to visual signals. Any unusual image will be perceived as a potential threat. On the other hand, what they can't see won't be a worry.
- When presented with a potential threat (e.g. a drover) outside their flight distance, cattle will stand and face the threat. When the drover approaches within their flight distance they will move away, if they can. If the threat is too close, and they cannot make an appropriate response, they may panic.

Figure 7.1 (from Grandin, 1998) illustrates the application of these principles to the movement of cattle through a curved race. Ideally the race should have solid sides with the outer side high enough that the cattle can see nothing beyond it. The inner circumference should be high enough that the cattle cannot escape but low enough to permit them to see the drover. A group of cattle (preferably not a

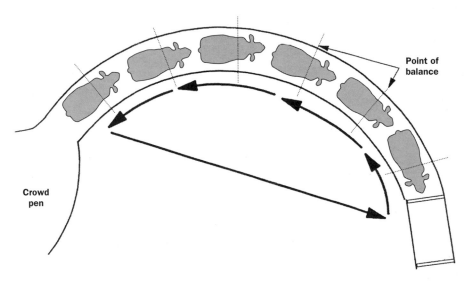

Figure 7.1 Handler movement patterns for inducing cattle to move forward in a curved race. Animals will move forward when the handler crosses the point of balance for each animal (from Grandin, 1998).

mixed group from different sources) may be crowded into the race through a forcing pen. Within the forcing pen, the animals are in the reassuring presence of each other and at this stage can move forward without fear since this is what the rest of the herd is doing. When in the race, they may be halted by procedures taking place at the far end. To move them on, the drover approaches the first animal to within its flight distance and forward of the shoulder. He then moves towards the tail of the beast. As he passes the point of balance at the shoulder, the animal moves forwards. He continues to walk down the line, against the flow of the cattle and they should move forward in orderly fashion. When he gets to the start of the race, he takes a direct line back to the front that is outside the flight distance of the animals so does not stimulate any action. The solid partition between cattle and drover is reassuring to both parties. The cattle view it as a barrier against aggression from the drover. All that is required is a few steps forward and the potential threat disappears. The purpose of the drover is not to drive but simply to provide information leading to appropriate action. It follows that the cattle will be more relaxed if drovers remain out of sight until action is required.

Although cattle can be moved through well-designed handling facilities with minimal distress, it is highly probable that when they get to the end they will be restrained and something more or less unpleasant will occur. The cheapest and easiest way to keep cattle moving forwards to the point where they can be restrained, whether for administration of medicines, foot trimming, or stunning and slaughter, is to make the end of the race appear like a point of escape; a well-lit area that appears to offer an unrestricted view of freedom. An alternative, high-tech, high-welfare option pioneered by Grandin for use in abattoirs is to walk the cattle onto a conveyor belt that rises between their legs and carries them forward on their briskets to the stunning point. It is a convenient (if somewhat disturbing) feature of the behaviour of ruminants in general and cattle in particular that when their capacity for escape is cut off, either through effective restraint, or because their feet no longer touch the ground, they very seldom struggle.

7.2.1 Pigs

Most of the essentials for the humane handling of pigs are similar to those for cattle. There are, however, some special features of the perception and behaviour of the typical farmed pig that can be exploited to minimise distress for all:

- Many pigs can learn to derive pleasure from human contact. This may be linked only to feeding time, but it can be strongly reinforced by gentling behaviour, such as back scratching. On a fully mechanised factory farm, however, there may be little opportunity for such reassuring contact.
- Pigs tend to be more inquisitive than fearful so are unlikely to become alarmed unless seriously disturbed. It should seldom be necessary to force pigs along well-designed passageways.

- Pigs have relatively poor vision. They can be guided using a portable 'pig board'. They are unlikely to spot visual threats at a distance. However, apparently minor and harmless novelties within their line of sight, such as a step, a drain or even a ray of sunlight, may halt them in their tracks.
- Pigs sent for slaughter are unaccustomed to walking any distance on the level and find it extremely difficult to ascend steep ramps. Loading and unloading facilities on the farm and at the abattoir should be designed with this in mind.

7.2.2 Sheep

The most obviously efficient way to drive and corral sheep at pasture is with a well-trained sheepdog. The dog operates according to a strict set of rules. The sheep face the dog and watch it carefully as it approaches. As the flight distance is reached the sheep turn and move away in a direction defined by the dog's angle of approach. The dog comes close enough to communicate the need to move but not so close as to cause alarm. An alternative method for small-holders and hobby farmers without a trained dog is to employ a 'bellwether'. This is typically an adult castrate male that has been hand-reared from birth and who has been maintained as a pet thanks to a regular supply of titbits during shepherding visits. The bell-wether should also by virtue of age and status be a dominant member of the flock. The theory has it that when the owner calls, the wether comes and the rest of the flock, hearing the bell, follow. I have seen it work in practice (even without a bell), but it does require a special sort of shepherd.

Because the signals mutually conveyed between dog and sheep are direct and unambiguous, it should, in theory, be possible to construct a robot sheepdog. Indeed, robots have been devised to control the movement of ducks in strictly confined circumstances and under strictly experimental conditions. Such experiments provide valuable information as to the rules of engagement. However, leaving aside the technical difficulties of devising a robot that can sprint over the hills of Scotland, I believe it could never capture perhaps the most essential feature for success, namely the eye of the sheepdog. This is not a fanciful belief. When the stationary sheepdog holds his flock in stationary suspense, he is just on the limit of their flight distance. His eyes are on them and their eyes are on his eyes. Sheep have an innate fear of dogs. They recognise a potentially severe threat and know that they may need to act on the instant to prevent this threat from becoming a reality. Before the robot can replace the dog we shall need to breed a race of sheep with an innate fear of robots.

The design of handling facilities for sheep once coralled presents no special problems. As always, the animals should be kept together whenever possible and moved in such a way that what they see ahead of them is either another sheep or the prospect of escape. The size and relatively harmless behaviour of sheep makes it possible for the shepherd to carry out many routine husbandry procedures (e.g. drenching, injections) on animals confined together in the race. Sheep are especially stressed by isolation and this should be avoided wherever possible. More-

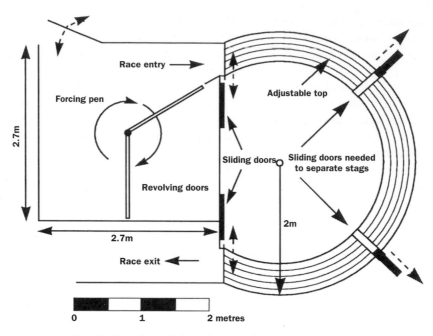

Figure 7.2 Handling facilities for red deer (from Matthews, 1993)

over, when they make a dash for freedom they dash together. When handling sheep *en masse* it pays to break them into relatively small groups to avoid large pile-ups, e.g. at the end of a long raceway.

7.2.3 Deer

All species of farmed deer (e.g. red deer, fallow deer, wapiti or elk) present special handling problems. They are innately more 'flighty' than traditionally domesticated cattle. Even in farmed deer reared in paddocks and regularly exposed to human contact, average flight distance is seldom less than 30 m, which means that they are likely to be alarmed by handling procedures such as those used for cattle and illustrated in Figure 7.1. Deer that are bottle reared from birth can be tamed and may come to a call. In theory this could be used to lead a herd between feeds or into a corral on the 'bellwether' principle. In practice, however, it is less likely to work for deer than sheep. The lead animal needs to be recognised as dominant by the herd. A dominant, adult male deer, whether castrate or entire, with or without antlers, that has lost its innate fear of humans is potentially dangerous.

The other big problem with deer is that they are much more athletic than cattle or sheep. When alarmed and in a position that offers a prospect of escape they can clear a 2-m-high wall or fence from a standing jump. They can also injure themselves, other deer or human operators in the attempt. It is therefore absolutely essential to design handling facilities that minimise both the risk of causing alarm and the risk of causing injury. Matthews (1993) has produced some very practical recommendations based on his experience of handling deer in New Zealand. In the example illustrated in Figure 7.2, the deer are herded as a mob into a forcing pen but handled in a semicircular race that is 600 mm wide and can be partitioned off with sliding doors to keep animals apart. The walls of the race and holding pen are 2.3 m high. They are solid to a height of 1 m to minimise risk of damage to limbs. However, above 1 m the outer walls are perforated with 10 mm diameter holes. It is not entirely clear why this works. Possibly the deer are attracted by an overall impression of light and space but unable to distinguish what is on the other side, or, indeed, it does constitute a barrier until too late. The race has an adjustable ceiling to prevent and dissuade animals from trying to jump out.

Matthews (1993) reports that his deer appear less inclined to develop aversion to repeated handling procedures on the farm than cattle or sheep. He suggests that deer may be less able to make the association between what goes on during the marshalling process and what happens at the end of the line (worming, injections, removal of antlers). An alternative explanation is that deer are more frightened by the marshalling process itself than by the procedure for which they were marshalled, which may be brief and presage release. In either event this habituation to handling is more likely to reflect the quality of the handling facilities rather than some innate 'tameability' of the deer. This provides a specific illustration of an important generalisation. If it becomes progressively easier to handle deer, cattle or sheep on repeat visits to a particular handling system, then the system is, by definition, non-aversive; or, at least, less aversive than the approaching drover. As the animals overcome their initial neophobia, they become progressively less stressed. If, on the other hand, a handling system becomes progressively more aversive, then it is, by definition, a bad system. The observation that deer are more likely to habituate to handling systems than sheep or cattle suggests that most handling systems for deer are well designed for the simple reason that they have to be. Many sheep and cattle may be handled badly simply because we can get away with it.

7.2.4 Poultry

For most poultry (broilers, ducks, turkeys, laying hens) handling means just that: picking them up and carrying them from one place of confinement to another. This may be done by hand or by machine. Potential stresses include fear, pain, injury and sudden death. The risks of incurring these stresses are determined by the difficulty in catching the birds, the physicality of the handling procedures, the emotional response of the birds to the procedures and their susceptibility to injury and shock (Table 7.2). Obviously the ideal way to carry any bird is individually cradled in your arms, comfortable but secure. This is not going to happen during the depopulation of commercial units containing many thousands of birds. The

Table 7.2 Potential welfare problems during poultry handling classified according to handling procedure and bird response.

Stress	Handling procedures	Bird responses
Fear	Rough handling	Wing flapping
	Insecure surfaces	Tonic immobility
	Innate fear of humans	
Pain and injury	Removal from cages (hens)	Fractures (osteoporosis)
	Catching and crating	Pain: hens with fractures; broilers
	Shackling	with leg weakness; heavy turkeys
Sudden death	Depopulating colony systems (hens)	Crushing, asphyxiation
	Depopulating colony systems (broilers)	Cardiac failure (ascites)

Welfare Codes for Poultry recognise that birds will be caught by the legs and carried in groups. They require that birds should be carried by both legs, primarily to reduce pain and injury. Broilers that are reluctant to stand for more than a few seconds at a time because of pain in their legs are likely to experience some pain when carried by two legs and greater pain when carried by one. Turkeys are less likely to experience leg pain during the rearing period, but these heavy birds almost certainly experience some pain when suspended upside down. Any pain and fear experienced while suspended upside down by the feet applies, of course, both during depopulation from the poultry house and when shackled onto the conveyor prior to killing at the abattoir (Gentle & Tilston, 2000).

Welfare problems during handling obviously increase in proportion to the difficulty in catching the birds. This has been recognised in caged layers, who are especially prone to fractures as a result of chronic osteoporosis. The problem of recent bone fractures in spent hens from battery houses has been greatly reduced through 'improvements' to the design of the conventional cage (particularly the front) to reduce the risk of injury during depopulation. However, the life of the conventional cage is drawing painfully to its close, in Europe at least. Alternatives to the conventional cage may be much more acceptable to hen and customer, nearly all the time, but they do present greater problems at depopulation. Hens plucked from enriched cages are more likely to be injured by the furniture. Large colonies of hens in barns with perches and nest boxes are inherently more difficult to catch. If they are seriously alarmed mass panic may occur, leading to deaths from crushing and asphyxia. The humane and efficient depopulation of large hen houses is a job that calls for a great deal of calm skill, acquired through training and reinforced through compassion. It follows that any farmer who markets high-welfare free-range or barn eggs must be able to demonstrate that this concern for welfare extends to the time of catching, transport and slaughter. The 'least worst' solution for the spent layers would be to experience unforeseen sudden death (e.g. by gassing) while still in the familiar environment of the hen house. Since the cash value of spent hens is so low, this could become an economically acceptable feature of high-welfare egg production. However, it almost certainly will not. The success of free-range eggs is based on the image of hens in green fields. It is hardly likely to be improved by images of the gas chamber.

Broiler houses are relatively easy to depopulate by hand for the simple reason that the birds are practically immobile. Catching turkeys is more difficult. However, a producer of value-added, free-range or barn-fed turkeys could certainly improve overall welfare by incorporating a well-designed non-handling system that allowed the birds to walk, without disturbance, onto appropriately designed vehicles, or even right to the point of slaughter. Several types of mechanical 'poultry harvester' have been developed, designed to gather broiler chickens from the floor of the rearing unit and deliver them to the point where they can be loaded into crates for transportation to the abattoir. There is convincing evidence to show that the birds experience less distress (Duncan *et al.*, 1986) and are less likely to be injured (Knierem & Gocke, 2003) when harvested by machine than by hand. It would also appear that they are less alarmed by the appearance of the harvester, and the actions of the harvester, than by the appearance and actions of a team of human catchers. This is probably because the machine moves them gently but firmly in a normal standing position. It may also reflect the fact that poultry have an innate fear of man but not of large machines.

7.3 Welfare in transport: what is wrong with going on a journey?

Current UK legislation, the Welfare of Animals (Transport) Order (WOTA) (1997), is based on the premise that transportation *per se* is a stressful experience for farm animals. The stress can be reduced by attention to vehicle design and by sensitive operation, but it is nevertheless a stress and one that should be kept within tolerable limits by imposing maximum journey lengths. Thus there are relatively few regulations on farmers driving their own animals less than 50 km. Anyone prepared to travel regularly on the London Underground has formally acknowledged that journeys in severe conditions of confinement and thermal stress are tolerable provided that the duration of the journey is short. Vehicles transporting cattle, sheep, goats, pigs and horses on journeys longer than eight hours must meet specified design standards. Regulations concerning journeys whose total time exceeds eight hours are summarised in Table 7.3. The first key point is that maximum journey length is defined by what is deemed tolerable to the animal, rather than by the distance between its point of departure and final destination. Thus, for pigs, maximum journey length is 24 hours provided that they have continuous access to liquid. If the animals are not at their destination by this time then they must be unloaded from the vehicle, fed and watered and rested for 24 hours* at an approved lairage whose accommodation is comparable to that which they have

---

* This limit may be relaxed in the event of unavoidable delays or for good reasons stated in the route plan.

Table 7.3 Regulations concerning journey times for animals transported within the European Union.

Species	First leg	Rest period	Second leg
Unweaned calves, lambs, kids, foals, piglets	Maximum 9 hours	At least 1 hour	Maximum 9 hours
Cattle, sheep, goats	Maximum 14 hours	At least 1 hour	Maximum 14 hours
Pigs	Maximum 24 hours with continuous access to liquid		
Horses*	Maximum 24 hours with liquid and food if necessary		

*Excluding registered horses

previously experienced on farm. The thinking behind the regulation for (weaned) pigs is that a period of 24 hours without food is acceptable, so long as water is available. A rest period when the vehicle is stationary is unnecessary since pigs can lie down to rest in relative comfort and security while the vehicle is in motion. Cattle, sheep and goats (except unweaned animals) may remain on the vehicle without food and water for a maximum of 29 hours, but the vehicle must stop to permit them to rest for one hour after the first fourteen. The logic of this is that these animals stand up while in transit, mainly through fear of being trodden on or crushed if they lie down, and it is more tiring to stand while a vehicle is in motion than when it is at rest. The maximum journey time for unweaned animals is set at 19 hours. One of the limitations of regulations is that they tell you what to do but do not explain why. In this case, the maximum journey length presumably reflects the reasonable belief that unweaned animals should be fed and watered more often. If this is so, then prolonging the journey with a compulsory one-hour rest period may do more harm than good, since all these young animals should be able to lie down to rest while the vehicle is in motion.

All this begs the question 'Why should travel necessarily be assumed to be a stress?' I have already pointed out that sheep and cattle, properly handled, become progressively easier to load onto vehicles with successive journeys. Once they have overcome their neophobia, transportation *per se* does not appear to be aversive. In *Eden I* (Webster, 1994), I wrote: 'Many of the stresses imposed on animals in transit are caused by the design of the vehicle and the handling of the animals and these stresses are not likely to be removed by legislation simply designed to restrict journey length. If the environmental conditions within a livestock vehicle could be made as good as those experienced by the animals on the farm then they could, in theory, stay on the lorry indefinitely. It follows from these arguments that legislation to improve the welfare of animals in transit should be based on the "carrot and stick" approach; proscriptive legislation to restrict journey lengths in conventional vehicles but special provisions for hauliers who can, by improved vehicles designs and journey plans, provide an environment that will allow animals to travel for extended periods without suffering'. The 1997 WOTA regulations go some way to meeting these objectives and, as I write, I anticipate further actions based on the European Council Regulation (EC) No. 411/98 which will set standards for road vehicles used for carriage of livestock on journeys exceeding eight hours. This formally recognises the principle that maximum journey times only become relevant when the vehicle is unsatisfactory (or badly driven). Journey times for horses (Table 7.3) do not apply to 'registered horses' transported to stud farms or between race tracks for the simple reason that we already take great care to ensure that these valuable animals travel in comfort and safety.

I am pleased to acknowledge that since I wrote *Eden I* there have been substantial advances in legislation designed to improve minimum standards for the welfare of animals in transport. Moreover this legislation encourages the intelligent application of both carrot and stick. It seeks to improve animal welfare both through proscription and incentives. In this regard, I believe that it can act as a model for future regulations that seek to achieve a fair deal for animals, producers, consumers and the living environment within the much broader context of good husbandry on the farm. It is, of course, inherently much easier to draft legislation to improve welfare standards on a single journey than it is to legislate to improve the lifetime welfare of all animals on all farms. However, the principles are the same. Legislation by proscription, use of the stick, can seldom do more than prohibit the most serious, systematic abuses of animal welfare. Legislation by incentive (here the incentive to design better vehicles) is inherently more flexible since it is designed to assist individual good shepherds to use their own initiative to improve the welfare of their own animals in the special circumstances of their own enterprises.

7.4 Welfare at the place of slaughter

The welfare of an animal at the point of slaughter must be defined by the totality of its experience from the moment it arrives at the place of slaughter until death puts an end to its capacity to suffer. For many years, legislation concerning welfare at slaughter concentrated on the principle that animals should 'be slaughtered instantaneously or rendered instantaneously insensible to pain until death supervenes'. This was admirable up to a point, but it did not take into account stresses of fear, pain, discomfort and exhaustion that animals may experience in the minutes or hours preceding the actual killing process.

The Welfare of Animals (Slaughter or Killing) Regulations 1995 is broader in scope. It now defines stunning as 'any process which causes immediate loss of consciousness which lasts until death'. The distinction between 'immediate' and

Table 7.4 Stunning and slaughter methods used internationally in abattoirs (from Gregory, 1998b).

	Cattle	Pigs	Sheep	Poultry
Stunning methods				
Electrical stunning	*	***	***	***
Captive bolt	***	*	*	
Percussion bolt	*			
Gaseous stunning		**		*
Killing methods				
Sticking after stunning	***	***	***	**
Cardiac arrest with bleeding			*	**
Sticking without stunning†	*	*	*	*

† Includes religious slaughter
*** main method, ** common method, * uncommon method

'instantaneous' is something of a semantic nicety. More constructive is regulation 4, which states: 'No person engaged in the movement, lairaging, restraint, stunning, slaughter or killing of animals shall:

(a)   cause any avoidable excitement, pain or suffering to any animal, or
(b)   permit any animal to sustain any avoidable excitement, pain or suffering'.

This command is clear and comprehensive. The question now becomes how to put it into practice.

7.4.1 Stunning and killing methods

The regulation that 'animals should be slaughtered instantaneously or rendered instantaneously insensible to pain until death supervenes' is so worded to permit slaughter by methods that kill the animal either 'instantaneously' or in a two-stage process whereby the animal is first stunned into unconsciousness, then 'stuck' so that it bleeds to death. Table 7.4 (from Gregory, 1998b) summarises the stunning and slaughter methods used in abattoirs around the world. Stunning followed by sticking is the most common practice for the slaughter of cattle, sheep and pigs. The purpose of the stun is twofold: (1) to render the animal unconscious so that it can be stuck and bled without causing pain or distress and (2) to immobilise the animal so that it can be bled conveniently and safely by the operator. Sticking also has a twofold purpose: (1) to kill the animal before it regains consciousness and (2) to remove blood from the carcass.

Bleeding out, to remove the blood from the carcass, is essential to meat quality. However, contrary to traditional thinking, a heart that continues to beat is not essential to the process of bleeding out (i.e. the amount of blood retained in the carcass). Thus there is no good reason why the stunning process should not also stop the heart. The most common stunning method for cattle is the captive bolt gun. When the cartridge is fired by pulling the trigger, or by contact with the head of the animal, the bolt shoots forward, penetrates the skull and stuns the animal by concussion. The percussion bolt gun has a blunt, mushroom-shaped end that does not penetrate the skull. Both methods, properly applied, meet the objective of rendering the animal instantaneously unconscious and insensitive to pain. The placement of the gun is critical. However, with both methods, the stunning is achieved by diffuse concussion, rather than penetration of the brain by the captive bolt. The percussion stunner has, in some Islamic communities, been pronounced acceptable for Halal slaughter. However, it is more difficult to use. It has a greater recoil and many operators consider that it carries a higher risk of failing to achieve an effective stun with the first shot.

Electrical stunning

Electrical stunning is the most common method for sheep and pigs. A current is passed through the brain with the intention of causing epilepsy. The current required to induce epilepsy is 1.25 amps for pigs and 1.0 amps for sheep and calves. Gregory (1998b) has described in detail the physiological consequences of successful and unsuccessful electrical stunning. In brief, an effective stun induces an epileptic seizure (almost immediately). It is assumed, not least, by analogy with humans, that a *grand mal* epileptic seizure causes unconsciousness. However, sheep and pigs start to regain consciousness within 40 seconds of the termination of the stun. By law therefore 'death should supervene', i.e. the animal should be shackled, stuck and bled out to the point of being brain dead within 40 seconds of terminating the stun. This is something which is almost impossible to guarantee even in the most well-run abattoir. The time from sticking to brain death, as assessed from loss of visually evoked responses (VER), depends on what blood vessels are cut and the size of the wound. If both carotid arteries of the sheep are cut in the neck, time to loss of VER is about 14 seconds. The time to loss of VER in pigs following a chest stick that severs the brachiocephalic trunk supplying both carotid arteries is about 18 seconds. If the stick fails to cut off the carotid arterial supply to the brain, time to loss of VER can be as long as five minutes. In cattle, the vertebral arteries carry a significant amount of blood to the brain. Time to loss of VER following section of both carotid arteries can approach two minutes. Electrical stunning, which is commonly used for young calves, should only be considered an acceptable practice if it is accompanied by chest sticking that effectively severs the brachiocephalic trunk.

The most effective way of cutting off all blood supply to the brain is to stop the heart. In most large poultry plants the birds are shackled at the legs and suspended upside down. Their heads pass through a water bath containing a submerged plate electrode. The voltage of this electrode is regulated to ensure that an electrical current of 120 mA passes through the bird from the head to the leg shackles, which act as the earth. This shock, when delivered with a 50 Hz alternating current, both stuns the brain and stops the heart thereby guaranteeing an 'instant' kill. The automated killing and bleeding process in poultry plants is entirely humane so long as it works. If the current is inadequate (and this is not a constant function of the applied voltage) stunning may be ineffective. It is moreover possible for a bird to lift its head and escape both the stunning and bleeding procedures, with consequences that are almost too awful to contemplate. It is essential to ensure competent human supervision of the whole process with remedial action as necessary.

The effectiveness of the stun and kill process for poultry depends on the fact that the current passes through both the brain and heart. A 'head-to-back' electrical stunner has been developed for use in sheep to induce epilepsy and cardiac arrest in sheep. However, placement of the electrodes is critical. A 'neck-to-back' stun can cause cardiac arrest without inducing unconsciousness. We can take it as read from human experience that this is extremely painful.

The simple, single-shock head-to-back stunner is not suitable for pigs. The current necessary to stun and kill is liable to induce (unconscious) muscular convulsions sufficient to cause broken bones. However, in abattoirs designed so that pigs are carried forward to the stunning point on conveyors so that they are unable to make any large movements, it is possible to apply a high-frequency (1500 Hz) shock to the head to induce epilepsy and a low-frequency (50 Hz) shock to the heart to induce cardiac arrest. This method carries the double benefits of reducing stress before stunning and eliminating the possibility of recovery between stunning and sticking.

Gaseous stunning

It is common practice to stun pigs with carbon dioxide (CO_2). This practice accounts for about half the pigs slaughtered in the UK and nearly all pigs in Scandinavia. The pigs are lowered into a pit containing carbon dioxide (CO_2) which is heavier than air at a concentration that must exceed 70% by volume in air. At this concentration CO_2 induces unconsciousness within 30–40 seconds, and with sufficient exposure time, the pigs will not recover before they have been stuck and bled to death. However, any animal (including humans) exposed to a high concentration of carbon dioxide experiences severe respiratory distress, expressed as a sense of breathlessness and asphyxia (or choking). Pigs display profound aversion to even the briefest exposure to CO_2. Thus the method does not meet the criterion of rendering the animals unconscious and insensible without avoidable pain and distress. It is, however, necessary to consider the method within the broader context of seeking to minimise any avoidable excitement, pain or suffering. Thus a period of some distress lasting perhaps 20 seconds could be viewed as acceptable if it were an integral part of an overall process that minimised excitement, fear and distress at the place of slaughter. The two methods commonly used to lower pigs into the pit are the gondola, fitted into a carousel and the dip-lift. In the gondola method pigs are advanced in single file and pushed or goaded onto the gondola, which then descends into the pit. The stress involved in goading pigs that are reluctant to move onto the gondola may be exacerbated because they sense a high concentration of CO_2 at the entrance to the pit. In the dip-lift process pigs move forwards in groups of about five animals onto the perforated floor of a lift, which then descends into the pit. Up to the point of exposure to CO_2 this is arguably the most humane process for handling pigs in the abattoir.

One of the most memorable experiments from the physiology course I took as a veterinary student over 45 years ago was to re-breathe air from a large 'Douglas' bag, thereby progressively reducing the concentration of oxygen and increasing the concentration of CO_2. In this simple experiment our breathing became more and more laboured until it became impossible to continue. We then introduced a chemical absorbent for CO_2 and repeated the experiment. This had to be performed under supervision. The subject was given a pencil and paper and instructed to keep writing. The supervisor terminated the experiment when the subject's writing became incoherent. The point of this demonstration was that it is the increasing concentration of CO_2 that induces heavy breathing (to the point of distress). The body shows little if any response to simple anoxia and can pass into unconsciousness without being aware of anything amiss – a well-documented fate of pilots and climbers at high altitudes. This being so, it is possible to induce irreversible unconsciousness in animals by exposing them to air without oxygen. In practice, this involves filling the stunning pit with the inert, heavier-than-air gas argon. Mohan Raj (1996) pioneered the experimental development of this technique. Poultry and pigs exposed to a gas containing a mixture of argon and atmospheric nitrogen so that oxygen concentration is 2% behave as I did as an undergraduate. They display no aversion and will pass into unconsciousness within about 45 seconds. Thus the killing method itself creates no excitement, pain or distress.

The 2001 Amendment to the UK Welfare of Animals (Slaughter or Killing) Regulations 1995 permits the slaughter of poultry using gas mixtures that contain: (1) argon, nitrogen or other inert gases, or any mixture of these gases in atmospheric air with a maximum of 2% oxygen by volume; or (2) any mixture of argon, nitrogen or other inert gases with atmospheric air and carbon dioxide, provided that the carbon dioxide concentration does not exceed 30% by volume and the oxygen concentration does not exceed 2% by volume. A gas mixture containing no CO_2 is guaranteed non-aversive and will induce unconsciousness within 45 seconds. The second method is based on the observation of Raj (1996) that turkeys displayed no significant aversion to gas mixtures containing no more than 30% CO_2. Carbon dioxide is cheaper than argon. Moreover the time to unconsciousness in this gas mixture was about 20 seconds, i.e. half that when argon is used alone. It has therefore been judged an acceptable killing method. The further attraction of gaseous stunning in poultry is that the process is carried out with the birds still in the crates in which they were transported to the abattoir. Thus the excitement, pain and distress caused by hauling the birds out of the crates and suspending them upside down on shackles has all been avoided. Birds will display convulsive limb movements after gaseous stunning, but in the confines of the handling crates they cannot move far enough to cause damage to their own carcasses or those of the other birds. There can be no doubt that the development of gaseous stunning for poultry has been one of the great leaps forward towards improved welfare. In accordance with my principle that any high-welfare production method for farm animals should imply high welfare from birth to death, I would suggest that any scheme for marketing high-welfare poultry meat or eggs should incorporate an insistence on gaseous stunning.

At present the stunning of pigs by anoxia using argon without CO_2 is not licensed for use in the UK. It has been shown experimentally to be as effective and non-aversive a method for inducing irreversible unconsciousness in pigs as in poultry. The incidence of carcass damage associated with post-stunning convulsions is unproven, but preliminary indications are that it does not differ in this respect from CO_2 stunning. However, pigs are aversive to gas mixtures containing argon and 30% CO_2 which makes this cheaper option unacceptable. The capital costs of converting a plant currently killing pigs by asphyxiation with CO_2 to one that used argon to insensibly induce unconsciousness through anoxia are very small. However, the running costs are higher, which puts the plant at a disadvantage unless the increased cost is met by retailing value-added high-welfare pork or it is enforced by law. It is valid to argue that gaseous stunning using CO_2 is in breach of existing law since it neither renders animals immediately insensible to pain nor avoids excitement and distress. A new EC regulation that permitted gaseous stunning only by anoxia rather than asphyxia would be fair to all plants using gaseous stunning and, following the McInerney argument illustrated by Table 1.5, should have a negligible impact on consumer prices. I offer this suggestion to those powerful lobby groups such as Compassion in World Farming who share my view that it is better to limp towards Eden step by step than to retire to the comfort of the moral high ground and cry havoc on all who live in the real world.

7.4.2 Killing fish

In Chapters 2 and 3 I presented both physiological and behavioural evidence to indicate that fish have some capacity to experience both pain and distress. It follows that we have a responsibility to prevent avoidable excitement, pain and distress in the fish we kill and eat for food (or simply catch and kill or maim to pass the time). The fish that is hauled out of the water and simply left to die may not experience pain, but, since its mechanism for respiratory exchange has been interrupted, it will experience both anoxia and hypercapnia (increased CO_2 concentration in blood). We should, by analogy, assume that the latter is a source of distress and we know that this may last for several minutes before the fish passes into irreversible unconsciousness. In this regard therefore the problem is worse for the fish killed by asphyxiation than for the pig stunned by carbon dioxide.

Gregory's (1998b) book *Animal Welfare and Meat Science* contains an excellent chapter that considers all aspects of catching, handling, stunning and killing fish, crustaceans and squid, whether from the open sea or on fish farms. I recommend this to those with a particular interest in fish welfare. The only point I feel the need to make in the context of this section is that the principles governing the welfare of fish at slaughter are exactly the same as those that appertain to mammals and birds. Stunning by a blow to the head, whether practised by the individual fisherman or the commercial salmon slaughterer wielding a 'priest', can achieve an instantaneous and irreversible stun. Stunning fish (e.g. salmon) in CO_2-enriched water can speed the time to death relative to asphyxiation in air. However, it induces violent activity in the fish, which may be assumed to be consistent with excitement and distress, and which certainly can lead to carcass damage. This is not an acceptable method. Electrical stunning is potentially humane but has not yet proved effective in practice since the muscular contractions it can induce in a powerful fish such as the salmon can break their backs. There is a real need for research into more humane, practical slaughter methods for fish and other sources of sea food.

7.5 Religious slaughter

The regulations for religious slaughter set down by the sons of Abraham, whether the Jewish sons of Sarah or the Ishmaelite sons of Hagar, were a worthy expression of best practice according to the standards of the time. The regulation that the animal should be unblemished at the time of killing was a powerful aid to improved meat hygiene, and the regulation that the animal be killed by a holy person after saying a prayer conveyed a sense of moral respect for the animal being sacrificed. The regulation that the killing should be achieved by an uninterrupted cut from a sharp knife (that severed both jugular veins, carotid arteries, oesophagus and trachea) sought to minimise distress by requiring that the killing should be done quickly and by a competent individual using effective equipment. The principles relating to meat hygiene and moral respect are as true today as they ever were. However, the argument that the method seeks to minimise distress is only sustainable by extreme sophistry either in the interpretation of what constitutes suffering or, indeed, in terms of what constitutes current UK law.

It was possible to argue that religious slaughter by the Halal and Shekita (or Shochetim) methods was consistent with the regulation that animals should be rendered 'instantaneously insensible to pain until death supervenes' on the basis that a rapid cut with an uninterrupted movement does not produce an immediate sensation of pain. However, as I argued in *Eden I*, the source of distress for the animal is not pain but the conscious awareness that it is choking to death in its own blood. The Welfare of Animals (Slaughter or Killing) Regulations 1995 'do not permit any animal to sustain any avoidable excitement, pain or suffering'. Religious slaughter clearly contravenes regulation 4 since, so far as the animals are concerned, excitement and distress associated with death by exsanguination and preparation of the animal for the rapid, uninterrupted cut can both be avoided. The Act therefore includes a Schedule 12 which overrides this regulation provided that animals are reasonably humanely restrained (not upside down at least) and their throats slit using 'rapid, uninterrupted movements' according to provisions set down for Shochetim slaughter.

This regulation that allows respect for traditional religious practice to override a concern for animal welfare that imposes a strict code of practice on the rest of the community has not met with the approval of the Farm Animal Welfare Council. They include the following recommendations in their 2003 *Report on the Welfare of Farm Animals at Slaughter or Killing: Part 1 Red Meat Animals*:

> 201. *Council considers that slaughter without stunning is unacceptable and that the Government should repeal the current exemption.*

> 203. *Until the current exemption which permits slaughter without pre-stunning is repealed, Council recommends that any animal not stunned before slaughter should receive an immediate post-cut stun.*

These recommendations concerning the slaughter of red meat animals exclude, by definition, poultry, and, of course, pigs. It is valid to point out that when poultry are slaughtered using a head-to-shackle electric shock, or sheep are slaughtered using a head-to-back stunner, this induces immediate stunning and cardiac arrest, leading rapidly to death. All that follows is the bleeding-out process. Thus both paragraphs 201 and 203 contain an element of ambiguity that could delight lawyers and hold up progress. Paragraph 203 is a nonsense; worthy but a nonsense nevertheless. Its clear aim is to reduce the time between cutting the throat and loss of consciousness, especially in cattle, where the vertebral arteries make a significant contribution to the blood supply to the brain. For those whose set of values calls for slaughter methods that prevent avoidable suffering, this clearly does not go far enough. Those whose set of values (the phrase 'mind set' is not appropriate) requires the animal to be unblemished at the time of slaughter are asked to eat meat from an animal that has, while still alive, been subjected to a procedure that would have been intolerable had it occurred seconds earlier.

Many Muslim communities have shown a flexible approach to reconciling the conflicting ethical demands of animal welfare and religious practice. In the UK this dates back to the 1930s when the Imam of Woking issued an edict permitting methods of pre-slaughter stunning that did not appear to cause physical damage (or marked distress) to the animal. Today many communities will accept as Halal meat from sheep and poultry bled out following electrical stunning. It is probable that gaseous stunning of poultry may also be acceptable if it is caused by anoxia, using inert gases, rather than asphyxia using CO_2, in which case Halal slaughter of poultry could become the most humane of methods.

Faced by those who are unprepared to consider any changes to traditional practice, then I offer my backing to the recommendation given in paragraph 201 of the 2003 FAWC *Report on the Welfare of Animals at Slaughter or Killing*. The Government should repeal the current exemption for religious slaughter contained in Schedule 12 of the 1995 Act, since this states quite simply that the regulation that 'no person engaged in the movement, lairaging, restraint, stunning, slaughter or killing of animals shall cause any avoidable excitement, pain or suffering to any animal' shall not apply. In accordance with my principle that the best legislation is that which achieves practical improvements through intelligent use of both carrot and stick, may I suggest the following: *whenever it is deemed necessary, on the grounds of established religious practice, to consume meat from animals that have been killed by exsanguination without experiencing prior physical damage, then the animals should be rendered unconscious and insensitive to pain by methods that do not cause physical damage.*

There is an element of sophistry in this too, but that is inherent to the debate. Electrical stunning is already acceptable to the leaders of many devout Muslim communities, although there are those who could argue that this technique damages the animals. Narcosis induced by anoxia with inert gases is reversible if stopped in time with no lasting signs of damage. Other 'harmless' techniques for inducing narcosis, such as the use of electromagnetic induction, are at the experimental stage. Those who commend the practice of religious slaughter should reinterpret their commitment to the principles of hygiene, humanity and respect in terms of the best current understanding as to how these admirable principles should be achieved.

Animals for Science and Biotechnology

Absolute morality is the regulation of conduct in such a way that pain shall not be inflicted.

Herbert Spencer (1820–1903)

The use of animals by man for 'scientific procedures' is a catch-all phrase that covers three quite distinct pursuits:

(1)   the use of live animals in experiments designed to advance the understanding and practice of science and medicine;
(2)   the use of live animals for toxicology testing of commercial products in order to meet health and safety regulations;
(3)   the biotechnological manipulation of animals in order to increase their value to man.

When I discussed these issues in *Eden I*, I gave little attention to the moral arguments for and against experiments on animals, and concentrated largely on their impact on animal welfare. This was justified on the basis that an animal's perception of its own welfare is uncomplicated by any concept of the purpose or justification of what is being done to it, an ethos robustly expressed as 'spare parts or sausages; it's all the same to the pig'. This argument still applies. However, it is impossible to ignore the fact that no animal welfare concern attracts more attention than the morality of using animals for purposes defined by the state as 'scientific procedures' and by the passionate as vivisection. In the UK the principles (and the law) that define these practices have been reformed by the Animals (Scientific Procedures) Act (ASPA) (1986), which replaced the 1876 Cruelty to Animals Act. In brief, these reforms may be summarised as follows:

- ASPA (1986) recognises that there is more to cruelty than pain alone and expands the definition to include 'pain, suffering, distress or lasting harm'.
- Every application to carry out a scientific procedure with protected animals must be subjected to a cost/benefit analysis to determine whether the cost (or

180

harm) to the animal can be justified in terms of its potential benefit to humans or other animals.

- The Act recognises that the welfare of the animals used in scientific procedures is defined not only by the procedures to which they are subjected but also by the quality of their living environment, so pays particular attention to day-to-day care.

- The final authority for animal welfare is given to the individual responsible for day-to-day care, reinforced by a named veterinary surgeon. These individuals can override the wishes of the Project Licence holder (the individual with the authority to carry out the specified procedures) if, in their view, any individual animal may be experiencing an unacceptable degree of suffering or harm.

The publication and implementation of ASPA (1986) represented an impressive step forward in the general direction of Eden for laboratory animals. However, it was only one step and it did little to lessen the debate, not least because recent advances in biotechnology made possible by our understanding of the biological basis of genetic inheritance have greatly increased the scope of what can be done to animals. The most obvious expression of this new biology is the genetic modification of animals using laboratory techniques, either to knock out specific genes or splice in new ones. The armoury of biotechnology is such that almost anything *can* be done to manipulate the structure, function and behaviour of animals. The debate therefore centres on what *should* be done; and this is a matter of morality rather than science.

8.1 Experiments with animals: the moral debate

My aim throughout this book is to achieve practical improvements in our understanding of animals and our treatment of animals. I have chosen to leave discussion of the moral status of animals to others such as Singer (1990) and Ryder (1998). Nevertheless it is self-evident that any procedure calculated to cause pain, suffering, distress or lasting harm to any sentient animal presents inescapable moral problems that do not have a clear-cut solution not least because moral conclusions are (rightly) based not on facts but on values. My review of the debate will be based almost entirely on reports published in the UK and dealing with the law and practice as governed by ASPA (1986). These include reports from bodies as disparate as the Banner Commission (Banner, 1995), the Royal Society (2001), Compassion in World Farming (2002), GeneWatch UK (2002), the House of Lords Select Committee (2002) and the Animal Procedures Committee (2003). I am aware that these are all UK publications, but I believe they cover the full spectrum of the argument, wherever it may occur and whoever may be involved. These disparate reports honestly review the same evidence and honestly use that evidence to derive different value judgements. This is perhaps the most telling illustration of the principle outlined in Chapter 1, namely that values are truly a matter of conscience. They may be informed by science, but they cannot be defined by science because they operate in a different dimension.

In recognition of the importance of ethics, the UK government has established the Animal Procedures Committee (APC) to advise the Home Secretary on matters concerning ASPA (1986), i.e. procedures 'which may have the effect of causing a protected animal pain, suffering, distress or lasting harm'. In particular it is required to review the elements of the ethical cost/benefit equation that weighs 'the likely adverse effects on the animals concerned against the benefit likely to accrue'. Use of the expression 'cost/benefit' in this context is, of course, philosophically suspect since the costs are borne entirely by the animals and the benefits accrue entirely to ourselves. The APC is currently chaired by Michael Banner, a philosopher and theologian. Its members include (by my categorisation) five scientists that use animals, six animal welfarists, three philosophers, two lawyers and two cross-benchers.

The ethical basis of existing law regarding the use of animals for scientific procedures has been stated succinctly by the House of Lords Select Committee (2002) in the following terms:

It is morally acceptable for human beings to use other animals but it is morally wrong to cause them unnecessary or avoidable suffering.

Implicit in this statement is an acceptance of the cost/benefit principle. The APC and the House of Lords Select Committee (2002) have suggested that the expression 'cost/benefit' should be replaced by 'harm/benefit', to be consistent with the 1986 Act which specifies that the severity of harm likely to be experienced by the animals must always be minimised and can only be justified in terms of the benefits likely to accrue to society (or other animals). However defined, this appears to be a strictly utilitarian argument that justifies costs to individual laboratory animals so long as they can be shown to be for the greater good. In fact, the argument never goes quite that far. Banner (1995) made a clear distinction between a minority of things 'which should not be done in any circumstances' and those things that may be done if they can be justified on the basis of a cost/benefit analysis. It follows that what *is* done is that which has been justified on this utilitarian basis.

A utilitarian analysis that seeks to measure the cost to animals of things we do to them when we use them for our own ends may quantify overall suffering in the following terms:

Total suffering = Individual suffering (Intensity × Duration)
    × Number of animals involved

On this basis, the total cost we expect laboratory animals to pay to meet our expectations of good health and high-quality medicine is miniscule in relation to the potential cost we are prepared to accept from the animals that we farm for food. To quote from *Eden I*: 'The average human omnivore who maintains a good appetite to the age of 70 years manages to consume 550 poultry, 36 pigs, 36 sheep and 8 oxen. At present we use approximately 3 million animals per year for scientific procedures. This corresponds to less than four laboratory animals per human lifetime'.

It is, however, necessary to make one clear distinction between animals farmed for food and those used for scientific procedures as defined by ASPA (1986). All experiments licensed under the terms of ASPA are, by definition, calculated to cause some degree of 'pain, suffering, distress or lasting harm'. Millions of farm animals may experience some degree of suffering, but if we exclude aberrations such as repeat elective Caesarians for the double-muscled Belgian Blue, there is no deliberate intent to cause suffering or lasting harm to a living animal. The premise that 'it is morally wrong [deliberately] to cause unacceptable or avoidable suffering' to animals used in science and technology implies, by definition, that some suffering is 'acceptable and unavoidable within limits that must be defined on the basis of moral, rather than scientific argument'. The moral question is therefore: 'Where should the lines be drawn?'

The call to abolish vivisection is based on Herbert Spencer's premise that 'absolute morality is the regulation of conduct in such a way that pain shall not be inflicted', i.e. that it is absolutely unacceptable deliberately to cause any pain or suffering to any animal. In practice, advocates of this absolute position tend to reinforce their argument with 'evidence' selected to demonstrate that the benefit to humans is trivial or non-existent. I cannot believe that those who claim that experiments with animals have contributed almost nothing to medical knowledge or the sum of human happiness have actually given any thought to what they are saying. Indeed, if one is equipped with the absolute moral belief that humans should not deliberately inflict any suffering on any other sentient animal then the cost/benefit argument has no meaning. It simply becomes propaganda designed to persuade others to support their absolute position.

It is, of course, futile to seek a debate with those who will brook no argument. However, it is valid to point out to those who will listen that the set of 'things which should not be done in any circumstances' can never be as absolute as it sounds. Even the most extreme example of this set, 'Thou shalt not kill', is applied with a fair degree of moral relativism. In practice, it is usually interpreted as 'Thou shalt not kill, unless directed by a higher authority to kill specified individuals, or unspecified individuals from specified nations deemed by that higher authority to present a threat serious enough to warrant action with extreme prejudice'. Thus expressed, the law reads to me like a copper-bottomed cost/benefit argument. Individuals may conscientiously object to taking part in the killing but have no power in law to override government policy. Those who oppose vivisection in any form are entitled to categorise themselves as in the same position as the honourable minority who conscientiously object to participating in war. When they claim that 'vivisection' (i.e. scientific procedures with animals) is unacceptable 'in any circumstances', what they are actually saying is 'in any circumstances acceptable to me and those who share my views'. Those who advocate this minority opinion may only justify it as a moral absolute if they are prepared to reject medication or any other benefit derived from experiments with animals (and *all* licensed medicines are tested on animals*) for themselves, their children or those in their care. Those who pronounce vivisection as absolutely unacceptable while in good health and without making this absolute commitment are themselves applying a highly personal cost/benefit argument. What they are saying, in effect, is 'I call on you to stop all experiments with animals on the basis that this will involve little or no cost to myself because (as I speak) I am currently deriving no benefit from these experiments'.

I suggest therefore that the cost/benefit analysis is an inescapable feature of the entire debate concerning the use of animals in science and technology. The harm done to the animals is defined by the numbers involved, the severity and the duration of the harm. Assessing the last two elements requires a knowledge of welfare science and the principles of good husbandry. The potential benefits to humans should be assessed on the basis of both science and values, and the weighting given to each will depend on circumstances. For example, the benefit to be derived from development of a vaccine against HIV/Aids, based on experiments that tested its efficacy first in primates and then in humans, may be defined almost entirely by science and the impact of science. If it works, the potential benefit to mankind would be enormous, since it would save millions of young lives. The moral value of saving young lives may be taken as read. The actual benefit will be determined by science and technology, namely the efficacy of the vaccine and the costs of production.

At the other end of the spectrum let us consider the scientific and technological development of hormone additives to promote the production of beef and milk from cattle. These drugs are licensed for use in the USA on the basis of scientific evidence which demonstrates their quality, efficacy and safety (for us, who consume the end product). Europe has decided to call a moratorium on the use of these drugs 'pending further scientific investigation'. On both sides of the Atlantic the word science has been hijacked to suit the value judgements of the people (or, more precisely, the legislators and those who influence the legislators). The science is not in dispute. The drugs do what they say on the box. The opposing judgements within the USA and Europe are not based even remotely on science but are entirely value judgements that reflect the relative political values given both to the right of the individual to prosper in an unregulated market and the responsibility of the citizen in a social democracy.

---

* I exclude herbal and homeopathic preparations that have not been submitted to testing for quality, safety and efficacy.

It is important to remind ourselves that 'scientific procedures', as defined by ASPA (1986), describe only those experiments calculated in advance as likely to cause pain, suffering, distress or lasting harm. ASPA replaced the 1876 Cruelty to Animals Act that 'did not disallow specified acts calculated to cause pain'. It is widely accepted as a massive improvement on its predecessor. However, in substituting the relatively bland expression 'scientific procedures' for the emotive (but honest) word 'cruelty', the legislators have, to some extent, created a rod for their own backs. One can achieve a great deal in biological science without recourse to experiments calculated to cause harm to live animals. Faced by a fundamental question in biology, or the need to address a specific problem of (e.g.) human health or nutrition, scientists should consider the extent to which they can address the question either without using animals at all, or on the basis of experiments that do no harm. This philosophy is most succinctly expressed by the principles of the '*three Rs*': *Replacement*, *Reduction* and *Refinement*, first advocated by Russell & Burch (1959). The sequence of the *three Rs* is critical:

(1)   *Replacement*: is it possible to achieve the scientific objectives without using live animals?
(2)   *Reduction*: if replacement is not possible, what is the least number of animals necessary to achieve the scientific objective? The answer to this question requires careful statistical analysis of the numbers necessary to test the hypothesis. If more animals are used than necessary, then some of the animals will have been wasted. If *less* animals are used than necessary to test the hypothesis then *all* of the animals will have been wasted.
(3)   *Refinement*: this question should be addressed last. Having achieved as much as possible by way of replacement and reduction, it is necessary to question the extent to which the experiment may be refined, either through the design of experiments calculated to cause less harm (or no harm) or through the use of animals that may suffer less.

8.2 Use of animals within the Animals (Scientific Procedures) Act

Table 8.1 summarises the use of animals in procedures licensed by the Home Office under ASPA in 1992 and 2002. These figures are drawn from the annual statistics published by the Home Office (www.homeoffice.gov.uk/docs/animalstats). The total number of procedures* reported in 1992 and 2002 were very similar (2.92 v. 2.73 million animals) and in both years the overwhelming majority of animals used were rodents (mainly mice). However, these broad similarities mask a number

---

* The expression 'number of procedures' may be read as 'number of animals'.

Table 8.1 Categorisation of scientific procedures using animals in 1992 and 2002.

	1992	2002
Total number of procedures (millions of animals)	2.92	2.73
Distribution of procedures (% of total)		
All rodents	79	84
Horses, dogs, cats and primates	<1	<1
Genetically modified animals		26
'Naturally' bred animals with harmful genetic defects	6.1	10
Toxicology studies	8.8	18

of radical changes that have occurred in the last ten years. In 1992, 6% of all animals were categorised as likely to suffer harm as a result of a genetic abnormality and these were produced almost entirely as a result of the 'natural' breeding of individuals carrying a gene known to be harmful or lethal in homozygous individuals. By 2002 the proportion of genetically 'abnormal' animals had risen to 36%, 10% produced by the natural breeding of animals with genetic defects and 26% produced by the new technology of genetic engineering – knocking out or splicing in genes (see Royal Society, 2001). The successful insertion or deletion of a gene is normally followed by the process of cloning to produce a genetically identical population of animals engineered specifically to study the biological function of that gene in health and disease. The number of animals (usually mice) involved in the creation and cloning of a transgenic line may be substantial. However, once established, the use of transgenic mice in scientific procedures meets the criteria of *reduction* and *refinement* because far less animals are required to address a specific problem when all the animals respond to the problem in an identical way.

The techniques used in establishing lines of genetically modified (GM) animals do involve surgical procedures that may cause some degree of pain or suffering. Once established and maintained by conventional breeding, the genetically modified animals may or may not experience lasting harm. In some cases the harm is obvious. Mice that are naked, or unable to coordinate their movements, or severely immuno-deficient are clearly unfit and liable to suffer. It is entirely proper that animals that have been genetically modified in such a way as to cause obvious harm should be recorded in the statistical returns of the Home Office, and that the cost/benefit of the genetic modification itself should be assessed according to the rules of ASPA in addition to the cost of any procedure to which they may be exposed during their working life. However, the inclusion of all genetically modified animals within the annual returns of scientific procedures implies, *a priori*, that all genetic modifications are likely to inflict lasting harm. In fact, within the protected environment of Home Office approved laboratory animal accommodation, it would appear that many transgenic animals experience little or no harm, which means that the statistics exaggerate the numbers of animals actually called upon to suffer for science. It is, however, necessary to acknowledge that any procedure involving genetic modification of a laboratory animal may compromise the fitness and feelings of that animal, not only in the way intended by the genetic modification but also in ways that were unforeseen in advance and may be too subtle to recognise in retrospect. One of the great priorities for welfare science as it applies to laboratory animals is to develop structured and sympathetic methods for assessing the fitness and feelings of genetically modified animals. I shall, of course, return to this topic.

The decision to replace the word 'cruelty' in the 1876 Act with the more anodyne 'scientific procedures' in ASPA (1986) was obviously intended to soothe public concern. In practice, however, the Home Office annual statistics of animals used in scientific procedures has contrived to give a misleading picture of the suffering imposed on animals used for science and technology. It is, moreover, a picture that can be exploited to effect by those whose opposition is absolute.

- By omitting scientific procedures with animals that are not calculated to cause harm the statistics give the impression that all procedures are harmful.
- By including all forms of genetic manipulation as scientific procedures, they imply, by definition, that all such procedures are likely to cause harm.
- By omitting to classify procedures according to their severity ranking, they hide the numbers where the severity is substantial but also fail to identify the great number of procedures in which the harm done to the animals ranges from the mild to the scarcely perceptible.

Those of us who adopt an experimental approach to the study of animal health and welfare obviously 'use' animals in a scientific way. However, much of this work is designed to cause no harm. In the UK, as in many other countries, it is deemed necessary to submit all experiments with animals to ethical review to decide first whether or not the experiments can be conducted without causing harm. It is proper to ask these questions and it is proper that experiments designed to cause no harm should not be included in the statistical returns as currently published. It is a shame, however, that there is no mechanism to demonstrate the extent to which scientists carry out experiments with animals that have been devised specifically on the grounds that such experiments will *not* cause any degree of pain, suffering, distress or lasting harm.

The decision of the Home Office not to publish numbers of procedures carried out within the three severity bands, mild, moderate and severe, has been criticised by both the House of Lords Select Committee (2002) and the Animals Procedures Committee (2003). Once again it appears that government, in its attempt to avoid alarm by concealing the numbers of procedures whose severity may give grounds for real concern, may be achieving the exact opposite of the desired effect, since it also conceals the vastly greater number of procedures (e.g. the taking of a single blood sample from a sheep) that would be seen by 'the reasonable man' as no more severe than that which he would experience during a routine visit to the doctor's clinic.

In recent years a number of regulatory developments have taken place, all within the spirit of ASPA and all designed to reduce the cost to animals in circumstances where the alleged benefits can no longer be justified (see APC, 2003). These include:

- a ban on the testing of finished cosmetic products on animals;
- a ban on the use of great apes (none had actually been used since the passing of ASPA 1986);
- a ban on the testing of alcohol and tobacco products on animals;
- a ban on the acute oral lethal dose 50% (LD50) test, save in exceptional circumstances.

All this is to the good. It is, however, depressing to record (Table 8.1) that the proportion of animals used for toxicological testing (which has little or nothing to do with science) has risen from 8.8% in 1992 to 18% in 2002. This category includes procedures required by law used in the testing of food ingredients, pharmaceuticals, industrial and agricultural chemicals and a few household products. There has undoubtedly been some refinement in the use of animals for toxicological testing. However, those who legislate for our protection in terms of health and safety, and their own protection in terms of litigation, have been far less parsimonious than the scientists in the matter of reduction and replacement.

8.3 Assessing the cost of scientific procedures

The costs imposed on animals involved in scientific procedures licensed by the UK Home Office under ASPA (1986) are defined as the adverse effects, i.e. pain, suffering, distress or lasting harm, likely to be experienced by the animals used during the course of a study. These costs include:

- Any material disturbance to normal health, physical, mental and social well-being. This includes disease, injury and physiological or psychological discomfort.
- Both immediate and long-term effects of regulated procedures, e.g. transient discomfort from an injection and the possible toxic effects of the substance injected.
- Effects arising from both acts of commission and omission, e.g. dosing or withdrawal of food and water.
- Procedures for generation and breeding of animals likely to suffer adverse effects. These include:
  - breeding animals with harmful genetic defects;
  - manipulation of germ cells or embryos to alter the genetic constitution of the resulting animal;
  - subsequent breeding of such genetically modified animals.

- Costs arising from the systems of housing and husbandry imposed on the animals from the time they are issued from stock until they are killed by an approved method or discharged (honourably) from the controls of the Act.

This list is satisfactory for the purposes of defining the elements of welfare that are embraced by the Act (i.e. practically everything). What it does not do is indicate how these procedures might compromise welfare nor how much suffering may be involved. It is not therefore of much practical use to scientists, day-to-day care persons, ethical committees or Home Office Inspectors seeking first to assess and then to minimise the potential costs to animals when planning a new experiment. To do this, I suggest, as always, that it helps to work within the comprehensive framework defined by the Five Freedoms. Table 8.2 presents examples of procedures (and husbandry practices) that may be defined by each of the freedoms and classifies them within the three severity bands, mild, moderate and substantial.

Let us consider, as a first example, the stress of hunger. Any deliberate denial of the nutrients necessary to support normal body function will cause some degree of distress and lasting harm. The distress imposed by prolonged starvation may be considered substantial. Deficiencies of specific nutrients such as the amino acid lysine, the vitamin biotin or the mineral zinc will, if prolonged, cause harm of at least moderate severity. In the shorter term, laboratory animals, especially rodents, deprived of specific nutrients may show no loss of fitness but may display signs of behavioural disturbance as they perceive that their food source is not meeting their physiological needs.

Table 8.2 Examples of the cost to animals incurred by scientific procedures.

	Severity		
	Mild	**Moderate**	**Substantial**
Hunger	Unbalanced diets		Starvation
Metabolic stress	Acute heat or cold		Swimming to exhaustion
Discomfort	Wire cage floors	Surgical implants	
Pain	Venepuncture (sheep jugular)	Venepuncture (mouse, retro-orbital) Recovery from surgery	Burns, fractures
Malaise	Mild infections, tumours	Toxicology Tumour chemotherapy	Fulminating infections, tumours
Acute fear	Acute isolation	Isolation, restraint and manipulation	
Chronic anxiety	Chronic isolation		Anticipated pain, exhaustion
Behavioural deprivation	Barren environments	Prolonged constraint	

It is, of course, imperative to minimise the pain arising as an immediate or long-term consequence of any scientific procedure. Anyone working with laboratory animals should be aware of the signs of pain, e.g. abnormal posture and movement, sensitivity to touch, vocalisation and depression (Morton & Griffiths, 1985; Wall & Melzak, 1994). However, in almost all experiments with animals, any evidence of lasting pain should be construed as a sign of failure in planning or execution. Every experiment that has the potential to cause pain or lasting harm must be planned in advance so as to prevent, or at least minimise, the appearance of pain, partly through judicious use of analgesia before, during and after any surgical procedure, but mainly through refinement of the procedures themselves so as to minimise lasting harm. This principle should apply to all procedures, even one as simple as taking a blood sample. The proficient withdrawal of blood from the jugular vein of a tame sheep using a fine-gauge needle is, I believe, a procedure that causes almost no immediate distress and absolutely no lasting harm. Taking a blood sample from a wild sheep may cause acute distress, due not to the venepuncture itself but to the necessary isolation and restraint. Procedures for sampling blood from a mouse will always cause some degree of lasting harm. Nipping a slice off the end of the tail will cause chronic pain at a sensitive spot. Blood sampling by retro-orbital or cardiac puncture will cause substantial (and sometimes lethal) damage.

Many scientific procedures licensed for the study of disease and technological procedures licensed for the testing of drugs, food additives and household products will cause animals to experience a sense of malaise (i.e. feel ill). This may, in law, be defined as 'unavoidable suffering'. It is, however, essential to consider ways whereby the sense of malaise associated with sickness can be minimised through a sympathetic understanding of the altered environmental and behavioural needs of the sick animal. These include an increased need to rest in a comfortable bed, sufficiently remote from other animals to avoid harassment, a disinclination to eat but an increased thirst. A good example of a sympathetic approach to these changed needs may be drawn from good farm practice. Many calf rearers construct 'sick pens' for animals with diarrhoea or pneumonia. Typically these pens are bedded with deep straw and furnished with an infra-red heat lamp to provide physical and thermal comfort. Water is freely available. Each pen will contain only one calf, so that it can lie in peace, but will be in sight, sound and smell of other animals. It is the farmer's belief that calves in these circumstances are less likely to 'give up' than when kept in complete isolation.

The generic message to be drawn from this specific example is that the physiological and behavioural needs of healthy animals for comfort and social contact may differ radically from the physiological and behavioural needs of animals that are suffering from chronic pain or malaise. A population of healthy mice may not suffer physical discomfort when housed in cages with wire floors and no bedding. However, when they are sick or in pain, their needs for comfort, security, peace and quiet become that much more intense. Any procedure calculated to cause lasting pain or malaise must, at the planning stage, make provision for these altered needs.

Costs listed in Table 8.2 within the categories of acute fear, metabolic stress and behavioural deprivation need little explanation. In general terms it may be said that their severity will depend on how well (or how badly) the animal manages to cope. A sheep or primate that is well housed, well fed and thoroughly tamed by regular affectionate treatment will habituate to a minor procedure such as repeated blood sampling to the extent where the stress (e.g. measured by cortisol concentration) is negligible or non-existent. If, on the other hand, an animal is subjected to procedures that are substantially painful or profoundly aversive (e.g. repeated electric shocks or swimming to exhaustion) then the acute stress at the time of the experience is likely to increase and the chronic anxiety induced by the expectation of future harm may become severe.

It is Home Office policy that individual animals should not be subjected to repeated 'scientific procedures' unless this is essential to an experiment of high scientific merit and potential value. The normal Home Office rule is therefore 'one animal = one procedure'. Applying, once again, the 'cost equation' Total suffering = Individual suffering (Intensity × Duration) × Number of animals involved, the Home Office policy of 'one animal = one procedure' achieves the aim of reducing suffering in all circumstances where the severity of suffering for the individual increases with each repeated procedure. Thus it is better that 20 animals experience a moderate degree of suffering on one occasion before being humanely killed, than that four animals should on five occasions experience a degree of suffering that proceeds from the moderate to the severe, perhaps because they become increasingly sensitive to pain or develop chronic anxiety. However, when tame animals habituate to repeated mild procedures (e.g. blood sampling from sheep) then the solution to the total cost equation becomes an overall reduction in suffering when the same animals are used for more than one experiment. A rigid insistence that animals must, in all circumstances, be used for one procedure only can sometimes be counterproductive.

8.4 Assessing the welfare of laboratory animals

This heading announces the reappearance of the big tune: namely, the creation and implementation of robust protocols for the assessment of animal welfare in practical circumstances (in this case, in the laboratory) and procedures for remedying problems as they arise. In the UK there are clear guidelines for inspection of premises licensed for laboratory animals to ensure compliance with standards laid down by the Home Office *Guidance on the Operation of the Animals (Scientific Procedures) Act 1986* (Home Office, 2000). Many of these relate to formal aspects of provision, such as stocking densities, temperature, humidity and ventilation and need no further discussion here. My contention, as always, is that every establishment housing laboratory animals should, in addition to meeting the standards of provision defined in regulations, develop a standard procedure for assessing the welfare state of its animals based on observations and records taken from the animals themselves. Whenever this assessment of welfare outcomes identifies a problem, this should then be traced back through the system to identify where the problem may lie, either in the matter of provision or in the animal itself, or some combination of the two. The need for this approach has been intensified by the great increase in the number of laboratory animals (mostly mice) that have been genetically modified, either through biotechnology or through selection of harmful mutants to maintain a line of animals better suited to the specific experimental needs of the scientist. Such genetic modification carries a high risk of compromising the ability of the animal to sustain fitness and meet its physiological and behavioural needs. It follows therefore that any newly created line of genetically modified laboratory animal needs to be assessed with great care for welfare problems. If the line is to be sustained, special husbandry provisions must be established to address any special problems. A record of these special problems and special needs should accompany these colonies and be available to the animal care persons wherever these animals are kept.

Table 8.3, following standard procedure, sets out a comprehensive but skeletal list of welfare concerns and fleshes it out with examples of observations and records that may be used to assess the quality of both provision and outcome with respect to these concerns. Some of the examples in this table require little or no further explanation since they relate to welfare problems that have been discussed elsewhere. I have, for instance, already stressed the need for the provision of special 'hospital care' for individuals that may suffer any degree of pain or malaise as a result of the imposed procedures.

One issue that does merit further examination is the provision of environmental enrichment for laboratory animals. Throughout the time that a laboratory animal is actually being used in an experiment it needs to be visible and accessible to test the primary and side effects of the imposed procedure. It is, moreover, necessary to keep a strict control on diet and the microenvironment. Home Office guidelines state that mice and rats should be kept at an air temperature of 25°C ± 2°. In fact, mice and rats do not *need* to live within such a narrow temperature range. Given sufficient food and shelter, both can thrive outdoors in the British winter. To be more precise, the animals act to achieve thermal comfort and regulate energy balance by selection and manipulation of their microclimate in order to control heat loss and adjustment of food intake to fuel heat production. Moreover, each will be inclined to seek its own way to achieve comfort and fitness. As a result, the metabolic rates of rats and mice maintaining themselves successfully in different 'satisfactory' environments may vary by a factor of 3 or more. A threefold difference in metabolic rate may be achieved with reasonable comfort by the animals, but it can make a nonsense of an experiment designed, for example, to measure the pharmacodynamics and metabolism of a new drug. It is necessary

Table 8.3 Outline of the provisions and outcomes necessary to assess the welfare of rodents kept under laboratory conditions.

	Provision	Outcome
Hunger and thirst	Chow only – chow plus vegetable supplements	Difficulty in eating; state of incisor teeth
		Condition: good – thin
		Pot bellied, staring coat
Comfort	Cage floor: wire v. solid with litter	Hair loss, skin abrasions
	Nesting substrates	Quality and cleanliness of litter
Security	Shelters: tubes, igloos	Stereotypies, wall hugging
Pain and injury	'Hospital care' for individuals in pain	Abnormal posture: hunched, shivering
		Sensitivity at wound site
		General hyperalgesia
		Vocalisation
Fitness and health	'Hospital care' for individuals with malaise	Alert – apathetic
		Nose, eyes: clear – discharge
		Neuromotor abnormalities
		Records: mortality, breeding success
Fear and stress	Background noises (music?)	Stereotypies
	Shelters?	Wall hugging
	Handling: sympathetic – rough	Response to handling
Natural behaviour	Environmental enrichment: gnawing material: wood blocks running wheels	Inquisitive behaviour
		Cage gnawing

to point out that the very strict limits imposed on air temperature, ventilation rate, etc. in the Home Office *Guidance on the Operation of the Animals (Scientific Procedures) Act 1986* (Home Office, 2000) are not primarily intended to ensure the welfare of the animals but rather consistency within experiments. There is, of course, a secondary welfare benefit from standardising the environment to minimise between-animal variability, namely a reduction in the number of animals necessary to achieve the scientific objectives. However, the environment necessary for animals actually on experiment (always visible for inspection in a standardised microenvironment) may be far from ideal when assessed according to freedom to express normal behaviour and freedom from fear and stress. Breeding stock and all other animals not currently involved in an experimental procedure should be accommodated wherever possible in more enriched environments that offer the security of individual shelters (igloos, tubes), the comfort of a well-littered solid floor and the behavioural satisfaction provided by some form of nesting substrate.

In Chapter 3 (Figure 3.3), I discussed how the primitive but necessary emotion of fear may, according to environmental circumstances, develop into either an adaptive response that favours survival in a challenging environment, or a non-adaptive state of chronic anxiety or learned helplessness. In brief, animals must learn to cope with fear, by learning to distinguish between real and imagined threats and what action to take when the threat is real. In the confines of the laboratory, animals are seldom given the opportunity to develop these skills, nor an environment wherein they can take effective action. Rats and mice kept from birth in cage rooms where almost nothing ever happens can display exaggerated alarm when startled by sudden sounds. This appears to be an acute expression of a chronic anxiety that can manifest itself as stereotypies or other forms of abnormal behaviour such as infanticide. It is common practice to play background music of the easy listening variety throughout the day in laboratory animal colonies. This does appear to soothe the animals. It would be nice to think that they enjoyed it, although it is more likely a matter of becoming habituated to the concept of meaningless noise.

8.5 Assessing the welfare of GM and mutant mice

The 'normal' breeding programme for a line of laboratory mice is to select couples for natural mating to sustain the desirable phenotypic traits within the line but without introducing problems arising from excessive inbreeding. Thus standard lines of laboratory mice maintained to a satisfactory state of reproductive fitness through careful selection and reared in satisfactory, suitably enriched environments should exhibit normal behaviour, i.e. that which enables them to cope without difficulty within the environment to which they and their ancestors have become accustomed*. Any departure from the normal programme for breeding for fitness, either through the selection of harmful mutants or through the use of biotechnology to create genetically modified (GM) lines, carries the risk of compromising fitness and the capacity of the animals to cope. Indeed, most GM lines and all harmful mutants are produced with the specific intention of impairing one or more of the genetic regulators of normal physiology so as to study the mechanisms involved. Although suffering is not an inevitable consequence of genetic modification, it should be assumed that every line of GM or mutant mice may carry its own specific welfare problems that will require special attention.

A great deal of thought has been given to the development of tests to identify the special behavioural problems of GM mice. As an introduction to further reading I suggest Crawley (2000), Wahlsten *et al.* (2003) and the website 'What

---

* In Manuel Berdoy's film *The Laboratory Rat: A Natural History* (www.ratlife.org), rats bred for over 200 generations in the laboratory reacquire, within hours, the skills necessary for survival in the wild.

is wrong with my mouse?' (www.mymouse.org). These authors describe a comprehensive and time-consuming series of tests that may be used to describe with precision that nature of a specific behavioural disorder which may then be related to both a specified gene and/or a defined region of pathology, e.g. within the central nervous system. The main purpose of this complex array of behavioural tests is, of course, to aid the scientific understanding of the specific problem, rather than to redress welfare problems as perceived by the animals. Those whose primary concern is for animal welfare (a list that includes the named veterinary surgeon, the day-to-day carers and, of course, the mice) may be better served by simpler but comprehensive cage-side protocols for assessing provisions and outcomes as listed in Table 8.3.

The two main categories of welfare problem likely to be induced by 'knock-out' techniques in GM mice are metabolic disorders due to loss of a single enzyme and behavioural disorders, leading to a failure to cope, brought about by some disruption of the process of recognition, interpretation and action taken in response to signals from the external environment. The diagnosis and redress of metabolic disorders is outside the scope of this book. What *is* relevant is to emphasise the need not only to identify behavioural disorders in GM animals but also to discover how and where these problems have arisen. Figure 8.1 explores the possible origins of abnormal behaviour in GM animals using the model previously illustrated in Figure 3.1 to outline how sentient animals perceive their world and act upon their perception. Two forms of stimuli are shown: those that elicit a simple reflex action and those that involve the higher centres of the brain. The latter category are first recognised, then interpreted always emotionally and sometimes cognitively to create a motivation to act. The conscious and reflex actions invoked in response to the stimulus will create a pattern of behaviour designed to cope with the stimulus. An animal with an abnormal phenotype (through GM or for any other reason) may fail to marshal an effective behavioural response through failure at any stage in this chain of command and action. Starting from the effector end, these include:

- failure to achieve the behaviour intended by the signals for action, e.g. muscle weakness, pain, inability to sustain normal posture and movement, no teeth;
- failure to transmit the correct signal for action, e.g. incoordination or disordered righting reflex;
- abnormality of motivation, e.g. reduction in exploration, hunger;
- abnormality of mood, e.g. anxiety, apathy;
- impaired cognition, e.g. loss of memory;
- impaired recognition, e.g. loss of sight, smell, hearing.

A GM mouse may 'fail' or perform badly in a behavioural test, such as learning its way through a maze, through knock-out of a gene directly involved in memory and the cognitive ability to create mental maps. It may also fail through a reduced physical ability to run the maze, attributable to pain or muscle weak-

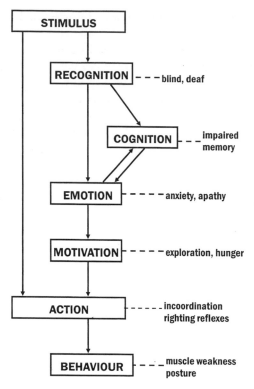

Figure 8.1 Possible factors contributing to abnormal behaviour in GM and mutant mice.

ness. Its motivation to attempt the maze may be affected by feedback from pain receptors or a resetting of its overall mood, in the direction of either apathy or paralysing anxiety. Finally, it might fail because its primary ability to recognise environmental stimuli has been impaired through loss of sight, smell or hearing. It is clearly important for the scientists studying the specific behavioural problem to identify its primary cause. Those responsible for day-to-day care also need to understand the nature of the problem in order to devise the most sympathetic ways of helping the animals to cope within the confines of the animal house. Consider, for example, a line of GM mice that appears to be having difficulty in eating enough to sustain normal growth and development. This could be due to a physiological failure to digest and metabolise the food. It could also be due to a failure to recognise the food, through loss of special senses, a reduced ability to gather the food, through muscular incoordination, or an inability to eat it, through impaired dentition or a complete lack of teeth. Impaired dentition is a relatively common unintended consequence of GM for other purposes (Wahlsten *et al.*, 2003). The hunger of mice that have difficulty in finding or gathering food may be assuaged by scattering dry food over a solid cage floor. An unavoidable problem arising from abnormal dentition may be redressed by providing a liquid diet.

To summarise this section: it may be unrealistic to run the full battery of bio-chemical and behavioural tests on every new line of GM mice, although some la-boratories are offering to provide this service (see www.mymouse.org). However all laboratories producing and/or rearing GM mice should institute formal proce-dures for identifying any welfare problems arising as a consequence of phenotypic abnormalities in GM mice, take steps to redress these problems, record the con-sequences of their actions and make their records of both problems and solutions available to all who may use (or contemplate using) these animals. In most cases the protocols can be based on relatively simple cage-side observations (Table 8.3). Where major difficulties in coping become apparent, these need to be explored in more detail using the approach illustrated in Figure 8.1.

8.6 Impacts of science and biotechnology on the food animals

The final topic that I wish to consider in this chapter is 'tinkering', namely the biotechnological manipulation of animals in order to increase their commercial value to man. The most dramatic and extreme examples of the use of science and technology to manipulate animals for our own economic ends have attracted a great deal of publicity, most of it adverse (Compassion in World Farming, 2002; GeneWatch, 2002). These include the use of hormones to increase growth or lactation in cattle, the insertion of the human growth hormone gene into pigs in an attempt to 'improve' the efficiency of growth, and the insertion of genes into sheep and cattle to alter the composition of milk. The aim of procedures designed to alter the composition of animal produce may be to improve the quality of the product assessed simply as food (e.g. to produce better cheese) or to produce 'phar-maceuticals', specific chemicals in animal produce that may be used to improve the health of the majority or treat individuals with specific genetic disorders.

Ten years ago the notion of engineering animals for profit created a major battleground between those who were absolutely appalled by the new biology and condemned the whole notion as 'Frankenstein farming' and those who were absolutely entranced by it and considered that anything that could be done was worth a try. Needless to say, I support neither absolute position and have argued that each case should be considered on its merits. Thus the use of recombinant growth hormone to increase milk yield in cows is unjustified because the cost to cows is significant but the benefits to society (or even the farmers) are minimal. Engineering growth hormone into a pig to make it grow faster becomes totally unacceptable when the cost to the animal is severe (it is crippled by chronic pain). On the other hand, production of a line of GM sheep that produce in their milk a specific chemical such as α-1-antitrypsin, which can be used to keep alive children suffering from a form of cystic fibrosis, appears to me to be ethically admirable. The biotechnological procedures needed to develop the GM line (embryo collection, gene transfer, abortions and abnormalities of fetal development) do constitute a significant cost for the first generations of sheep. However, once the line has been established and is breeding normally, the long-term costs to the sheep are negligible when set against the potential benefits in terms of human health and happiness. Moreover, animals capable of producing such a high-value product (relative to milk considered simply as a food) are likely be treated with the same degree of care as the goose that laid the proverbial golden eggs.

I developed this argument at greater length in *Eden I* and shall not reprise it here. This is partly because the ethical argument has not changed and partly because the whole topic of engineering animals for profit has rather gone off the boil. Consumer resistance has undoubtedly contributed to a general loss of enthusiasm for engineering animals for profit, but this is by no means the whole story, not least because there is no single consumer and attitudes differ greatly, e.g. between Europe and the USA. The biggest deterrent to investment in biotechnology designed to manipulate whole sentient animals for profit in the production of either food or 'farmaceuticals' seems to be that the profit simply is not there. Even projects that appear most ethically sound and most likely to add value (e.g. the production of α-1-antitrypsin in sheep milk) have been put on the back burner rather than taken into fully commercial production.

This raises a more general, and to scientists an even more worrying, question: 'What use is science to the commercial business of producing healthy food from animals in a sustainable environment?' There can be no doubt that the international animal production industry has succeeded in its aim of producing lots of food of consistently high quality at a reasonable price. We must, however, honestly address the questions 'How much of this progress is a direct consequence of animal science and how much would have happened anyway?' Table 8.4 presents a critical review of the extent to which elements of conventional animal production for food, namely nutrition, reproduction, growth, lactation, health and welfare, may or may not have been influenced by three drivers: practical technology, systems science and laboratory science. Each heading is further subdivided according to whether the impact of the drivers has been *directive* (it has directly advanced production) or *remedial* (it has been used to address problems thrown up by technological progress) and each example is scored from 1–3 for its impact, whether positive (+, ++, +++), negative (−, −−, −−−) or non-significant (n.s.). The examples selected for inclusion reflect my personal interests and I would not expect you all to agree with them all. Table 8.4 does not pretend to be comprehensive. It is intended as a guide to constructive review of what animal science is *for*.

8.6.1 Nutrition

One of the great simple truths of animal nutrition is that there is far more to be achieved from manipulating the nutritive value of the (plant) food we give to animals (and ourselves) than there is to be achieved through attempts to

Table 8.4 Analysis of the impact (or lack of impact) of technology, systems science and laboratory science on the productivity, health and welfare of the food animals. (n.s. Not significant).

	Technology	Systems science	Laboratory science
Nutrition			
Directive	Feed processing ++ (Crop improvement +)	Feed evaluation +++ Nutrient requirements +	Microbial metabolism + (Genetic engineering of crops ++) Intermediary metabolism n.s.
Remedial	n.s.	n.s.	Deficiency disorders ++
Reproduction			
Directive	Artificial insemination +++ Embryo transfer +/−	n.s.	Endocrinology + Molecular biology n.s. Cloning n.s.
Remedial		Ethology +	Endocrinology +
Growth			
Directive	Genetic selection ++	Population genetics ++	Endocrinology +? Genetic engineering of animals −− Bone and matrix biology ++
Remedial			
Lactation			
Directive	Genetic selection +++	Population genetics +++ Nutrition ++	Endocrinology +? Cloning n.s.
Remedial	Milking machines		
Health			
Directive	Intensification −−− (+?)	n.s.	Vaccines and chemotherapeutics ++
Remedial		Epidemiology + Population genetics +/−−	Vaccines and chemotherapeutics +++ Genetic resistance to disease +
Welfare			
Directive	Intensification −−− (+?)	n.s.	n.s.
Remedial	Humane slaughter +	Ethology + Motivation analysis ++	Neurobiology n.s. Bone and matrix biology ++

manipulate the efficiency with which animals digest and metabolise the food we give them. Plant breeding and conventional technology (e.g. fertilisers) have done a great deal to increase the yield of crops, although relatively little to improve their composition and nutritive value. Laboratory science (e.g. genetic engineering) has not yet done much to improve crop value for animals and man, but the potential to engineer crops more suited to animal needs (e.g. better grass for cows) is enormous. However, this is plant science, not animal science. Moreover, the development of genetic engineering in plants is also bogged down in debate that has become a confusing mish-mash of science and quasi science, ethics and quasi-ethics, commercial opportunism and self-indulgent outrage. (I shall stay out of it.) 'Systems' animal science, directed towards better understanding of nutrition rather than new discovery, has achieved a great deal towards improving both health and efficiency by attaining a better match between nutrient supply and demand. Laboratory animal science, designed to explore the dynamic biochemistry of nutrition, has led to a great improvement in our understanding of what happens inside the animal but has not, in all honesty, had much impact on the way we feed animals in practice.

8.6.2 Reproduction

Most of the advances in the breeding and reproduction of farm animals can be attributed mainly to a few, relatively simple pieces of practical technology. Artificial insemination (AI) has been of immense benefit to animal production because it can be used to achieve genetic improvement through selection of superior sires at relatively little economic cost. In more recent years newer science has generated more sophisticated procedures to achieve breeding objectives, such as MOET (multiple ovulation with embryo transfer) and cloning. Although these procedures may be more technically impressive than AI, they have had nothing like the impact of AI on animal production for food for the simple reason that they seldom give value for money. Perhaps the most useful technological aid to reproduction in farm animals has been the use of ultrasound for pregnancy diagnosis, especially in sheep. The technology is not only effective, but also cost effective, since it can pay for itself several times over by making it possible for pregnant sheep to be housed and precisely fed according to the number of lambs that they are carrying.

Laboratory science, in the form of endocrinology, has, I suggest, had minimal direct effect in *improving* reproductive performance in healthy animals. It has, however, been successful in improving the treatment of problems of obstetrics and infertility. Thus its primary contribution has been remedial rather than directive. However, the need for such remedial science is increasing. In Chapter 5, I discussed the extent to which selection of dairy cows for production traits is progressively compromising fitness measured in terms of fertility and longevity. The old adage 'Evolution will always be more successful than the cleverest scientist' is never more true than in the matter of reproduction.

8.6.3 Growth and lactation

We have witnessed spectacular increases in growth rates in the meat animals, especially poultry, and milk production in the dairy cow. A large part of this has been achieved through simple genetic selection for production traits, i.e. the technological application of established procedures. The science of population genetics has helped to refine this technology. However, I suggest that it has been more useful in identifying and seeking to remove correlated responses to selection for performance that may compromise animal fitness and welfare. Thus, here again, I suggest that the best science has been remedial rather than directive. Similarly, new genetics, e.g. marker-assisted selection, may also prove to be more effective in preventing harmful consequences than simply accelerating productivity *per se*.

In theory (I repeat) the most promising directive role for genetics, old or new, in this area of food production, is in manipulating the composition of meat or milk. There is great potential for the development of 'designer' meat and milk products that promote good health, or are perceived to promote good health – which will sell just as well. Unfortunately such developments, however rational, tend to rub against the grain of human sentience. On the one hand, we do not like to feel that the animals we eat have been 'messed about'. Moreover, as confirmed by countless consumer surveys, we also believe that the healthiest food is natural food. These two beliefs have effectively killed off commercial interest in the 'scientific' manipulation of meat and milk, at least in Europe. As an aside, I must say that I am wrily amused by the successful marketing of 'scientific' dog foods: specialist canned diets designed to prevent diseases from renal failure to brain ageing (yes, really). Whereas food such as dairy produce for humans tends to be promoted by images of contented cows in green fields, canned food for dogs is promoted by images of clean-limbed scientists in sparkling white coats. Such products appear to retail very well within the same affluent market that will seek organic food for themselves and their children. The dogs, of course, will eat anything they are given.

8.6.4 Health

All health science may, in the broadest sense, be defined as remedial, i.e. it is directed towards the prevention and treatment of disease. However, I have also made it clear that health science had a major (indeed arguably *the* major) directive impact on the intensification of animal production (Chapter 5). The two main drivers of intensification were mechanisation and antibiotics. Suitable bulk-handling machines were available in the 1930s, but intensification did not really take off until the 1950s when the availability of antibiotics made it possible to confine large numbers of young animals at a high stocking density without incurring unacceptable losses from bacterial infections. Since then new discoveries of antibiotics and anthelmintics, together with the development of vaccines against viruses and bacteria, have continued to sustain the health and productivity of the food animals. These vaccines and chemotherapeutics have also made it possible for farm animals to survive and grow in environments that are unacceptable on welfare grounds. This is not always the case and it would be fatuous to extrapolate this argument to a blanket condemnation of the use of drugs for the control of health in the food animals. Pharmaceuticals have been very good for animal production. Nevertheless, new, real concerns are emerging; especially problems of drug resistance with both the antibiotics and anthelmintics. Thus the new science of therapeutics and alternatives to therapeutics in food animal production will once again be remedial rather than directive.

The new molecular sciences (genomics, proteomics) hold great promise for human and animal health (and glittering prizes for scientists) through identification of the key vulnerable steps in the life cycles of pathogens and the aetiology of disease in their hosts. I believe that this branch of molecular biology is currently the 'hottest' and most exciting area in all science. One has, however, to pose the question 'Is it likely to have much impact on production and health in the food animals?' With some regret, I predict that the impact may be quite small. I can envisage the successful further development of poultry with genetic resistance to specific diseases. The structure of the poultry industry and the genetic turnover time of poultry make research of this sort an economically attractive investment. However, the major disease problems of cattle, sheep and pigs are not particularly suited to genetic control. Endemic infectious diseases such as mastitis and enteritis tend to be associated with a multiplicity of potential pathogens, such that exposure to infection is the natural state and disease usually reflects a loss of equilibrium between host and pathogen. There is undoubtedly a genetic component in other major categories of multifactorial production disease in intensively managed food animals (e.g. metabolic disorders and lameness). However, the most promising approach to their control is through systems science (including epidemiology) and systems management.

8.6.5 Welfare

Table 8.4 includes, for completeness, a category for science in the service of animal welfare. I shall not recapitulate here themes that I have discussed throughout the book. I would say only that the aim of farm animal welfare science has always been remedial, either through a better understanding of animal needs or through the redress of welfare problems systematically induced through intensification. I have no option but to give the technology of intensification a three-minus score in the welfare box, but I also add a single opposing plus to remind you that intensification *per se* is not automatically a dirty word. Some forms of intensification, like the housing of ewes at lambing, have been good for welfare. At this point I must also restate my belief that the highest priority for welfare scientists is to put our understanding into practice through the development and implementation of effective protocols for assessing and implementing animal welfare on farm.

8.7 Are animal scientists failing society?

Here I shall draw a clear distinction between the discipline of science and the people who practise science. Science, *per se*, has arguably been our most effective route to understanding the world and (when correctly applied) a massive contributor to our health and happiness. However, since the whole moral argument in this chapter revolves around the cost/benefit equation as it applies to the use of science and technology as it applies to the animals we use for our own purposes, it is necessary to ask the more specific question: 'Is animal science succeeding or failing in its aim to meet the needs of society?' In the case of science as applied to animal production the answer to this question is probably 'No'. Unlike medical science, which we trust to keep us alive, most of us believe that food and farming were fine before scientists came along to mess it up with things like BST and BSE. I know this perception may be irrational, but perceptions arise from feelings not thought. More careful inspection of the evidence would indicate that most of the major developments in animal *production* have arisen through the unstoppable progress of market-led technology. Where animal science has been most useful is in protecting us and the other animals from the worst consequences of rampant technology. It follows from this that the best and most important animal science will be done by those who are paid to serve the common good, rather than by those who choose to be the mistresses of industry.

It is terribly easy to mock scientists. Though science itself may be disinterested and rational, scientists are just ordinary people; sentient, feeling creatures, powerfully motivated by the desire to feel good about ourselves. We feel ourselves to be misunderstood by society and so become pathetically eager for the respect of our peers and tangible expression of that respect in the form of research grants. From the moment we embark upon our PhDs we are directed by our peers (though not by society) to 'focus'. Three years into a Post-Doctoral Fellowship and this focus is likely to have narrowed into a severe case of tunnel vision. I am not quite suggesting that too much science makes you go blind, but sometimes it gets close. Undoubtedly many of the great advances in biology have been achieved by highly focused work done in the laboratory or, in the case of Crick and Watson, by thinking about highly focused work done in other people's laboratories. However, the greatest of all the biologists, Darwin, developed his vision on the basis of deep thought about simply everything. Reductionist science is appropriate to the business of new discovery; but the greatest need for animal science is not new discovery but a better understanding of how animals best fit into strategies for sustainable production from the living environment. I include the word production because the living environment must produce things of value to us, otherwise we cannot afford to sustain it.

Currently I believe that animal scientists (in common with many others) are failing society. We are too interested in our own interests and most happy when talking to each other. While we scientists talk to each other in our own increasingly arcane language, society at large shies away from the stern discipline of evidence-based scientific reason into the mushy embrace of such things as homeopathy and herbalism. I illustrate this point with three remarks heard or read recently.

- 'This cooking pot is organic because it contains no chemicals.'
- 'This herbal preparation cannot be harmful because it contains only natural ingredients.'
- 'We believe that creationism should be taught in schools (in the UK!) because students should be exposed to different opinions.'

The truly terrifying feature of this last remark (which paraphrases our current Prime Minister) is that creationism and evolution should be classified simply as conflicting matters of opinion, to be given equal time in debate. This school debating society attitude becomes especially dangerous when it is dumbed down to three-minute fragments for broadcasting purposes. Typically the first 90 seconds is given to a tongue-tied scientist, overwhelmed by the weight of evidence at his or her disposal. He/she is then confronted by a highly articulate polemicist who presents the case for the opposition with the supreme confidence engendered by a Teflon Belief System; totally non-stick to all messy substances like facts. It pains me to say that in most such quasi-debates scientists are absolutely hopeless. This matters a great deal because issues such as animal welfare, the quality and safety of food from animals, and proper stewardship of the living environment desperately need good science carried out by good integrative biological scientists who can understand the whole through a profound knowledge of all its working parts. The approach should be holistic in aim but analytical in execution.

Finally, I must, once again, restate the obvious. We need better two-way communication. It is right that scientists should communicate to society not only the facts but also the moral virtue of a discipline based upon evidence and reason. It is also right that scientists should be made to listen to those whose appreciation of values and the true needs of society gives them a clear ethical understanding of the difference between what can be done and what should be done.

Animals for Sport

The last temptation is the greatest treason, to do the right thing for the wrong reason.

T.S. Eliot

This series of chapters headed by the words 'Animals for . . .' has dealt so far with our use of animals to provide our needs for food and clothing, medicines and the practical benefits of scientific discovery. It now changes tack, and turns to a review of our use of animals for the pleasures of life. I would remind you that my use of the selfish phrase 'Animals for' is deliberate. It is intended to ram home the message that whenever we come into close contact with animals, we use them for our own ends and (with the admirable exception of cats) control their lives to serve these ends. This chapter will consider how we use animals in sport, the next how we use our pets. I shall not reconsider our use of animals for entertainment in zoos and circuses; since not much has changed in this particular regard in the last ten years, I am content to stand by what I wrote in *Eden I*.

This bald introduction needs some qualification. We do not all 'need' animals to provide us with food. It is relatively easy for a non-lactating adult to thrive on a vegan diet and possible, though more difficult, for a growing child. A lacto-vegetarian diet that permits cheese but not beef is entirely compatible with good nutrition and health. However, I would be amazed if anyone who has read Chapter 6 could sustain a case for denying themselves beef but continuing to eat dairy products on the grounds of animal welfare. It is perfectly valid to claim that we need the pleasure we derive from our pets and from those animals we use for recreational purposes every bit as much as we need to eat beef or cheese. It is clear, however, that the phrase 'unnecessary suffering' enshrined by the Protection of Animals Act (1911) defines the acceptable limit to the amount of suffering we may cause to an animal by 'doing or omitting to do any act' according to the extent of our need, defined not by each individual but by the perceived need of society as interpreted by our legislators. Society will inevitably tend to draw the line between 'necessary' and 'unnecessary' suffering at a different level according to whether the animal in question is being used for science, for food, for sport or simply for companionship. Thus I have addressed the welfare of animals on the farm and in the laboratory on the pragmatic basis that society in general will always consider these needs to be essential. The question 'Should it be done at all?' may carry impeccable moral credentials in terms of personal ethics but is unlikely to have much impact on general practice. The more useful question is 'How should it be done?' within an ethical context that gives proper recognition to all parties worthy of respect, namely the consumer, the farmer, the animals and the living environment (Table 1.4). Similarly my review of the welfare of pets and our responsibilities to pets has to be written on the basis that pets too will be with us always. The legal and ethical rules of engagement become very different when we consider the use of animals for sports such as horse racing or fox hunting, or entertainments such as circuses or bullfights. Bullfighting is permitted in Spain but not in the UK. As I write, hunting with dogs is banned in Scotland and by the time of publication it may also be banned in England. Hunting *without* dogs remains legal. Indeed, hunting foxes *with* dogs is legal in Scotland so long as the fox is killed by a bullet from a gun rather than a bite from a hound. If you detect a note of cynicism, this is once again deliberate and intended to convey the message that the law and the ethical basis of the law concerning the killing of animals for sport is in a mess. In this chapter I shall refrain from telling you what practices I think should and should not be permitted. My aim is to judge the evidence and leave it to you, the jury, to reach your own verdict. However, before beginning an examination of the various uses of animals for sport and entertainment on a case-by-case basis I should make clear my own terms of reference:

(1)   The review will seek to give respect to the welfare of all sentient creatures affected by the sport. Thus, when reviewing fox hunting, I shall consider the welfare of both the prey species and other sentient animals within the area covered by the hunt.
(2)   The case for the animal 'used' for sport, whether it be the hunted fox or the horse used for hunting and steeplechasing, will be assessed on the basis of welfare over its entire life. The mode of dying will be treated as important but not all-important.
(3)   The pleasure that some people derive from sports that involve killing animals (and others derive from sabotaging these pursuits) will never (well, hardly ever) feature in my argument.

My decision to neglect this third principle needs some explanation. The first two rules of engagement are central to my overall aim, which is to do the best we can for all sentient animals within our dominion out of respect for their intrinsic value. Throughout this book and its predecessor I have advocated the case for the animals on the basis that their (lifetime) welfare is determined by how well they cope within the environment and circumstances in which they find themselves. Since suffering is defined by the failure of an animal to cope with stresses such as pain and fear, then our aim in all circumstances must be to minimise suffering at all stages of life. Cordelia (Figure 1.1) stands as a reminder that the nature of suffering experienced by a sentient animal such as a rat will be the same whether we keep it as a pet for use in the home, keep it in the laboratory for use in science, or keep well away, treat it as vermin and exterminate it if it gets too close. When we *do* choose to exterminate a rat (or a fox), it is of no consequence to the animal whether we derive pleasure from the act, or disgust, or allocate the task to someone else and try not to think about it at all. What matters is the intensity and duration of its own suffering and this may well be greater when it is poisoned than when it is killed quickly by a highly enthusiastic terrier towing an almost equally enthusiastic man in a flat cap. To be personal for a moment (and a moment only) I am on the side of those who feel the whole concept of killing animals for pleasure to be morally objectionable (and I do not do it). Nevertheless death is a fact of life and the means of death is an inescapable part of our responsibility to those animals within our dominion, whether we classify them as farm animals, pets, game or vermin (a categorisation that the animals may only infer from our behaviour towards them). If, for example, we legislate to ban the hunting of foxes with hounds on the grounds that we believe that no man has the right to inflict any degree of cruelty for pleasure, and if (and here I emphasise the word *if*) as a consequence of this legislation, the total sum of animal suffering is increased through neglect – leading to overpopulation, starvation and mange in foxes, increased losses of lambs through predation, and increased losses of ground-nesting birds, both through predation and loss of habitat – then we shall have done more harm than good. I shall marshal the evidence in relation to this and similar issues later. For the moment, let me acknowledge that this is once again a strictly utilitarian (and therefore limited) argument. Each of us will have a category of things that we believe should not be done in any circumstances and this list will be based on principles of autonomy and/or justice. We may believe that it is simply not right to kill any animal, such as a hare or even a spider, for no good reason. We may believe that it is not right to degrade a tiger by compelling it to perform in a circus. We may believe that it is unfair to confine a tiger or a pet rabbit in a cage. We will all have reasons to justify each item on our individual lists. The argument that follows is offered as an aid to reviewing your own personal list.

My approach will be to follow the principles of the ethical matrix as set out in Table 1.4. I shall identify the parties worthy of respect, and examine how to reconcile their often conflicting rights according to the principles of wellbeing, autonomy and justice. This approach has much in common with the scientific method. It analyses the elements of the problem as it stands, reviews the evidence, including the scientific evidence, poses a series of 'what if?' questions, and then, and then only, seeks to direct the jury towards conclusions and value judgements on the basis of the evidence. Let us begin by analysing and categorising the games people play with animals.

9.1 Games people play with animals

When we play games with animals we are using them for our sport. Whether they find the experience distressing or delightful is an important question, but it does not alter the fact that they are being used as instruments to give us some form of satisfaction or reward. So far as humans are concerned, the primary motivation for taking active part in any sport is the thrill of the contest and the more thrilling prospect of winning. This argument is as relevant to fishing as it is to football. The fly fisherman who justifies his pastime with the claim that salmon is good food is, deliberately or otherwise, dodging the issue. There are cheaper and easier ways of acquiring salmon.

Most humans, of course, draw their excitement from animal sports not as participants but as spectators. This applies equally to those who arrive at a horserace in a four-wheel-drive vehicle and those who follow a fox hunt on horseback. Whatever other arguments are advanced for and against the control of foxes by hunting with hounds, it is an inescapable fact that the majority of the riders streaming cross country in full cry are entirely superfluous to the business at hand. The hunt is conducted by the hounds under the (nominal) control of the Master of Foxhounds and his immediate assistants. Those who follow the hunt on horseback or in an off-road vehicle cannot justify their presence on the grounds that it is necessary since they are no more than mobile spectators. In common with the fly fisherman, they must accept at the outset that the only reason they do these things is because, to them, it is good fun.

All sports involve an element of competition. Animal sports are based on competition between animals or competition between animals and humans. Where they differ is in the costs (or benefits) to the animals of the contest itself and the penalties of losing. Thus, to a racehorse the race itself may carry little cost (it may, indeed, be a pleasure) unless it is unlucky enough to be injured, and there would appear (to the horse) to be no immediate penalty for losing. In a fox hunt, the cost of the event to the fox depends on how hard is the chase and the penalty for losing is death. The sociobiologist who seeks evolutionary links between the behaviour of man and animals would argue that the motivation to play is driven by the primitive need to develop life skills and improve evolutionary 'fitness'. Hunting, whether with hounds, rod or gun, has undoubtedly evolved from the primitive human need to ensure fitness by acquiring food and maintaining control over other animal species competing within the same habitat. It would be specious to claim that this is the primary motivation for hunting today, but equally specious to deny that this motivation has been essential to the evolution of the human species and is, by this definition, 'natural'. Other sports, such as sheepdog trials and rodeo, have ritualised and celebrated skills essential to farming and ranching. At first sight (to us) sheepdog trials may appear far more humane than bareback bronco riding. The animals may see things differently. The sheep are always harassed and usually lose (they end up in a pen). The bucking horse is also harassed but (to its mind) always wins, since no cowboy stays on for more than about eight seconds.

The lure that attracts the greatest number of people to participate in animal sports is entirely vicarious, namely the lure of gambling. The emotions of gambling – the excitement of the wager, thrill at winning, despair at losing – are the same whatever the contest, be it horse racing, greyhound racing, cock fighting or dog fighting. Organising races between animals to satisfy the punters is legal, organising fights between animals is not.

9.2 The Protection of Wild Animals Act

All UK legislation designed to protect wild and domestic animals from unnecessary suffering is still derived from the Protection of Animals Act 1911*. It is worth restating the essence of Article 1:

> *If any person shall cruelly beat, kick, ill-treat, over-ride, over-drive, over-load, torture, infuriate or terrify an animal, . . . or shall, by wantonly or unreasonably doing or omitting to do any act . . . permit any unnecessary suffering to be so caused to any animal . . . he shall be guilty of an offence of cruelty within the meaning of this Act.*

Article 1 of the Wild Mammals (Protection) Act 1996 states: 'If, save as permitted by this Act, any person mutilates, kicks, beats, nails or otherwise impales, stabs, burns, stones, crushes, drowns, drags or asphyxiates any wild mammal with intent to cause unnecessary suffering he shall be guilty of an offence'. Article 2 then goes on to state that a person shall not be guilty of an offence under this Act by reason of:

- attempted killing as an act of mercy;
- killing in a reasonably swift and humane manner . . . if he shows that the wild mammal had been injured or taken in the course of either lawful shooting, hunting, coursing or pest control activity;
- any act made unlawful by section 1 if the act was done by means of any snare, trap, dog, or bird lawfully used for the purpose of killing or taking any wild mammal;
- the lawful use of any poisonous or noxious substance.

Both the 1911 and 1996 Acts interpret cruelty as 'the intent to cause unnecessary suffering'. The 1911 Act recognises that this may be caused 'by doing or omitting to do any act'. The Protection of Wildlife Act (1996) excludes the omission

---

* The 1911 Act is under review as this book goes to press. In July 2003, DEFRA published a draft Animal Welfare Bill that proposes to redefine the offence of cruelty and impose on animal owners a duty of care. The Bill will not, however, deal specifically with wild animals.

clause on the reasonable basis that it is not an offence to neglect the welfare of any wild fox, pigeon or rat that strays onto one's land. It is, however, somewhat disingenuous in that which it prohibits and permits under the heading of lawful killing. For example:

Illegal	*Legal*
Stabbing	Shooting
Crushing	Snaring
Drowning	Poisoning
Use of a dog (Scotland)	Use of a bird of prey

Any good advocate for the wild animals could dismiss these distinctions as facile. An animal killed by a stab wound may take longer to die than when shot. However, an animal is more likely to escape but suffer chronic injury when shot from a distance than when stabbed while restrained at close quarters. A wild animal may not be crushed to death relatively quickly by a hooligan but may be crushed to death slowly by a legal snare. A wild animal may be asphyxiated by poison but not by drowning. Finally, and most bizarrely, it is permitted to use a bird of prey to kill a wild mammal but not (in Scotland) a dog. The law is riddled with inconsistencies, but one can understand what it seeks to achieve. In brief, its intention is to prevent wanton cruelty and ensure that the killing of wildlife, whether for population control and/or for sport, is in the hands of 'responsible' people (in the view of legislators), and regulated either by law (e.g. traps and poisons) or by internal regulatory bodies, such as the Masters of Foxhounds Association (MFA), or the more recent Independent Supervisory Authority on Hunting (ISAH).

The clear and simple intent of the 1996 Act is to punish the infliction of unnecessary suffering through wilful intent to commit acts that result in the death or mutilation of a wild animal. The problem with this is that no act that causes the death or mutilation of an animal used for sport can be strictly described as 'necessary'. By this definition, any person who deliberately commits any act that causes an animal to suffer or significantly increases the risk that it *might* suffer in the name of sport should be guilty of an act of cruelty. Strict interpretation of this principle could prohibit as unnecessary all the 'killing sports', i.e. hunting with or without hounds, shooting game, falconry and fishing. It could also prohibit any sport that exposed animals to a significant risk of severe injury or death such as National Hunt racing and Eventing. Once again, this illustrates the inadequacy of the phrase 'unnecessary suffering'. I suggest that it would be better to use the phrase 'unjustified suffering' as a basis for both ethical and legal judgements. This would permit exceptions to Article 1 of the Wild Mammals (Protection) Act 1996 only in circumstances where the practice could be justified, and strictly regulated, as part of an overall strategy to control or manage a population of wild animals used for sport in a way designed to minimise suffering through all acts of commission and omission throughout life, rather than simply at the point of death.

9.3 Ethical principles

It will be useful here to recapitulate briefly the principles of practical morality or 'common-sense ethics' outlined in Chapter 1. All ethics is based upon the principles of *right thought and right action*. Textbooks of moral philosophy tend to be written by thinkers and so emphasise right thought. However, I repeat the words of Thomas Carlyle: 'The end of a man is an action and not a thought, though it were the noblest'. Beauchamp & Childress (1994) have identified four principles for right action in the context of medical ethics: *beneficence, nonmaleficence, autonomy* and *justice*. In Chapter 1 the first two principles, 'do good' and 'do no harm', were condensed into *beneficence*, the single utilitarian responsibility to promote the wellbeing of animals in our care, with proper respect for the individual but, in many cases, action taken at the population level. Since in all sport hunting, whether with dog, rod or gun, there is a deliberate intention to do harm to some animals, this must be included as a separate column in the ethical matrix. The principle of autonomy implies respect for the intrinsic right of the animal: the right of a fox to live like a fox. I have argued already that whereas it is possible to apply the principle of 'do as you would be done by' to other people (who matter greatly in the overall ethical analysis), it is difficult to apply to non-human animals who have no mechanism that enables them to participate in such a reciprocal contract. The principle of autonomy as applied to wild animals within our dominion may be best interpreted by a policy that seeks to leave them well, alone. In practice, this means providing them with the habitat and resources to live their own lives in such a way that their needs conflict as little as possible with our own.

The concept of justice is more straightforward. Justice equates to fairness; in particular, fairness to those, like the animals in sport (all sports, not just killing sports), who do not volunteer for or stand to gain from the exercise (Rawls, 1972). Is it, for example, fair:

- to kill an animal or directly cause it to suffer simply to obtain personal pleasure?
- to use an animal for one's own recreational purposes, then kill it (humanely) when it has outlived its usefulness?
- to use an animal for one's own recreational purposes, then, when it has outlived its usefulness, sell or otherwise dispose of it to a destination where its welfare can no longer be assured?
- to increase the risks of injury or behavioural abnormalities in an animal in the interests of improving its sporting prowess?

I am aware that I am being drawn further than I intended into an ethically limited cost/benefit analysis. Nevertheless these are questions that cannot be dodged. These questions may appear at first sight to be no more than a list of strictly utilitarian concerns that weigh the costs to one party (the animals) in terms

Table 9.1 A comparison of the ethical principles involved in the use of animals for a variety of sports and for food.

	'Do good'	'Do no harm'	Autonomy	Justice
Fox hunting with hounds	Protects (e.g.) lambs, ground-nesting birds	Acute fear, pain	Freedom	None
Deer hunting with hounds	Provides food for people Provides food for deer Culls 'sufferers'	Fear, exhaustion	Freedom	Ranging rights
Deer stalking	Provides food for people Culls 'sufferers'	Injured escapees?	Freedom	Ranging rights
Coarse fishing	None	Fear, pain, exhaustion	None	None
Rearing pheasants	Provides food (for some)	Injured escapees?	Reasonable freedom	Feeding
Rearing broiler chickens	Provides cheap food	Pre-slaughter stress	None	None

of the benefits accruing to another party (us). However, they should not simply be evaluated in such terms since the principles of utilitarianism and justice do not always give the same answers. For example, the defence of hunting with hounds is usually based on (selected) utilitarian principles, namely that hunting preserves the habitat and therefore the fitness of the fox population. A more honest utilitarian argument would be that all animals but the fox are having a thoroughly good time: hounds, horses, huntsmen, even the hunt saboteurs. On strictly utilitarian grounds, the fox does not stand a chance. However, no moral argument can ignore the concept of justice. The key question, simply stated, becomes 'Is it just to kill foxes in this fashion?'

Table 9.1 uses these ethical principles to compare some of the ways we kill animals whether for sport or in the business of food production. The first set of examples compare the sports of fox hunting with hounds, deer hunting, either with hounds or by stalking and shooting, and coarse fishing. Next I compare the rearing of pheasants to be shot for food and fun with the rearing of broiler chickens to be killed with grim efficiency. Let us first examine the most contentious of all, namely hunting with hounds.

9.4 Fox hunting with hounds

The image of fox hunting in the eyes of those who follow the hunt, those who oppose it and those who simply look at hunting prints on pub walls is of a spectacle of horses and riders engaged in a mad gallop cross-country in pursuit of a

Table 9.2 Fox hunting statistics for England and Wales (2002/2003) prepared by the Independent Supervisory Authority on Hunting.

	Numbers	'Success' (% roused)	Allocation of kills (%)
Total days hunting	9072		
Number of foxes roused	48208		
Number of foxes hunted	31837	66	
Number caught in open field	5307	11	57
Number 'dug out'	4020	8.3	43

pack of hounds who are themselves in pursuit of a fox which they run down, kill and tear to pieces. Viewed simply as a spectacle, this image can arouse a variety of emotions ranging from exhilaration to abhorrence. While this is an accurate image of what happens in some hunts some of the time, the overall picture is rather more prosaic. Table 9.2 summarises some of the results presented in the first draft report on hunting practice published by the Independent Supervisory Authority on Hunting (www.isah.co.uk). This report is based on information provided by 147 hunts for the season 2002/2003. It includes nearly all the packs that hunt primarily for sport over the 'shires' of the English countryside. Very few reports were received from the hill packs of upland England and Wales. Table 9.2 reports 9324 foxes killed by these hunts, of which 57% were caught by the hounds in open field and 43% dug out of their earths and shot. The practice of 'digging out' is viewed with particular abhorrence by the opponents of hunting (see Burns, 2000) usually on the grounds that it is 'unfair'. The Masters of Foxhounds Association (MFHA) counter this criticism by stating that they will only permit 'digging out' and killing as a utility service at the written request of the landowner, normally because the fox presents a specific threat to the farmer's animals, such as newborn lambs or young pheasants. Some hunts have also used terriers to dig out and kill foxes suffering from starvation and hypothermia as a result of mange. This is a humanitarian service. Thus the practice of digging out and killing foxes is performed as a utility not as a sport. Although the hill packs have not yet provided detailed evidence, they claim that their primary purpose is to exterminate (often by shooting) foxes that present a specific threat to game birds and lambs.

Prior to drafting a Bill for the Regulation and/or prohibition of hunting with dogs, the UK government sought evidence from which to decide what practices (if any) could be justified on the basis of *cruelty* and *utility*. The Burns report (2000) on *Hunting with Dogs* had previously suggested that the use of dogs in hunting foxes (and other species such as mink) could be justified if it could be shown that the killing was necessary and that the participation of the dogs in the hunt was consistent with the aim to avoid wilful cruelty. This aim would be met if it could be shown that the contribution of the dogs either reduced the period of acute suffering prior to death and/or reduced the numbers of animals that suffered from chronic injury and pain following a non-lethal shot.

The pursuit of hunting that leads to the killing of foxes in open country by a pack of hounds followed at great expense by a herd of horses and riders could never be justified on the grounds of utility within the conventional economic sense of the word. It is, however, more valid to interpret utility within the context of a policy of efficient, sympathetic management of the living countryside that respects and gives due value to all sentient creatures, both animals with extrinsic value (e.g. lambs and pheasants) and wild animals with intrinsic value (e.g. foxes and ground-nesting skylarks). It is an undeniable fact of life that those who hunt the shires of England afford a high extrinsic value to sustaining a controlled population of healthy foxes (that give 'good sport'). Indeed, had the English countryman not enjoyed chasing the fox over the past centuries, the species would have been harried to extermination within the English shires, and its habitat plundered, with the consequence that the countryside would be less green and pleasant than it is today. It is equally undeniable that those who hunt over the shires for sport today are motivated by self-interest to preserve the fitness of the fox population by pre-serving habitat and helping to avoid overpopulation. This is a statement of fact, not a moral case. The moral argument states that we should seek to preserve the fox for its intrinsic value. This may involve some form of humane population control, but this should not depend on a killing method that is significantly cru-eller than other methods of population control.

This brings us to the nub of the debate: 'How cruel is hunting with hounds?' This is close to being an impossible question, but I shall attempt a partial answer. A fox may be harried by hounds for hours, but those that are killed in open country are run down after a final full-speed chase seldom lasting more than a minute. During that last minute we must acknowledge that the fox will experience both fear and pain. Ideally, death should involve no fear or pain. However, for a sen-tient wild animal (or human) a death that involves no more than a full minute of fear and pain must rank as one of the least distressing ways of dying. Instant death, following a successful shot, is even better, but a slow death after an unsuccessful shot much worse. The next question then becomes: 'How much do foxes suffer during the hunt prior to the final seconds?' Here the figures in Table 9.2 are of interest. The number of foxes caught and killed in open field was 5307 from a total of 48 208 roused and 31 837 hunted (i.e. actively pursued by the hounds). The percentages of roused and hunted foxes killed in open field were 11% and 17% respectively. Expressed in betting terms, the odds against a roused fox being killed in open field were 10:1, the odds against a hunted fox being killed were 6:1. Thus most of the time the fox escapes, and those that do not escape are killed only once. The logic that I have used throughout this book suggests that those foxes that survive the hunt learn by experience to cope with the stress of the hunt, expect to escape, and thus *may* not experience the distress arising from the perception that they are failing to cope until the very last seconds.

This argument is not intended as a justification for hunting foxes with hounds. It is, however, valid to conclude that the distress experienced by a fox that is dug out and shot having gone to earth will be far more prolonged than for one run down in open field. Thus, so far as the fox is concerned, death by hounds in open field in the interests of human sport is likely to be less distressing than death following the prolonged business of digging out for reasons of utility. It also follows that the more foxes killed in open field, the less will need to be dug out. The killing of foxes for fun may be a highly expensive and inefficient contributor to overall population control, but the evidence would suggest that the killing method itself does not, on balance, involve more and may involve less suffering than other, more utilitarian methods. This conclusion does not address the other element of the moral argument, namely that population control in a civilised society should not depend on people killing foxes for fun. If the (extremely good-looking) fox were rarer it would undoubtedly become a protected species. However, the absolutely amoral fact remains that one of the main reasons why the fox has not become an endangered species is that it carries a high extrinsic value for those who hunt. Speaking strictly as an advocate for the fox population I therefore advance the argument that those who derive value from the entertainment of the hunt should also carry the responsibility to repay that value by contributing positively to the lifetime welfare of the fox and other wild living creatures that coexist on the land over which they hunt.

The Independent Supervisory Authority on Hunting (of which I am a member) has established a protocol for the supervision and regulation of hunting with dogs. This protocol is based on the central principle of respect for all life in the countryside and founded on three pillars, namely humanity, utility and stewardship:

(1) *Humanity*: avoidance of unnecessary suffering.
(2) *Utility*: effective management of the quarry species.
(3) *Stewardship*: sensitive management of the living environment.

The parliamentary proposals for the regulation of hunting (with dogs) were designed to achieve least suffering and utility specifically in relation to the method of killing the quarry species. The ISAH protocol has a broader remit, expressed in the Burns report (2000) as the impact of hunting 'on the rural economy, agriculture and pest control, the social and cultural life of the countryside, the management and conservation of wildlife and animal welfare'. The impact of hunting (or a ban on hunting) on the rural economy is not relevant to the present argument. What is important is that the ISAH protocol calls the hunting communities to account for their stewardship of the whole living environment in the area over which they hunt. Because it is in the long-term interests of the hunting community to conserve and enrich the natural habitat, it should also become the responsibility of that community to make a long-term commitment to this end. ISAH is already exploring how the hunting communities can work with other environmentally conscious groups to enrich habitat and monitor the consequences for all wild creatures.

In suggesting that it might on balance be better for the animals not to ban hunting but to encourage poachers to become gamekeepers, hunters to become wildlife conservationists, I expect to arouse moral outrage in many of the animal welfare community. I do not feel too morally pure about these suggestions myself. Nevertheless, my aim is to encourage those who live in the countryside to do more to promote the quality of the living environment for all sentient life, and wild animals in particular. If this can be seen to work at ground level, then it matters little to me what is the view from the moral high peaks.

In summary therefore, I return to the ethical principles as outlined in Table 9.1. The practice of hunting the fox (by any means) can be said to do good because it protects other animals that may fall prey to the fox. It fails the test of 'do no harm', but it is valid to argue that the harm done to a fox killed in open field 'for sport' is not significantly worse than other forms of population control. A policy for regulation of hunting that incorporates the preservation and enrichment of habitat does respect its autonomy, its *telos*, the essential foxiness of the fox. As to justice for the fox, there is none. The regulation of fox hunting (*de jure*) is based on the premise that the fox is vermin so that the only permissible actions are those intended to keep the fox population down either by killing animals or by driving them away. In the hills, this is probably a fair reflection of what actually happens. In the shires those who seek to manage the fox population in such a way as to protect property but sustain good hunting are prohibited from making any direct positive contribution to fox welfare, whether by feeding them or the creation of artificial earths, but encouraged to contribute indirectly to their welfare through preservation of natural habitat. The principle is, of course, that the fox should be hunted 'in its natural state'. Enriching the natural state is consistent with the principle of *telos*. Hunting half-tame foxes for no good reason is not.

9.5 Deer hunting

The ethical rules of engagement governing the hunting of deer differ in many respects from those relating to the hunting of foxes. For a start, dead deer are eminently eatable. On this basis it is neither more nor less acceptable to kill a deer than to kill a broiler chicken. Deer are classified as game rather than vermin, which means that their 'owners' (those who permit red deer to graze their land) may provide them with food to sustain them prior to death whether by stalking and shooting in the highlands of Scotland or hunting with hounds on Exmoor in South-West England. This may, in extreme circumstances, involve carrying hay out onto the hill. However, for most practical purposes it involves giving the animals access to pasture that might otherwise have been used to support strictly commercial farm animals such as cattle and sheep. Thus according to the ethical principles of respect

Table 9.3 Welfare comparison of managing red deer by farming, stalking and hunting with hounds.

	Farming on lowland pasture	Stalking highland deer	Hunting with hounds
Nutrition	Generally good	Chronic hunger in winter	Generally good
Thermal comfort	Generally good	Cold stress on open moors	Generally good
Physical comfort	Generally good	Generally good	Generally good
Pain and injury	Treatment available	Culling possible	Culling available
Infectious disease	Controllable	Low incidence	Low incidence
Parasitism	Controllable	External parasites	Some risk
Natural behaviour	Restricted	Total freedom	Freedom
Fear and stress	Transport and slaughter	Natural incidence	Fear and exhaustion during hunt

(Table 9.1), the management of red deer meets the criterion of beneficence both because it provides food for (a few) people and because it seeks to preserve a population of healthy animals not only fit enough to hunt but also fit enough to eat. It may also help to reduce suffering by culling individuals suffering from chronic pain or disease. During their life, deer on open range have far more autonomy than any intensively managed farm animal. Moreover, permitting these wild animals to range on private property may be said to be fair. So far, so good. However, the biggest problem for deer hunters, particularly those who hunt with hounds, is to justify the method of killing. It is not enough to claim that natural death in the wild, e.g. through starvation or chronic disease, is likely to be much worse; it is necessary to demonstrate that when deer are 'used' for sport, both the chosen method of killing and the attention to lifetime welfare are consistent with the principle of least suffering.

Table 9.3 compares the welfare of farmed deer on lowland pastures with deer stalked and shot from a distance in the highlands and deer hunted with hounds to the point where they stand at bay and can be shot at close range. Farmed deer on lowland pastures are generally well fed and comfortable except in the most extreme weathers. Parasitism and infectious diseases are controllable and treatment or humane culling should be available for any individuals seriously injured or in acute pain. Natural behaviour is somewhat restricted but (so long as grazing is available) not to the point of causing distress. The problem for farmed deer comes during handling, transport and slaughter (see Chapter 7). Although the actual killing process may be humane, the duration, if not the intensity of stress imposed on farmed deer in the period prior to killing, greatly exceeds that experienced in either of the 'sporting' practices. By contrast, the practice of stalking and shooting highland deer is designed to kill the animal instantaneously (or produce loss of consciousness within a few seconds) as the result of a successful shot to the head or chest that hits the animal before it becomes aware that it is being stalked. As a method of killing, this is self-evidently more humane than the practice of rounding up farmed deer and transporting them for slaughter at an abattoir. It would appear more natural to allow red deer to range freely over the Scottish Highlands than to farm them in small paddocks in southern England. However, it does not necessarily improve their quality of life. Deer in the highlands are managed very extensively if at all. Moreover the harsh highlands of Scotland do not constitute a natural habitat for the red deer, which evolved in a more sheltered forest environment. A high proportion of highland deer die as a result of cold (especially in their first winter) and malnutrition. Thus stocking the bleak highlands with red deer for the purpose of sport may offer them the prospect of a better death, but it does not necessarily offer them a better life.

The population of red deer hunted by hounds on the moorlands of South-West England coexist with domestic ruminants in a milder environment and with easy access to improved pastures. This is undeniably a fit population. Moreover individuals that are suffering from chronic disease or injury are more easily spotted than in the highlands and can be culled by the hunt on humanitarian grounds. Indeed, the 2002/2003 report to ISAH revealed that 44% of the deer killed by the hunt were identified as casualty animals. Nevertheless, the use of hounds to hunt deer to bay does give serious cause for concern. A typical hunt begins when a small group of 'tufter' hounds are sent in to flush out an individual or group of deer preselected for hunting on that day. The first response of the deer is to run away. Since it can outrun the hounds, this strategy works, at first, and the deer stops to rest at a spot perceived to be safe. At this point the entire pack may be let loose to follow the scent line, catch up with the deer and harry it to move on. Eventually, after several escape runs covering in total 10–30 km and lasting from one to four hours, the deer will run no further and turn 'at bay' to face the hounds, often having made its last run downhill into water. At this point it is possible for one of the hunt staff to approach the stationary animal and shoot it with the high probability of ensuring (at last) a quick kill.

The key difference between a fox hunt and a deer hunt is that the fox is usually caught by the hounds while fresh and running at full speed, whereas the hounds only catch up with the deer when it can, apparently, no longer run fast enough to escape. This suggests that deer will only turn and stand at bay when they are physically exhausted, which implies that in the latter stages of the hunt deer will suffer both from physical exhaustion and profound fear arising from the knowledge that they can no longer cope with the physical demands of escape. This poses the vital question 'How long do they suffer?' Two groups have made physiological measurements on samples of material taken from deer after hunts of short and long duration. Bradshaw & Bateson (2000) addressed this question on behalf of the National Trust. Harris (1998) and colleagues were sponsored by the Countryside Alliance. Both groups made similar measurements with similar rigour and both, unsurprisingly, obtained similar results. However, this did not dissuade their sponsors from coming to diametrically opposed conclusions as to the intensity and duration of suffering experienced by the animals and therefore the acceptability or otherwise of the practice (National Trust = no; Countryside Alliance = yes). The results from both groups demonstrate conclusively that the deer turns at bay only when its muscles are glycogen depleted and can no longer sustain high-speed anaerobic metabolism so that it can no longer outrun the hounds. Where the two groups differ is in their estimate of the actual clinical damage to muscle and other tissues at this time, and therefore whether there will be prolonged suffering in animals allowed to escape. What neither can conclude from their data is how long the deer may have suffered the physical effects of extreme fatigue before it elects to stand at bay. The Harris group, moreover, do not address the more important problem of mounting fear in an animal that becomes progressively aware that its attempts to escape are in vain.

When asked to defend the practice of hunting deer on humanitarian grounds, its advocates contend that the duration of suffering (failure to cope) is not excessive. It is considerably longer than any suffering caused by an accurate shot from a stalker. However, they argue on utilitarian grounds that when unsuccessful shots that wound but do not kill are taken into account, the totality of suffering may be greater when deer are shot at from a distance without having first been brought to bay. The strength of this argument depends, of course, on accurate knowledge of wounding rates in different circumstances. Current estimates advanced by opposing sides of the debate range wildly from <2% to >15%. None is convincing.

To return to the overall welfare equation as illustrated by Table 9.3, red deer on Exmoor are effectively 'ranched' in a relatively gentle climate and in a way consistent with the Five Freedoms throughout most of their lives. In life, their freedom of natural expression is superior to farmed deer and their overall physical fitness probably better than that of highland deer. Prior to death they will suffer, although, when it comes, death is swift and certain. The intensity of suffering is likely to be much greater than in deer transported for slaughter in an abattoir, although the duration of suffering will be less. However, it is impossible to 'score' the two killing methods on the basis of the equation for overall suffering (Intensity × Duration × Incidence) since we simply do not have the evidence either for wounding rates in shot deer or how long hunted deer suffer from the physical and mental sensation of failing to cope. This debate could run and run and generate an infinite succession of 'scientific' studies that would, I fear, totally fail to alter the value judgements of the pros and antis at the opposite poles of the argument. As always, I suggest the moral case for any form of killing, whether for sport or utility, has to be based on the principle of least suffering. The case against deer hunting with hounds can be made on the basis that the animal's suffering may be not only unacceptably long but also unnecessarily prolonged in the interests of ensuring a good day's hunting. The only defence open to the deer hunting community is to declare their intent to manage the hunt so as to bring the deer to bay as quickly and efficiently as possible and to provide evidence from hunt records to demonstrate their success and continuing improvement in this respect.

9.6 Hare coursing

The sport of hare coursing is, in essence, a competition between greyhounds. Bets are taken. Hares are driven onto the course. Two greyhounds are unleashed and points awarded to the one that gives best chase (with marks for stylistic impression). Most hares escape, but some are killed. The number of hares harmed may be small relative to those chased, but the fact remains that harm is done and this can only be justified if it is set against some good, e.g. efficient wildlife management, enrichment of habitat, etc. I am unaware of any evidence to this effect.

9.7 Shooting game birds

Birds such as pheasant, partridge and grouse are defined as 'game'. They are managed and in some cases reared by professional gamekeepers to service the sport of game shooting. It is undeniable that the meat from these game birds is a delicacy and that the quality of the meat reflects in large part the natural habitat in which the birds spend all (or some) of their lives. Nevertheless the value of the meat makes a trivial contribution to the cost of maintaining habitat and paying the gamekeepers. The extrinsic value of these birds is conferred by those who pay a lot of money for a day's shooting.

Most pheasant shooting involves animals that are farmed for the purpose. Young birds are reared artificially, then turned out into an enriched, essentially natural woodland environment, before being put up before the guns by beaters with dogs and given a 'sporting chance' to escape. Not all shot birds will be killed outright, but the presence of retriever dogs ensures that badly wounded animals are likely to be retrieved. Death, for most birds, is likely to involve much less suffering that that experienced by broiler chickens during catching, transportation and shackling prior to slaughter*. Moreover, the quality of life for the game birds is undeniably superior to that of the intensively reared broiler chicken. I believe that no one who eats broiler chicken can sustain a moral argument against the practice of rearing and shooting game birds. Indeed, shooting game birds may be cited as a classic example of the T.S. Eliot moral paradox 'doing the right thing for the wrong reason' since it does what I have advocated throughout this book, namely afford a much higher value to the animals that we kill and eat.

---

* Shooting game birds falls unequivocally within the category 'hunting with dogs'. The springers increase utility by flushing the birds towards the guns. The retrievers increase humanity by capturing injured birds.

9.8 Fishing

It has been a common and honestly held belief amongst fishermen that hooked fish do not feel pain or, at least, do not suffer distress in a way similar to ourselves or even, perhaps, the fox. The Medway Report (1979) on welfare aspects of shooting and angling quotes Gathorne-Hardy: 'I do not believe that salmon feel very acutely, a reassuring theory for the tender-hearted fisherman. The desperate struggle of the fish to get free confirms the same view. Not all the instinct of self-preservation would induce a man to put a strain of even a pound if the hook were attached to some tender part of his flesh'. This assertion makes an excellent subject for scientific and ethical debate. Is the violent struggle of the fish to escape:

- instinctive, involving no element of consciousness whatever?
- consciously deliberate but forceful because the fish feels no pain from the hook?
- genuinely 'desperate' because the fish experiences both fear and pain, but the intensity of fear is the greater?

If the first premise is true, then hooking and catching a fish involves no suffering whatsoever. If the second is true, then the fish may experience some distress but no pain. If the last is true, then the distress induced by capture is so great that it forces the fish to submit itself to extreme pain in its efforts to escape. Gathorne-Hardy's comment that 'Not all the instinct of self-preservation would induce a man to put a strain of even a pound if the hook were attached to some tender part of his flesh' is clearly the assertion of a man who has never been put to the test. Not only snared foxes but also a trapped mountaineer have made the decision to hack off a trapped limb in order to survive.

Most of the 'scientific' literature has, until recently, tended towards uncritical support for the presumption that fish feel no pain, based largely on the quite invalid premise that the fish brain does not contain the zone known to be involved in pain perception in man (e.g. Rose, 2002). Even without its own limited scientific context, this argument is invalid, given what is now known about the plasticity of information processing within the brain. The more obvious criticism is, of course, that it makes the presumption that fish feel no pain without actually asking the fish.

In *Eden I* (Webster, 1994), I described the study by Verheijen and colleagues at the University of Utrecht designed to discover whether freshwater carp experience pain and fear-like sensations when hooked and captured. These experiments involved hooking alone, hooking and 'playing' (applying tension to the line), electrical stimulation by telemetry to the roof of the mouth and triggering alarm responses by release of pheromones from damaged skin. Fish showed physiological and behavioural responses indicative of alarm to all stimuli. When the hook was left in the mouth but there was no tension on the line, the response diminished. When the line was pulled and the fish sensed that it was captured, the alarm response was greatest. This evidence is entirely consistent with the conclusion that these fish exhibited a graded emotional response to stimuli known to cause fear and pain in sentient animals. Whether or not this involved a cognitive element is immaterial to the question of suffering, for reasons given in Chapter 3. Recent elegant studies by Sneddon *et al.* (2003) have reinforced the conclusions of the Utrecht team in regard to lasting pain induced by injection of a nociceptive chemical. They have demonstrated the existence of pain-sensitive neurones in the mouth and behavioural changes indicative (at least) of chronic discomfort. The balance of evidence is therefore in favour of the last premise, namely that the response of the hooked fish is genuinely 'desperate' because it experiences both fear and pain, but the intensity of fear is the greater.

It follows from this that anyone who elects to fish for sport must accept the fact that it almost certainly does cause some degree of suffering. This brings it into exactly the same category as hunting the fox or deer and forces the question 'Can this suffering be justified?' This at once creates a distinction between catching fish once, to be eaten (game fishing and sea fishing), and coarse fishing for species that will not be eaten but stored in a keep net, weighed, maybe photographed and then thrown back to be caught again another day. At first sight, catching without killing may seem the more humane alternative. However, the fish that is hooked, played, landed, stored in a keep net, then thrown back in the water at the end of the day has been hurt by the hook, frightened by the capture, bruised by contact with the keep net, then returned to the water in an injured state, probably to be caught again at a later date. Such fish are likely to suffer longer and more often than those caught and killed for food.

9.9 Horse riding

Horsey sports evolved from the fundamental need of humans to select and breed from animals deemed superior, according to our needs; horses that ran faster, stayed longer or responded better to control. On the grounds of autonomy, it may be argued that animals should have the right not to participate in sport if they do not want to. However, most sporting events with horses (except polo and bull-fighting) are based simply on exploitation of the animals' natural motivation to run and jump. Horses (and greyhounds) appear to participate in running sports as enthusiastic amateurs. No one forces a greyhound to race and there are strict penalties for excessive use of the whip in horseracing. Moreover horses have to be trained as amateurs. Unlike human athletes, they cannot be persuaded to run through the pain barrier again and again, in the expectation that this will improve their performance in a critical race six months hence. It is reasonable therefore to conclude that when horses are properly trained for the running and jumping events, this can be done without directly compromising their wellbeing.

However, horse riding is a risky business for both horse and rider. In justice, therefore, it is fair to ask the question 'Do horses experience fear during, or in anticipation of events such as a steeplechase?' Riders do for certain. This does not stop them competing, but they do, at least, have freedom of choice. How is it for the horses? I once heard a very famous event rider refer to the 'Badminton virgins', young horses who took on the entire cross-country course, even in the most appalling conditions, with great enthusiasm, but who sometimes, if their memory of the event was really bad, never again managed to recapture that first fine careless rapture. This implies that they acquired, by experience, an element of fear; not necessarily sufficient to cause suffering but sufficient to introduce an element of caution when next they faced the course. In short, they had learnt to cope.

The main moral issues concerning riding events with horses are likely to arise from consequences of the event rather than from the event itself. These include:

- risks of death and injury incurred during competition;
- risks of injuries attributable to racing thoroughbreds at a very early age (two- to three-year-olds);
- suffering attributable to lack of care in animals that have outlived their usefulness.

Sudden death, e.g. a horse that falls and breaks its neck in a steeplechase, is not a cause of suffering; in fact it may be the most humane death possible, equivalent to the old man dropping dead on the golf course. However, is it fair to submit a horse to increased risk of sudden death? If the horse was fit and running with enthusiasm at the time of the accident, I do not see any injustice. If the horse was unfit to start, or clearly needed to be pulled up, that is another matter. Injuries (to horses) associated with riding events range from (e.g.) immediate, severe conditions such as bone fractures to chronic states of unsoundness attributable to tendon injuries. The designers of cross-country courses have an obligation not to 'wantonly or unreasonably' incur risk to life and limb of horse and rider, but they are also under pressure to make their courses more demanding for the competitors and more thrilling for the spectators. When injury does occur, the main welfare problems for the animal are pain and incapacity to behave as normal. It is important to distinguish between acute and chronic pain. Much has been made of the argument that horses (and other athletes) appear to be insensitive to acute pain in the period immediately following a severe injury such as a fracture of the lower limb, for reasons that are usually attributed to secretion of endorphins (the natural opiates). While this may be so, there is overwhelming evidence that horses experience chronic pain in a similar way to humans. Moreover, the chronic pain that accompanies lasting injury does not appear to be eased by endorphins. Indeed, it is often associated with a state of hyperalgesia, or increased sensitivity, which increases the intensity of the conscious sensation (Wall & Melzack, 1994; Whay et al., 1998). It may be morally acceptable to enter horses for events that carry a significant risk of causing pain through injury. It is not morally acceptable to ignore the long-term painful consequences of any such injury.

If we elect to use any animal for our lasting entertainment then we should, in justice, assume responsibility for its entire life. If we can arrange for our old horse to live out its retirement in comfort and the good company of other horses, then that will not only make us feel good, but also be morally right. If we cannot manage this, then we can only guarantee that it will not suffer if we arrange for it to be killed humanely. It is an injustice to sell off a horse that has become surplus to requirements with no thought for the quality of its future life.

9.10 Greyhound racing

Most of what I have written about horse racing applies to greyhound racing. I note here only two points of difference. Greyhounds running (without a jockey aboard) are indulging voluntarily in the most natural of behaviour. Retired greyhounds make excellent companions and are therefore worth saving. (Readers should note that there I am employing neither autonomy nor justice in that last sentence.)

9.11 Bullfighting and rodeo

What these sports have in common is that they both involve violent competition between man and animal. The differences are differences of degree, but they are substantial. Consider, for example, contests between man and cattle. These include:

- Bullfighting:
  - Spanish style: the bull is fought and killed, unnecessarily slowly and after incurring both injury and exhaustion.
  - Portugese style: the bull is fought but not killed. It is, however, injured by the banderillas which have to be removed after the contest.
- Rodeo:
  - Bullriding: a bull is goaded out of the shute and spurred by the cowboy, whom it attempts to remove. After eight seconds the bull wins (according to its terms).
  - Calf roping: a young calf is lassoed by a cowboy on horseback, pulled over and trussed up.
  - Steer wrestling: a cowboy leaps off a horse across the horns of a yearling steer and attempts to wrestle it to the ground.
  - Chilean rodeo: two men on horseback first control the movement of a young ox within an arena, then charge it on horseback so that the horse knocks the ox to the ground.

Odberg (1992) reviewed the welfare implications of bullfighting (for bulls and horses). It is undeniable that both forms of bullfighting cause unnecessary suffering. The legal justification for the suffering differs, of course, in different countries. However, since it is most unlikely that bullfighting will ever be permitted in any society other than those where it is already embedded within the culture, I shall not dwell on it further here.

Most of the events in rodeo are based on skills that were (and often still are) essential to the cowboy managing semi-wild beef cattle on the open range. All the events listed above plus, of course, riding and spurring bucking broncos (horses) are designed to cause the animals some degree of stress. The first question, as always, is does this imposition of stress cause the animals to suffer? Calf roping, which is arguably the most functional of events, may be the one most likely to cause suffering. The young calf is isolated, forcibly thrown down and trussed up. Clearly this is an aversive experience. The degree of suffering will depend on how aversive the experience and how often the same calf is used.

Bucking horses and bulls used for the riding and spurring events are used again and again. A systematic study of their behaviour would reveal just how aversive this activity was (or was not) for different individuals. My own limited experience would suggest that most broncos stand quietly in the shute before release and leave the arena quietly with other horses after parting company with their rider. Bulls frequently attack their dismounted rider and have to be distracted by the rodeo clowns (but then trot back to their pens and resume feeding). What one does not see are signs of reluctance to enter the arena or learned helplessness. I am satisfied that these animals are stressed during the events but do not suffer. Moreover, they are maintained in a state of high fitness. The rodeo bull, in my opinion, receives a fairer deal from man than the dairy bull that spends its entire adult life within the confines of a bull pen.

Chilean rodeo, which uses two horses to control the movement of an ox, also celebrates the traditional riding skills of the herdsman. However, the final pass, in which the ox is knocked over twice against a (cushioned) barrier appears distressing and entirely pointless to me (and most Chileans). This is, in my opinion, only acceptable provided the oxen are used no more than once. Steer wrestling is just silly. Some of the steers may be hurt sometimes. The cowboys hurt themselves all the time.

9.12 Conclusions

It is an act of cruelty to cause unnecessary suffering to an animal by 'doing or omitting to do any act'. Since death is the end of suffering, what matters most is what we do (or do not do) to animals while they are alive. Although animals do not volunteer, they do partake in most competitive (non-killing) sports as enthusiastic amateurs. Some of these sports carry a significant risk of pain and injury.

Whenever we choose to use an animal for our own sporting entertainment we must, in justice to that animal, assume the responsibility for its wellbeing (health and happiness) for life.

'Field sports' (hunting, shooting and fishing) are based on the deliberate intention to kill or injure another animal. The fact that some humans derive pleasure from killing some animals raises profound questions about the nature of human morality but is of no direct concern to the animals; what concerns them is the manner of their own life and death. A case can be made for field sports on the utilitarian grounds that they help to preserve the habitat and fitness of the hunted species (whatever the means of killing). Justice, however, decrees that, whatever other arguments may be in play, each individual animal should be killed by the most humane method possible.

Animals as Pets

10

Dogs have owners, cats have staff.

Anon.

For the sake of those approaching this book in non-linear fashion, I must point out (again) that our approach to the animals we keep as pets (or 'companions' if you will) is fundamentally the same as our approach to those animals we use for food or for science. Most people love their pets, care for them to the point of death or terminal illness and are prepared to spend a great deal of money on veterinary services. Nevertheless, the fact remains that when we choose a pet, we select for our special attention an individual from a species compatible with our wishes, and usually from a breed that has been modified by us in a way that satisfies our personal whims. We then introduce it to an environment designed primarily for our convenience and interact companionably with it at times of our own choosing. Applying the rules of ethics, we can acknowledge that owners do seek to promote the wellbeing of their pets on a day-to-day basis (utilitarianism). Moreover most owners commit themselves to care for their pets for life. This reflects the fact that love for one's pet carries a very high extrinsic value. It also (up to a point) recognises the principle of autonomy by accepting that one's pet has an equal right to a full life span as oneself. A strict utilitarian would see no more problem in humanely killing a pet dog than a dry cow once it had lost its utility (e.g. it had become inconvenient to keep). However, no category of animal keeping has greater potential to compromise the autonomy, the *telos*, of an animal than keeping it in human company and denying it the company of its own kind.

In this chapter I shall review the principles of husbandry and ethics as applied to the keeping of pets, with special reference to the welfare of dogs, cats, horses and rabbits as examples of four very different categories of pet.

- The dog has adapted through evolution to life within a hierarchy that may involve a pack of other dogs, or humans and will acknowledge the 'ownership' of the pack leader, who will, in the case of pet dogs, be a human.
- The cat is naturally adapted to doing as it pleases. It will, however, amiably and affectionately interact with its human staff provided that they meet its needs. If not, it will probably push off.

- The horse is naturally adapted to life grazing the open plains within a herd of other horses. It can be trained, by breaking or gentling, to adapt its natural behaviour to suit human wishes, but, unlike the dog, it does not view itself as one of the family.
- Rabbits, guinea pigs, hamsters and other small animals that may be categorised as caged furry pets appear to enjoy human contact when being petted. However, when not being petted (i.e. most of the time) a solitary rabbit in a cage within the house or garden is rather worse off than in the average zoo, where it should, at least, be able to experience social contact with others of its kind.

In reviewing the welfare of these four categories of pet animal I shall assume for the most part that their owners have made proper provision for feeding, housing and health care. In these circumstances welfare problems are most likely to result from an imposed lifestyle that is inconsistent with natural patterns of behaviour. Deliberate cruelty to pets, whether by act of omission or neglect, is a separate subject that I shall consider later, with special reference to what may be deemed in law to constitute unnecessary suffering.

10.1 Behavioural problems in pet animals

Table 10.1 identifies five potential categories of behavioural problems: disturbances of oral behaviour, maintenance behaviour, social behaviour (animal-to-animal and animal-to-human) and, finally, sexual behaviour. Within these categories it lists examples of behavioural problems for the four classes of pet – dogs, cats, horses and rabbits. Disturbances of oral behaviour are mostly linked to inappropriate systems of feeding. Disturbances of maintenance behaviour may be attributed to

Table 10.1 Potential behavioural problems associated with keeping dogs, cats, horses and rabbits as pets.

	Dogs	**Cats**	**Horses**	**Rabbits (etc.)**
Oral behaviour	Stealing food	Faddiness	Oral stereotypies, e.g. crib-biting, wind sucking	Overgrown incisors
Maintenance behaviour	Separation anxiety Stereotypies, e.g. tail-chasing		Movement stereotypies, e.g. weaving, box walking	Movement stereotypies
Social behaviour animal-to-animal	Fighting	(Fighting)	Isolation anxiety	Fighting
animal-to-human	Aggression			
Sexual behaviour		Exhaustion		

an unsatisfactory physical and social environment. Disturbances of social and sexual behaviour are commonly linked to inadequate social contact with other animals and humans, especially during the critical 'socialisation' phase of early development. I shall consider the problems faced by each category of pet in turn. Blank spaces in Table 10.1 imply that a particular category of abnormal behaviour does not present a significant problem for a particular species (although some individuals might be affected).

10.2 Dogs

The natural oral behaviour of dogs is to 'wolf down' large meals at high speed and relatively infrequent intervals. The physiological and behavioural needs of the wild carnivore are to consume as much as possible in one meal, then rest to digest and conserve energy before the next hunt. Thus adult dogs will adapt readily to one large meal per day which they will consume with great enthusiasm and apparently little regard as to its constituents. Growing puppies will, of course, need to be fed more often. It is natural for the healthy dog to be greedy and it will, if given the chance, solicit and consume treats or scraps from the table in amounts greatly in excess of its needs. Thus the pet dog is naturally predisposed to obesity. Nevertheless it is even more natural for the dog to go for many hours without food so that once-daily feeding should not be associated with behavioural problems.

Stealing food can present a problem. Strictly speaking, stealing is a meaningless concept for non-human animals since they have no sense of property. If food is available and there is no obvious obstruction or penalty involved in obtaining it, then the natural instinct of any animal will be to take and eat it. For any pet animal other than the dog, the owner will have the good sense to keep food out of sight and out of mind except at meal times. However, many owners are able to train their dogs to the point where they can trust them to display complete obedience to their wishes (and remember what those wishes are) even when presented by extreme temptation in the form of a piece of chocolate or chicken. Clearly, a dog, in common with any sentient animal, can be trained to forego an immediate reward if it expects this to be associated with an immediate and more severe punishment. However, I believe (without firm scientific evidence) that dogs, perhaps uniquely among the animals in my experience, do display an emotion that can best be described as guilt. The trained dog that has stolen food or urinated within the house will typically display signs of extreme anxiety and appeasement even when the punishment that it has come to expect from its owner may be no more that a stern look or word. The parsimonious evolutionary biologist may be correct in asserting that such behaviour is simply a primitive emotional response in an animal that promotes fitness by placing a very high value on the approval of the pack leader. However, it is also possible that the old incontinent dog that has urinated in the house displays signs of extreme distress because it may be able to imagine not only how its owner may act but also how he/she may *feel*. I repeat I have no sound scientific evidence to support this suggestion, which is a shame because it touches on one of the most exciting and unresolved questions in animal psychology, namely the 'theory of mind' (Sodian *et al.*, 2003). This theory addresses the question 'In what species and in what circumstances can human and non-human animals put themselves into the mind of another individual, guess at what it is likely to do (or feel) and modify its behaviour accordingly?' To date, most 'theory of mind' studies in non-human animals have been based on the ability to practise deception; the deliberate intention of one animal to manipulate the mind of another towards making the wrong choice. Moreover most of these studies have involved apes in captivity (e.g. Povinella & Vonk, 2003), chosen presumably on the basis of an argument recognised as fallacious by Darwin, namely that apes are closest to humans and have therefore evolved 'furthest'. Even here the evidence in favour of the 'theory of mind' is equivocal. I have no evidence to confirm my intuition that a dog knows how its master feels, not least because most people are reluctant to 'do science' with dogs on the basis that both the dogs and their handlers would get too emotional if made to participate in the sort of psychological tests routinely imposed on rats. Nevertheless I suggest that dogs, by virtue of their extremely close emotional attachment to humans, would make excellent subjects for studies of complex patterns of feeling and cognition and expressed by behaviour such as guilt and deception. Dogs are ubiquitous and demonstrably enjoy doing things in response to human bidding. Some 'scientists' may claim that it is only possible to study a dog scientifically in the laboratory rather than in the home. If so, they are not very bright (the scientists, not the dogs).

Some of the most important behavioural problems in dogs may arise from breeding and training programmes that are based not on the exploitation of natural motivation (e.g. like the motivation of the horse to run) but on the frustration of normal behaviour. Many dogs are bred and trained to hunt but not attack (e.g. working sheepdogs) or gather food without eating it (e.g. retrievers of game birds). When a dog has been trained to distort its natural patterns of behaviour on command, it should not be a surprise when it appears to overreact to this frustration when not under control. There is much anecdotal evidence that retrievers find it particularly hard to overcome the motivation to 'steal' food and that working collies are particularly prone to display misplaced aggression to humans, other dogs or seriously stupid targets such as motor vehicles.

The category of maintenance behaviour identified in Table 10.1 is, in this context, intended to cover all routine activities in the dog's day other than those related to eating and drinking, social and sexual behaviour. Thus it includes activities related towards normal behavioural needs such as running and playing, grooming, resting and investigative behaviour (sniffing, searching) motivated either by expectation or by signals of an important event, such as the return of its owner, or simply by inherent curiosity. During a typical day a typical dog will be variously motivated to seek the following rewards: rest and sleep, lively activities broadly similar to those involved in hunting (like running and chasing sticks) and especially the joy they experience at the appearance of their owners. Thus the dog who senses and confidently anticipates the arrival of its owner will experience a pleasurable form of anticipation. The dog that is distressed following separation from its owner and not confident of his or her return may experience anxiety.

10.2.1 Separation anxiety

Separation anxiety is a major welfare problem among dogs isolated all day while their owners are at work. Evidence of separation anxiety visible on return from work includes chewed furniture and scratched doors. A video recorder (or a neighbour) may observe a wide range of abnormal behaviours during the period of separation including extreme restlessness, barking, whining, compulsively repeated (stereotypic) visits to doors and windows and possibly more injurious activities such as self-mutilation.

The aetiology of separation anxiety in dogs is complex (Schwartz, 2003). There are breed and strain differences in susceptibility. The overall anxiety of the dog may be profoundly influenced by its social contacts during early development and by the extent to which it has become dependent upon a particular individual. However, the primary cause of separation anxiety is undoubtedly isolation from contact with other members of the social group (dogs, adult humans and children). The symptoms (and the distress) can sometimes be reversed by habituating the animal to progressively long periods of absence starting at about 30 minutes. This approach can be reinforced if the dog is fed a bulky meal before leaving the house. This will motivate the animal to sleep so that it will not experience a sense of panic on its owner's departure, and wake, hopefully, in a relaxed state and adapted to spending some time on its own. It is equally important not to make too much of a fuss of the animal on one's return, so that the acts of both going away and coming home become far less emotional. Anxiolytic drugs may also be used, preferably in association with behavioural therapy. Separation anxiety is a significant source of suffering for many dogs. All responsible dog owners should ask themselves the question: 'Is it fair to keep an animal for my pleasure if I am unable to provide the physical and social resources necessary to ensure that it is not subject to unnecessary suffering?' Moreover the word 'necessary' needs to be viewed from all angles. The owner may justify the necessity to leave the dog alone while he/she goes to work. It may be less easy to justify the necessity of continuing to keep a dog in circumstances that cause it to suffer on a daily basis.

10.2.2 Aggression

Aggression is an entirely natural part of the behavioural repertoire of any sentient animal, since it is consistent with evolutionary fitness and, in the case of the breeding male, almost always a prerequisite for evolutionary fitness. In nature, however, most aggressive encounters (except perhaps between males in the breeding season) tend to be restricted to non-injurious rituals of posture and display designed to maintain the stability of the hierarchy. Many well-trained, well-socialised dogs have adapted these rituals to encounters with other dogs in the park and with visitors to the home. Uncontrolled, injurious aggression may not strictly qualify as a welfare problem (for the aggressor), but it is undoubtedly a social problem that may be attributed, at least in part, to abnormalities of breeding and environment imposed by humans. Some breeds (e.g. Dobermann, Rottweiler) have been bred for aggression in the interests of protecting humans and their property. Others (e.g. terriers) have been bred for aggression with the specific intention of increasing their ability to kill and maim other animals (e.g. ratting, digging out foxes, organised dog fights). Uncontrolled or misdirected acts of aggression in such breeds may present problems for these dogs and their owners, but they are not, in the strictest sense, abnormal. More serious are the problems of pathological aggression which can have a variety of causes ranging from dominance – the animal that seeks to establish and maintain itself as leader of the pack – through to fear – the animal that is so unsure of its place in the hierarchy that it nips strangers, then runs away.

Because this is a book on animal welfare not animal behaviour, it is not the place to discuss in detail all the neuroses that may afflict the modern domesticated dog. However, the common thread that runs through all these problems is that too many dogs are bred and kept in a fashion that seriously compromises their freedom to perform natural behaviour. Those of us who derive great joy from the companionship and sheer fun of owning a dog will normally find it easy to apply the ethical principles of beneficence and autonomy; we shall give respect to our duty of care and the dog's right to life. However, in the name of justice, we must always ask ourselves the question 'Are we being fair?'

10.3 Cats

My list of welfare problems for the domestic cat (Table 10.1) is refreshingly short. This is largely because most cats have accepted a form of domestication that interferes as little as possible with their natural behaviour. Most domestic cats, except in the most urban of environments, come and go as they please and succeed in their aim of doing what it takes to feel good most of the time. Indeed, I can confidently assert that the neutered, but free-ranging, domestic cat has a far better life than the sexually entire feral cat. I am less sanguine about the case of the cat that is kept permanently indoors in a small apartment and may have had its claws removed to stop it from damaging the furniture*. Denying cats the opportunity to explore, hunt, mate and sharpen their claws all constitute a breach of the fifth freedom – to perform natural behaviour. However, I have already argued that for

* Not permitted in the UK.

all of us, this should be interpreted as the freedom to perform most socially accept-able, non-injurious forms of natural behaviour (which many would argue should exclude promiscuous sex and murdering birds). As always, the more important question is not 'Is this animal in a natural environment?' but 'Is this animal in an environment to which it can adapt without suffering?'

Any mutilation is, by definition, an insult to the *telos* of any sentient animal and it may be argued that mutilation of the organs of reproduction constitutes the most profound insult of all. However, the ethical matrix will always require us to balance our respect for the autonomy of the animal with whom we share our life with our duty of care for its daily wellbeing. When assessed by the welfare crite-ria of 'fit and feeling good', neutering obviously destroys fitness in strictly evolu-tionary terms, but, on balance, for the cat, it should make a positive contribution to feeling good. The evolutionary reason for the mating urge in animals is to ensure the genetic inheritance. Nevertheless their *motivation* towards all behaviours con-ducive to survival and reproductive success is not directed by an understanding of Darwinian principles but by the emotional need to feel good (at the time) and this is most obviously true for sexual behaviour. When the motivation for sex is high so too is the potential for sexual frustration. The sex urge differs from the sensa-tions of hunger or thirst in that it does not *have* to be satisfied. Male dogs, cats and horses have the potential to be aroused at any time but the motivational stim-ulus to action appears to be largely external: the presence of a female in oestrus or, in the case of confused dogs, a fetishistic object such as the leg of a chair or neighbour. Most female animals are only motivated towards sex around the period of ovulation. In female dogs this usually occurs for two periods of the year, amounting to about four weeks in all. Given also that most pet dogs only leave the house when under the control of their owners, keeping a bitch sexually entire should not present any special problems to either dog or owner.

Circumstances for the cat are entirely different. The cat that is free to roam is practically guaranteed sexual contact. Cats normally have two breeding seasons, in spring and autumn. During this time they will come on heat repeatedly. More-over ovulation, which naturally concludes the period of heat, only occurs in response to mating. If they do not mate, these heat periods may last up to ten days. Thus most sexually entire female cats may spend most of their adult lives either 'calling' (on heat), pregnant or lactating. In these circumstances female cats cer-tainly fail to sustain fitness and I believe they suffer feelings of exhaustion. Male cats do not have to bear the long-term consequences of copulations past, but they are compelled to fight for the right to continue. Given that most neutered cats maintain their enthusiasm for outdoor pursuits such as hunting, in between long, hedonistic, entirely natural periods of sleep in the warmest spot in the house, and given that neutering makes it possible for them to carry out these pursuits without becoming sexually compromised, I am convinced that the quality of life of the free-ranging domestic cat is positively enhanced by neutering.

The cat that is confined indoors all day, every day (with or without claws) is denied a very wide range of natural expression of behaviour. According to the limited utilitarian principle of responsibility to prevent suffering, it is reasonable to argue that the intermittently isolated housebound cat is less likely to suffer than the isolated dog. Behaviours indicative of separation anxiety have been reported in cats, but the incidence is low relative to that for dogs, not least because cats are far less emotionally bound to their owners. As always, the question for any potential owner contemplating keeping a cat in such confinement must be 'Is it fair?' I would not do it myself. However, my advice to those wishing to keep cats in a high-rise apartment or similar circumstances where going out is not an option is: (1) keep two cats (at least) so they can benefit from the company of their own kind, and (2) if any cat develops disturbed patterns of behaviour indicative of suffering, then the owner must assume the responsibility to find the cat a better home or, failing that, destroy it.

Table 10.1 lists 'faddiness' as a potential problem of oral behaviour for the domestic cat. Almost every owner will recognise the problem of the cat that absolutely rejects a food preparation that it consumed with apparent relish yesterday. One instructive way of passing the time in a supermarket is to study anxiety behaviour in cat owners wandering vaguely among long shelves of cat food offering a stupefying variety of brands and flavours and wondering what Pussy might fancy today. It is probable that many cats are spoiled for choice. There are, however, features of the metabolism of the cat, an obligate carnivore, that suggest a more fundamental problem. Cats evolved on a diet of small wild animals, which consist mostly of protein and water. The amount of protein they would naturally consume is far in excess of that which they require for the specific purpose of synthesising and maintaining their own protein reserves. Most of their dietary protein is used as an energy source after deamination and excretion of the excess nitrogen as urea. There is good evidence from many animals that an accumulation of urea or other intermediary products of protein oxidation may create a feeling of malaise and this may create an aversion for the food that has produced this feeling. Thus it is entirely possible (although unproven) that a cat will suddenly reject a particular brand of food because last time it ate it, it felt ill. On the safe grounds that the cat that absolutely rejects its meal is either (1) off its food or (2) playing a trick on you, then the correct action is to remove the food and replace it with something very different, not now, but at the next meal.

Many cats are also reluctant to drink tap water and this can present special problems when dry food constitutes most or all of the diet. Most water 'fresh from the tap' contains enough chlorine to deter a cat and the problem is exacerbated when the 'fresh' water comes in a plastic dish. Water that is contained in porcelain and exposed to the air for some time, as in the toilet bowl, is much more palatable to cats. However, genuinely fresh rain water is to be preferred. Urban cat owners may wish to contemplate ways of gathering rain water. Failing that they could always hunt the supermarket shelves for a mineral water of choice.

10.4 Horses

Horses managed professionally – on a stud farm, in a racing stable or a livery yard – should have a good chance of achieving most of their physiological and behavioural needs. These include provision of appropriate food and water, reasonable physical and thermal comfort and prompt attention to problems of health and injury. They can also expect regular social contact with other horses and the satisfaction of daily grooming from devoted attendants. Nevertheless, despite the amount of time, care and money lavished on these high-value animals, welfare problems do occur. The welfare implications of injuries experienced by horses employed as athletes for the business of sport were discussed in Chapter 9. If we leave aside obvious cases of cruelty and neglect, the most serious welfare problems for stabled horses are those that manifest as stereotypic behaviour: the prolonged, obsessive performance of apparently purposeless activity. The traditional name for all horse stereotypies was 'stable vices'; a thoughtlessly anthropomorphic phrase that suggested 'horses behaving badly' whilst under our authority. It is now clear that stereotypic behaviour in the horse, as in any other sentient animal, is usually a consequence of some failure of provision; in other words, a system of environment and management that is out of tune with the animal's physiological and behavioural needs. The horse that constantly 'weaves' or circles its stable is displaying a similar pattern of abnormal behaviour to the compulsive pacing of the lion in its barren cage or the rocking and head banging of the autistic or socially deprived child. Most stereotypies in humans and other sentient animals are associated with a barren environment and/or a failure of the individual to respond normally to environmental stimuli. Stereotypic behaviours in horses are common (which means there is a serious welfare problem) and complex (which suggests a complex aetiology). It is useful to distinguish two categories: (1) movement stereotypies, e.g. weaving, box walking, and (2) oral sterotypies, e.g. crib-biting, wind sucking.

The movement stereotypies, weaving and box walking, probably do arise, in the first instance, from boredom or frustration in a barren environment. Weaving from side to side probably reflects frustration of the motivation to run in a horse confined for most or all of the day in a stable. Box walking typically involves repeated circuits of the box, pausing (very briefly) each time at the door. It is reasonable to interpret this as a ritualisation of the motivation to escape the confines of the stable. There is a perennial argument amongst ethologists as to whether such behaviour is a sign that the animal has learnt to cope or has failed to cope with the problem of barren environments (see Chapter 3). If the former interpretation is true then stereotypies are a measure of adaptation, albeit at some cost. If the latter is true then the horse is suffering. In either event they suggest (though do not confirm) a failure of husbandry provision at some stage of the horse's life. I advise caution before blaming owners for all stereotypies since some horses in stables may pick up stereotypies like weaving and tongue rolling simply from

watching others. This suggests that a certain amount of repetitive, apparently purposeless behaviour may, in fact, serve the function of instilling some degree of satisfaction in an individual with little to do (chewing gum and jogging may be
presented as examples closer to our own experience). The welfare problem arises
when the stereotypic behaviour becomes compulsive, excessively prolonged and
emancipated from its original environmental trigger. The animal that spends hours
of every day weaving or box walking loses condition (thereby compromising its
fitness). It also appears less able (or inclined) to marshal a normal emotional and
cognitive response to environmental stimuli. In a word, it becomes less sentient.
Such an animal may or may not be suffering. What is certain is that it has a welfare
problem.

Oral stereotypies such as crib-biting and wind sucking (grasping a fixed object
with the teeth and swallowing air into the oesophagus) are usually assumed to
reflect lack of oral satisfaction in an animal physiologically adapted to grazing
short grass for many hours a day but confined in a stable and fed a limited ration
of concentrates and hay that may meet its nutrient requirements but leave it
for hours with nothing to do with its mouth. This 'vice' is perceived as a welfare
problem because crib-biting ruins the incisor teeth and swallowing wind is thought
to cause colic. In some cases these oral stereotypies can be avoided or inhibited
before they become emancipated from the triggering stimulus and thenceforth
untreatable, by providing the animal with sufficient fibrous and non-fattening food
like hay or chaff to keep it orally occupied for much of the day. There is, however,
new evidence (Nicol *et al.*, 2002) to suggest that crib-biting and wind sucking
may arise not as a simple consequence of lack of oral activity but as a response to
abdominal discomfort. This pattern of behaviour is commonly seen for the first
time in foals around the time of weaning (whether stabled or at pasture). To
prevent a check in growth, the foals are likely to be given concentrate feeds based
on starchy cereals at this time and this may predispose them to abdominal discomfort and gastric ulceration. By biting and swallowing air into the oesophagus
(little if any air passes lower down the digestive tract) horses and foals are able to
stimulate salivation and accelerate rhythmic contractions of the stomach and intes-
tines. Thus, in the first instance, this pattern of behaviour may not be a stereotypy
at all but an adaptive behaviour designed to alleviate abdominal discomfort. There
may well be an association between wind sucking and colic, but colic may be the
cause, not the consequence.

It is not yet possible to make firm recommendations as to the prevention and
control of stereotypic behaviour in horses. Some degree of pointless behaviour in
stabled horses would seem to be 'normal' and, in most cases, it should be possible to prevent stereotypic behaviour progressing to the point where the horse loses
condition (and sentience) through careful attention to diet and management. A
question that I cannot resolve concerns the welfare implications of devices and
procedures designed to prevent horses from performing stereotypic behaviour.
These include anti-weaving bars on stable doors, anti-wind-sucking collars and,

most extreme, surgery to sever the neck muscles used to swallow air. Surgery is a transiently painful mutilation and will chronically compromise both abnormal and normal behaviour (swallowing food). Anti-wind-sucking collars appear uncomfortable and once again compromise normal behaviour. Anti-weaving bars do not involve direct interference with the horse. Moreover they only compromise abnormal behaviour. On these grounds, anti-weaving bars may be considered an acceptable constraint to stereotypic behaviour. What is not known is the extent to which a horse that has developed stereotypies may experience distress when it is prevented from carrying out the behaviours it has developed as a means to feel good (or less bad) in circumstances where it has difficulty in meeting its physiological and behavioural needs. My clinical opinion (which means I am speaking as a vet who needs to provide an answer even when none is available) is that preventive measures that do no direct harm (e.g. anti-weaving bars) should not be seen as the only remedy but may be used in association with other changes in diet and management designed to discourage stereotypies and prevent them from progressing to the emancipated, irreversible stage.

Welfare problems considered so far are those that may arise in a well-equipped, well-run stable yard, where the horses get regular expert attention and can enjoy the security and social intercourse that comes from 'natural' life within the herd. Let us now consider possible welfare problems for a twelve-year-old pony, the beloved pet of a girl of the same age. She spends 75% of the year at boarding school. The pony spends 95% of the year isolated in a small paddock with a stable box in the corner. Using, as always, the Five Freedoms as a check list, we can identify:

- Nutrition and oral satisfaction: erratic. Too much grass in the spring; risk of obesity and laminitis.
- Comfort: should be satisfactory provided the pony has adequate shelter and bedding.
- Health: high risk of intestinal parasitism (controllable with diligent attention to worming); unfitness due to irregular exercise; risk of muscle damage (azoturia) when exercise is resumed.
- Fear and stress: chronic insecurity and separation anxiety.
- Natural behaviour: minimal opportunity for social interactions with other horses.

I do not intend to elaborate on these potential problems since most of them are self-evident. It is, however, necessary to stress that it is profoundly unnatural to expect a single horse or pony to spend most of its life in a single field. At best, the seasonal growth of grass bears no relation to the constant nutrient requirements of the animal. In the spring the grass is likely to be too rich and plentiful and this may lead to obesity and possibly laminitis. Repeated grazing of the same pasture by the same species will inevitably lead to a build up of intestinal parasites. The horse will instinctively act to reduce this risk by discriminating between areas for grazing and areas for dunging. If there is no provision to manage the pasture properly through (e.g.) mechanical topping, conservation for hay or grazing by sheep, then it will, in a very short time, disintegrate into a useless mess of weeds and docks, providing little more than the occasional pair of oil drums and painted stick for jumping over. I know that many horses kept as family pets are cared for very well, but many are not. It should hardly need saying that any person who assumes the responsibility of care for a horse, whether for their own pleasure or for that of their children, must acknowledge that this is a 365-day-a-year commitment. This principle applies to ownership of any pet animal. However, one simply cannot apply the same standards when addressing the question 'Shall we buy a horse or pony?' to those we apply when asking 'Shall we buy a cat or dog?' A house and garden can provide a satisfactory environment for a dog or cat that gets its food from a bowl. A stable and field do not provide a satisfactory environment for a single horse or pony. Humans as the only species available for social intercourse may be satisfactory for the dog that thinks itself one of the family, adequate for the cat that walks by itself, but seriously lacking for a horse that needs the herd for friendship and security. Horses kept as pets will be happier in a livery yard than 'at home'. Love is not enough; one has to be fair.

10.5 Rabbits and other caged pets

The responsibility of the pet owner for day-to-day care applies, of course, just as much to the owner of a rabbit or guinea pig as it does to the owner of a dog or horse. However, caged pets are easier to overlook, particularly when the cage is at the bottom of the garden. The caged rabbit that is fed and watered daily but gets mucked out and perhaps a five-minute cuddle once a week has a pretty mean life. There is little point in enumerating the behavioural problems that might occur. Physical problems may include difficulty in eating as a consequence of overgrown incisor teeth and difficulty in locomotion due to overgrown (and perhaps ingrowing) claws. Such an existence may not qualify as cruelty in law, but, once again, it simply is not fair.

10.6 Breeding for fashion

Much of this section will be very similar to that in *Eden I*, since the welfare problems associated with breeding animals to suit our whims of fashion in defiance of the principle of natural selection for fitness are the same now as then. When man first domesticated animals such as the cow to provide food, the horse to provide work and the dog to aid in the hunt, he discovered that he could improve their utility by arranging matings between animals that appeared phenotypically superior according to traits that suited him: more milk, harder work, greater obedience. This selective breeding progressively altered the phenotype from that which was best adapted to the wild state when animals had to make their own choices of diet, habitat and sexual partner within the resources available. However, selective breeding under domestication did create animals that were more functional in terms of human needs, and usually better adapted to the domestic environment. Thus breeds were born. These animals were of such use to man that they helped him to progress from a life of constant toil to one where leisure time became available and with it the opportunity for play. Those with land to spare and time on their hands began to breed domestic animals not merely for their utility but for their amusement value. This practice saw its greatest flowering among the landed gentry of England, individuals whose mission in life was to devise elaborate rituals for passing the time without actually working. These rituals included 'field sports' such as hunting with hounds and shooting, which required the selective breeding of hounds to follow the scent of a fox or deer, spaniels to spring game birds from cover and retrievers to gather up the dead and wounded. Small aggressive terriers were bred to attack foxes and rats in small holes, and even that achondroplastic dwarf the dachshund was bred originally to pursue a badger into its set. Other dogs were bred to be 'toys' or fashion accessories. The strong standard poodle was shrunk to the dimensions of a toy that could be carried, crimped and coiffured. The pug, Pekinese and Chihuahua were not only shrunk but also reshaped to produce big eyes that stare straight into your face like a human baby. All this may be seen simply as an innocent game. However, all games should be played by the rules and the first rule for this game must be that one should seek to do no harm.

The variation (and distortion) of the 'natural' or wild phenotype achieved through artificial selection is most conspicuous in the dog. An alien would be unlikely to recognise the St Bernard and the Chihuahua, or the Borzoi and the bulldog, as animals from the same species (the dogs themselves have no such problems). It may be that the dog genome is particularly well equipped to achieve such phenotypic variation. It may simply be that humans have spent much more time messing around with the dog to totally non-functional ends than they have with the horse or cat. Indeed, there are depressing signs (the Falabella horse, the Ragdoll or Munchkin cat) that other breeders are following suit. The chic are threatening to inherit the earth.

The effects of selective breeding on dog welfare may be assessed according to the same rules as those used in respect to the artificial breeding of animals for food or science, by any means: natural mating, artificial insertion of semen or of fertilised embryos, or genetic engineering. The Farm Animal Welfare Council defined the following potentially harmful consequences of artificial breeding: 'the manipulation of body size, shape or reproductive capacity . . . in such a way as to reduce mobility, increase the risk of pain, injury, metabolic disease, skeletal or obstetric problems, perinatal mortality or psychological distress'. The Animals (Scientific Procedures) Act (1986) permits procedures (including artificial breeding) that carry

Table 10.2 Some abnormalities in dogs associated with selective breeding.

	Abnormality	**Susceptible breeds**
Accidental	Retinal atrophy	Red setters, springer spaniels
	Epilepsy	German shepherds, dachshunds
	Gout	Boxers, Great Danes, German shepherds
Unfortunate	Hip dysplasia	German shepherds, Old English sheepdogs
	Osteosarcomas	Giant breeds: Great Danes, St Bernards
	Slipped lumbar discs	Dachshunds
Deliberate	Locomotor disorders	Bassets, bulldogs
	Ectropion and skin disorders	Bassets, bulldogs, bloodhounds
	Breathing difficulties	Bulldogs, boxers
	Obstetric problems	Chihuahuas

the possibility of causing 'pain, suffering, distress or lasting harm' only if the risk and severity of harm can be justified in terms of a potential benefit to humanity (or other animals). Anyone who, in the interests of science, sought, by genetic engineering, to turn a greyhound into a bulldog would need to give an extremely good reason (like a cure for cancer) to justify the deliberate imposition of so much harm: restricted mobility, respiratory distress, increased risk of skin and eye infections (Table 10.2). Furthermore, if such a procedure were permitted, the laboratory would no doubt be picketed by animal rights activists, many of them dog lovers.

Table 10.2 lists some examples of abnormalities in dogs that can be attributed wholly or in part to selective breeding. I identify three categories:

(1) *Accidental:* abnormalities arising from the 'chance' emergence of recessive genes within inbred populations.
(2) *Unfortunate:* abnormalities that were not foreseen but that can be linked, at least in part, to deliberate selection for a body shape that is inconsistent with fitness.
(3) *Deliberate:* abnormalities that have been deliberately induced by selective breeding because they are thought to be aesthetically pleasing, or simply different.

Some of the accidental congenital abnormalities, such as progressive retinal atrophy in red setters, have been shown to be linked to single recessive genes. They emerged through inbreeding, but, having emerged, breed societies do try to identify the carriers and breed them out. Other accidental abnormalities such as epilepsy in dachshunds and German shepherds have a strong familiar predisposition, but the genetics is less clear cut so they are more difficult to breed out (Foley *et al.*, 1979). I have called the second category the 'Unfortunates' because the problems have arisen as an unforeseen (although not unforeseeable) consequence of selection for a body size or shape that has proved inconsistent with fitness. The sloping top line favoured by judges of German shepherds has predisposed to hip dysplasia. This partial or complete dissociation of the ball joint of the femur from its socket in the pelvis can cripple affected animals at an early age. Hip dysplasia is not simply a matter of genetics, but its prevalence can be controlled through careful attention to selection.

Another major welfare problem that falls within the 'Unfortunate' category is the high incidence of osteosarcomas (bone cancers) in giant breeds of dog such as the Great Dane, Newfoundland and St Bernard. These conditions are probably not inherited in the strictest sense of the word since there appears to be no familial association. The cancers develop at the points of the limbs where the bones are subjected to the greatest mechanical stresses. These abnormal stresses cause chronic and repeated damage to the bone tissues and predispose them to the errors in cell replication that give rise to bone cancer and its sequelae: pain, immobility and premature death.

The third category of 'Deliberate' abnormalities are those where breeders have continued to select for traits that they find amusing in the full knowledge that the animals they breed carry a high risk (or certainty) of experiencing pain, suffering, distress or lasting harm. Breeds that have been selected to carry an excess of loose skin and deep wrinkles on the head are especially prone to chronic inflammation and secondary infection of the skin and eyes. Bulldogs and bassets have seriously reduced mobility. Brachycephalic breeds like the bulldog, boxer and pug experience respiratory distress because their nose is distorted and their soft palate too large for their throat. Chihuahuas have an abnormally large incidence of obstetric problems, caused not by their size but by their shape. Fashion has decreed that they should have large domed heads and these are often too big to pass through the birth canal.

It should be clear that I find many of the more grotesque breeds of dog objectionable and the deliberate creation of such monsters a profound insult to the *telos* of a wonderful animal. Nevertheless, what matters is not my sensibilities but the welfare of the animals. I am satisfied that dogs do not possess the self-awareness necessary to be concerned about their physical appearance *per se*, although they may be sensitive to their owners' reactions to any departure from the way in which they are normally perceived. Thus a toy poodle may accept it as normal practice to be dressed in a coat before being taken out of doors. A dachshund will not feel ashamed to be seen as a dwarf. However, a dog who submits to having (e.g.) a bow tied around its neck or tail and then has to witness the consequent scenes of hilarity and mirth amongst its onlookers may well be distressed by the action *because* of its consequences. Thus I do not believe that it is an abuse of welfare to breed a dog that no longer looks like a dog. It is, however, an abuse of welfare deliberately to breed an animal in a manner likely to cause suffering from painful physical infirmities, irritating afflictions of the skin, or repeated, premeditated Caesarian section. This, bizarrely, places the Chihuahua in the same category as the Belgian Blue cow (Chapter 6). In the following section I discuss the possibility that acts 'likely to cause unnecessary suffering' might come to be considered an act of cruelty. If so, then breeding of the bulldog or Chihuahua could become a criminal offence.

10.7 Ownership: the duty of care

That excellent saying 'A dog is for life, not just for Christmas' makes the point that anyone who assumes the ownership of a pet animal commits him or herself to a duty of care that should extend for the natural life span of that animal and that this should be curtailed only by extreme senescence or disease. In other words, we are responsible for that life so long as it is a life worth living. Breach of this contract may involve an act carried out with the deliberate intention to cause the animal to suffer pain and fear or, more commonly, a wilful omission, i.e. neglect. Both may be considered in law to constitute cruelty under the Protection of Animals Act (1911). Section 1a of the Act states that it is an act of cruelty to 'wantonly or unreasonably do or omit to do any act causing unnecessary suffering to any animal; or cause, procure, or, being the owner, permit any such act'. The full legal implications of the 1911 Act and subsidiary legislation have been given a very comprehensive and thoughtful review by Radford (2001). I am not equipped to review the human acts and omissions that may be deemed in law to constitute cruelty. My brief is to consider the consequences of allegedly cruel acts and omissions, i.e. what may or may not constitute unnecessary suffering in a sentient animal. Nevertheless, before I proceed, it may be useful to dissect the elements of the key clause in the 1911 Act:

- *Animal* means any domestic or captive animal 'which is tame or which has been or is being sufficiently tamed to serve some purpose for the use of man'.*
- *Wantonly* implies that the act of direct cruelty (e.g. beating a dog to death) or the omission (starving a pig to death) has been carried out in full awareness of its likely effects on the animal.
- *Unreasonably* implies that the act of commission or omission is one that would be deemed cruel 'by a reasonably competent and compassionate individual'. It is no defence for the owner to claim that in his or her opinion a dog will not suffer in consequence of chronic beatings or starvation.
- *Do or omit to do* covers actions involving either direct cruelty or neglect.
- *Unnecessary suffering* implies, once again, that in the eyes of a 'reasonably competent and reasonably compassionate person' the degree of suffering experienced by the animal was unnecessary and/or unavoidable.
- *Being the owner, permit any such act* establishes the principle that the owner of an animal has the ultimate responsibility for the way it is treated. It is no defence to claim that the animal was in the hands of someone else at the time.

* Separate provision is made for wildlife, e.g. the Wildlife and Countryside Act 1981.

Radford (2001) states (his italics) that ownership *'carries with it a positive, continuing, non-delegable, legal duty to exercise reasonable care in order to prevent the animal suffering unnecessarily'*. In justice to the animals in our care, we have a duty to prevent suffering. It follows that it is an injustice to behave in a manner that is likely to cause suffering. However, according to existing law, 'likely to cause suffering' is not normally considered sufficient grounds for prosecution and it is necessary to establish that an animal has already experienced an unnecessary degree of suffering. There is one exception to this rule. The Abandonment of Animals Act (1960) makes it an offence to abandon an animal (for an unspecified period of time) in 'circumstances likely to cause the animal any unnecessary suffering'. Radford (2001) has argued that the 'likely to cause suffering' clause should become the rule rather that the exception in new animal welfare legislation. The UK government is currently reviewing the legislation relating to the welfare of all domestic animals with a view to regulating the responsibilities of those who keep animals as pets in similar fashion to those who keep them for food production or other licensed commercial activities in (e.g.) kennels or riding establishments. The spirit of the debate would seem to be moving towards regulations that require owners not simply to refrain from acts or omissions likely to cause unnecessary suffering but actively to promote the welfare of the animals in their care. It is clearly a good idea to commit owners to do more than simply refrain from cruelty. It is important, however, to avoid phrases like 'ensure the welfare of animals in their care'. Nobody can ensure the welfare of all their animals all the time. Disease, accident and injury occur in the best of homes. The responsibility must be to make provision for welfare through proper attention to husbandry and preventive medicine, competent and regular evaluation of the welfare state of the animals in their care and prompt action to resolve problems as they occur, with professional (veterinary) advice and assistance as appropriate.

Any prosecution for cruelty to a domestic animal will inevitably devote an unconscionably long time to matters of law rather than justice. However, the success or failure of any prosecution will depend on the quality of evidence concerning the nature and severity of suffering in the animal concerned and the extent to which that suffering may be considered unnecessary or avoidable. Here the expertise must be provided by veterinarians and others who are demonstrably competent in matters of animal welfare and animal care. It is for them to provide the evidence that will determine whether or not a pet animal, e.g. a dog 'rescued' by the RSPCA on the grounds of alleged cruelty, has experienced an unnecessary or avoidable degree of suffering. It is not sufficient simply to identify and describe signs of suffering in the dog. The evidence must also establish that the suffering was due to a wanton or unreasonable act or omission on the part of its owner, and could not reasonably be attributed to more innocent causes. This will require a series of thorough clinical assessments of the physical and mental condition of the animal, first at the time of rescue, then on more than one subsequent occasion after transfer to a place of safety. The assessment of welfare state should be made according to the usual rules. I list below the five categories, and illustrate each by way of example.

(1) *Malnutrition:* Assess body condition and identify its likely cause. An emaciated animal may be malnourished or suffering from chronic disease. A malnourished dog (unless in an extreme state) will probably devour food with gusto and recover rapidly. A chronically sick animal may be anorexic and deteriorate further.

(2) *Comfort:* A filthy coat, hair loss, skin abrasions and open sores *may* indicate that the animal has been housed in conditions of squalor. They may also reflect chronic infestation with external parasites and/or self-mutilation, which may or may not be associated with living in squalor.

(3) *Health and injury:* Malaise, loss of body condition, hair loss, respiratory distress (etc.) may indicate poor welfare due to disease. These symptoms may be severe enough to constitute suffering. A sick animal is, of course, no proof of a cruel owner. However, the owner may be guilty of an act of cruelty if he/she does not act promptly to seek veterinary action to cure the disease or at least reduce the severity of the symptoms.

(4) *Fear and distress:* A dog chronically subjected to acts calculated to provoke acute fear and distress is likely to express signs of extreme anxiety, presenting either as withdrawal or as aggression when it first encounters its 'rescuer'. Other dogs may display extreme aggression to any stranger but genuine affection to their owners. It is important to determine the behaviour of the animal both in the presence of strangers and with its owner.

(5) *Denial of natural behaviour:* It is easy to demonstrate denial of natural behaviour, e.g. in the case of dogs kept permanently in a cage or a closed and squalid room so that they have no option but to urinate and defaecate close to where they lie. It is less easy (but possible) to assess at what point the severity and duration of this denial may constitute suffering. Once again, it can be best assessed from observation of behaviour after rescue. In my opinion the most convincing evidence for this form of chronic abuse is provided by signs indicative of learned helplessness, such as apathy, indifference to where they pass their motions, abnormal grooming behaviour, etc.

The written evidence presented by the rescuer and subsequent carer should be detailed and explicit as to the clinical and behavioural signs observed at the time of rescue and the subsequent changes in its physical and mental condition during recovery. In cases of direct cruelty, such as the infliction of severe injury from a beating, this should be straightforward. Cases of alleged neglect may be more difficult to prove. If the evidence fails to establish beyond reasonable doubt that the animal's suffering could have been avoided by the actions of a reasonably competent and reasonably compassionate person then it will not survive cross-examination.

10.8 Striving to keep alive: the responsibility of the veterinarian

One of the most difficult and distressing dilemmas for all those responsible for the care and welfare of a pet animal, whether as owner or veterinary surgeon, arises when it reaches a state of chronic distress or infirmity through disease or old age and the decision must be taken as to whether or not to terminate its life through euthanasia. Below I reproduce a check-list drawn up by Edney (1989) designed for vets faced by the decision whether or not to recommend euthanasia to the owner of a seriously sick, infirm or injured animal:

(1) Is the animal free from pain, distress or serious discomfort that cannot be effectively controlled?
(2) Is the animal able to walk and balance itself reasonably well?
(3) Is the animal able to eat and drink enough for maintenance without much difficulty and without vomiting?
(4) Is the animal free from tumours that cause pain or serious discomfort and are considered inoperable?
(5) Is the animal able to breathe without difficulty?
(6) Is the animal able to pass urine and faeces at normal intervals and without serious difficulty or incontinence?
(7) Is the owner able to cope physically and emotionally with any nursing and medication which may be required if the decision is taken to 'save' the animal?

This is a very good check-list provided that it is not interpreted too zealously. Chronic pain (for example) with no hope of recovery can become intolerable and may be sufficient reason for euthanasia. However, many old pets and many more old people learn to cope with chronic pain by adapting to a severely restricted lifestyle, aided by pain-killing drugs. The old dog and the old man, both nearly crippled with arthritis, may still be able to derive joy from each other's company and dignity from sharing each other's suffering. For those who consider the word dignity is inappropriate when describing the emotional state of a dog, I would ask you to consider the condition of the old dog who can no longer control its bowels or bladder. The compassionate owner will not punish the dog and may indeed commiserate with its distress; but distressed it will be and, in the absence of any punishment, this distress would appear to me to arise from a loss of dignity.

The vet's dilemma at this time is compounded by the fact that he/she has to consider the welfare of not one party but three and this generates three inescapable questions.

(1) How much will the animal suffer if I elect to prolong its life?
(2) How much will the owner suffer either from the death of the loved pet or from the physical, emotional and financial problems of striving to keep it alive?

Table 10.3 Kidney transplants – the ethical dilemma.

Respect for	Benefit	Cost
Recipient cat	Improves/prolongs quality of life 'Right to life'	Prolonged suffering – post-operative complications – relapse
Donor cat:		
non-survival	None	'Telos'
survival	Adoption?	Post-operative suffering
Owner	Defers the sorrow of loss Respect for life	Cost of treatment Prolonged distress
Vet	Good income Professional satisfaction	None?

(3) How much money could I/should I make from attempts to prolong the animal's life through surgery and/or prolonged medication?

All three questions must be addressed because all three parties are worthy of respect. The questions are not new, but they have in recent years become progressively more difficult as approaches to surgery and therapeutics have become progressively more sophisticated and more expensive. Vets and pet owners are increasingly presented with cases where three options are available: prompt euthanasia, palliative treatment followed by euthanasia when the animal has deteriorated to the point where quality of life becomes unacceptable, or heroic and expensive surgery followed by prolonged and expensive post-operative care. This dilemma has been most dramatically highlighted by the debate within the veterinary profession over kidney transplants for cats and I shall use this as an example. However, the ethical issues are not unique and apply to all complex and expensive procedures designed, in that crude but catchy phrase, 'to prolong the suffering of geriatric pets'.

10.8.1 Kidney transplants in cats
Let us consider the good and harm that may be involved for the various parties concerned in the matter of kidney transplant surgery for cats. The issues are raised but not resolved in Table 10.3.

The recipient cat
Successful renal transplants have been reported to extend the life of cats for several years*. However, the survival rate after one month appears to be below 70% even when the best-trained surgeons operate in the best-equipped hospitals. Complica-

---

* Kidney transplants in dogs have been abandoned at the experimental stage because of insurmountable problems of tissue rejection.

tions thereafter include acute episodes of rejection, malignant hypertension (33%) and central nervous disorders (15%). Thus some recipient cats will enjoy years more high-quality life, but for a high proportion the operation will either fail or produce prolonged periods of distressing ill health. In a strictly utilitarian sense the operation does more harm than good to day-to-day welfare for the greater number of cats. The justification for the recipient must therefore lie in its inherent 'right to life' and this, of course, must be considered quite separately from its value to the owner. It would be absurd to suggest that cats are troubled by the desire to achieve longevity *per se*. Thus euthanasia is not a welfare problem for the cat because being dead is not a welfare problem. If it curtails a good life, then this may be a moral problem for the owner, but death is always the end of suffering.

The donor cat

If kidneys are removed under proper surgical conditions, just before or even immediately after the euthanasia of a cat that has already been condemned to death, then the procedure does not impose any added cost. (I stress, this does not make it 'right', it is simply part of the overall ethical analysis.) If one has respect for the *telos* or intrinsic value of every cat as an individual, then it is proper to question whether it is right to destroy the life of one cat to satisfy the wish, not of another cat, but of its owner. The alternative procedure adopted by the Feline CRF (chronic renal failure) Information Center, USA (www.felinecrf.com), is to perform a transplant only on the basis of a contract whereby the owners of the recipient will adopt the donor. In this way, it is claimed, two cats are saved, not one. The subsequent medical prognosis for the healthy donor is good. Moreover, it is highly probable that owners prepared to spend a small fortune on one cat are likely to lavish care on another that they willingly allow to enter their home.

The owner

Whether or not the owner has a form of pet insurance, the financial cost of agreeing to a kidney transplant will be large. Figures from the University of California at Davis suggest an initial cost of between $3500 and $13000, with a continuing annual cost of approximately $2000 for immunosuppressive therapy, laboratory tests and back-up visits. I have two delightful cats in my house, but I would not personally be prepared to pay that much for either of them, even if I thought (which I do not) that it was in the interests of their welfare. Some people, however, are prepared to put that price on the sentimental value of their pet. Thus any veterinary surgeon who discusses the option of a kidney transplant with the owner of a cat should acknowledge that the prime object of the exercise is to make the owner feel better; *and should say so!* Since the owner is likely to outlive the cat, surgery will only defer the sorrow of loss. This principle applies to all circumstances where euthanasia is a proper option for the vet whose constant endeavour [in the words of the oath sworn by each new UK graduate before admission to the

Royal College of Veterinary Surgeons (RCVS)] is 'to ensure the welfare of all animals committed to my care'. Having honestly explained the prognosis and all the complications of surgery, the veterinary surgeon should pose the question 'Do you believe that it is fair to your pet to run the risk of prolonging its suffering simply to reduce your distress at this time?'

The veterinary surgeon

We must finally consider the moral position of the veterinary surgeon as a stakeholder in any exercise that involves heroic surgery and expensive post-operative care. If it succeeds, even for a while, not only does the vet stand to make a lot of money but also there is the satisfaction of success in a complex and delicate operation. Neither of these is an inherently improper aim for a professional person working to support him or herself and his/her family. However, the *only* potential cost to the veterinary surgeon is the risk of ignominious failure. Thus implicit in any decision to proceed with a kidney transplant or other comparably heroic form of surgery is the conscious or unconscious acknowledgement that self-interest has overridden all other concerns. In my opinion, a vet faced by a client desperate to save his or her cat with failing kidneys should never recommend a kidney transplant *a priori* but attempt to persuade him/her that palliative therapy leading to euthanasia at the appropriate time would be the kindest solution for the animal. If the owner insisted upon a transplant, then the honourable decision would be to seek the 'least worst' solution. This would almost certainly involve referring the case to a hospital with a proven record of success (should such a one exist). It would never be right to pocket the bill and hope for the best.

In this, as in all ethical issues, my intention is to review and judge the evidence but leave it to readers to come to their own verdicts. There will be those who will 'instinctively' conclude that such radical surgery falls into the category of those things that should not be done in any circumstances. However absolute and immediate that gut feeling may be, it will inevitably have involved some element of judgement as to benefit versus harm. Thus you may conclude that it is a wrong thing to do, but it is not wrong to contemplate doing it. I understand the reasons, at least in law, why the RCVS has agreed to permit kidney transplants subject to (limited) ethical and clinical guidelines. I would not do it myself, but that is easy for me to say because I never sought to make a living from small animal practice.

Limping Towards Eden: Stepping Stones

The end of a man is an action and not a thought, though it were the noblest.

Thomas Carlyle

The path of duty lies in what is near, and man seeks for it in what is remote.

Mencius

I have taken the liberty of prefacing this final chapter with two quotations. The first, from Thomas Carlyle (1795–1881), repeats that which prefaced the final chapter of *A Cool Eye*. In both these books and throughout 30 years of professional work in animal welfare my aim has been not just to study the subject but also to help to get done the things that should be done, and can be done. This dual aim, described in *Eden I* as 'right thought and right action' has been founded on the philosophical principle of the 'middle way', which has its basis in the 'noble eightfold path' of Theravada Buddhism, namely 'Right views, right attitude of mind, right speech, right action, right means of livelihood, right effort, right mind control and right serenity'. Having thought more about the nature of sentience in us all, I have at last become aware that the noble eightfold path gives proper regard both to cognition (right views) and emotion (right attitude of mind, right serenity) in the motivation towards right action. I now concede that right action cannot come from right thought alone.

The second quotation from Mencius (a Chinese philosopher from the third century BC) neatly describes the second pillar of my philosophy. *Limping Towards Eden* is not a title that suggests that my goal is to achieve all the Five Freedoms for all the animals all of the time, whatever the cost to the rest of society. I have always argued that the cause of animal welfare is not helped by 'impossibilists': those who make strident calls from the high moral ground for actions that cannot be enforced. *The path of duty lies in what is near.*

In Chapter 1, I identified the elements of right thought, right feelings and right action that may be used as stepping stones on the long and difficult road towards improved standards of welfare for sentient animals. These were:

- a clear definition of animal welfare ('fit and happy') and a systematic approach to its evaluation (the Five Freedoms);
- a sound ethical framework which affords proper respect for the value of animals within the broader context of our duties as citizens to the welfare of society and the living environment;
- comprehensive, robust protocols for assessing animal welfare and the provisions that constitute good husbandry;
- an honest policy of education that can convert human desire for improved welfare standards into human demand for these things;
- realistic, practical, step-by-step strategies for improving animal welfare within the context of other, equally valid aspirations of society.

I have considered the nature of animal welfare, sentience and suffering, outlined protocols for the identification of welfare problems that can occur in the home, on the farm or in the laboratory, and suggested case-specific remedies. In this final chapter, I shall review the broader issues and try to set out a series of 'rules of engagement' for those who seek to improve animal welfare within the real world, where animal welfare has to compete with countless other priorities.

11.1 Right action

Action to improve animal welfare needs to be considered at two levels.

(1) The animal level: here the aim is to identify and remedy specific problems for individual animals or groups of animals in specific circumstances in the home, on the farm or in the laboratory.
(2) Within society: here the aim is to promote the cause of animal welfare within the context of the multiple aspirations of society.

Although I am generally happier with specifics than with abstractions, I believe that it is useful to identify certain properties of 'right attitude of mind' as precursors to right action, provided that they are clearly defined within context. Anyone who has a direct impact on welfare at the level of the individual animal or group of animals should be:

- *Competent*: This requires a proper understanding of what is meant by animal welfare (i.e. 'fit and happy') and a structured, comprehensive approach to its evaluation (e.g. the Five Freedoms).
- *Compassionate*: This requires a proper sense of empathy with the animal(s) in question. This can be sought through an acceptable form of reverse anthropomorphism. Ask not 'How would this cow feel if it were me?' but 'How would I feel if I were this cow?'

- *Informed*: This can be achieved by proceeding systematically through a comprehensive protocol for assessing welfare state and diagnosing welfare problems in an animal or group of animals.
- *Effective*: To be effective, and to be seen to be effective, any actions taken to resolve a specific problem in animal welfare must meet all of the following criteria:
  - correct diagnosis and treatment to reduce suffering in affected animals;
  - identification of failures of provision at critical control points and action to redress these failures;
  - records of actions taken to address failures of provision and subsequent audit of their impact.

Also anyone who seeks to promote the cause of animal welfare within society at large should be competent, compassionate and informed, although not necessarily to the level of professional expertise required to deal with a specific problem such as lameness in dairy cows or feather pecking in free-range hens. Such people also need a split personality. They must be passionately and tirelessly committed to their cause, but they also need a second pair of cool eyes able to view their arguments and their actions from the perspective of other reasonable people. No individual has the absolute right to assume that his/her value set is intrinsically superior to that of another individual in different circumstances. Libertarianism is a fundamental element of the principle of autonomy. It is perfectly proper to campaign passionately for one's set of values on the basis of scientific and ethical argument, but every case has to be made. Simply proclaiming 'I am right and you are wrong' is not right action. Our goal should be *justice* for the sentient animals. Since justice, by definition, implies fairness to all concerned parties, it follows that wherever there is an honest conflict of interest, the just solution can never (well, hardly ever) be achieved without *compromise*.

11.2 Sentience, suffering and wellbeing

Before attempting to identify and prioritise actions that could, should and must be done to promote animal welfare, it is necessary to revisit the nature of sentience, suffering and wellbeing: to consider what things matter to a sentient animal as it seeks to meet its physiological and behavioural needs, how much they matter, how far it is able to adapt to environmental pressures, and what may be the consequences when it fails to cope. The working definitions to which I have referred throughout are as follows:

- Sentience = feelings that matter. Sentient animals care how they feel and so should we.
- Wellbeing = fit and feeling good.
- Suffering = difficulty or failure in coping with stress.

I use the term 'wellbeing' rather than welfare to define the state of being fit and feeling good since 'welfare' is used in common parlance in reference to a state of body and mind that may vary over the entire spectrum from healthy and happy to sick and desperate. An animal will experience a sense of wellbeing (thus its welfare will be good) when it is physically fit and feels good because it can, without difficulty, meet its physiological and behavioural needs within a particular environment. It may be easier for the animal to meet these needs if the environment is similar to that which helped to shape its phenotype. However, provision of a natural environment is not a prerequisite for wellbeing. The animal simply needs access to appropriate resources and the freedom to exploit its full behavioural repertoire to exploit these resources. As a rule, physiological adaptation to the environment, e.g. shivering in the cold, sweating in the heat, concentrating urine in a drought, is the second line of defence to environmental stress and an indication that the act of coping is being achieved at some cost. The sentient animal exposed to the hot sun will be motivated to seek shade, if it can, rather than simply stand there and sweat.

Suffering occurs when an animal fails to cope, or has difficulty in coping, with stress because the stress itself is too severe, too complex or too prolonged, and/or because the animal is prevented from taking the constructive action it feels necessary to relieve the stress. Possible sources of suffering in any sentient animal include primitive stresses such as hunger and thirst, heat and cold, pain, malaise exhaustion, fear and anxiety (Table 3.3). They may or may not include 'higher' feelings such as boredom and frustration, loss and loneliness and depression and present as apathy or learned helplessness.

Immediately before being admitted to the Royal College of Veterinary Surgeons, new graduates are required to swear an oath, the last line of which reads 'my constant endeavour will be to ensure the welfare of all animals committed to my care'. Anyone committed to care for animals is, by definition, required to promote their welfare. Justice and the Codes of Welfare for Farm Animals (which do not carry the force of law) require animal owners and stock-keepers to take active steps to promote wellbeing. As I write, the law itself offers no more than the most restricted of guarantees to those animals that we take into our care. The Protection of Animals Act (1911) only protects animals from the offence of *cruelty* arising when an owner causes an animal unnecessary suffering by wantonly or unreasonably doing or omitting to do any act. It is, at present, almost impossible to convict an individual or an organisation for systematic disregard of their responsibility to promote wellbeing. However, UK legislation concerning the welfare of all domestic animals is under review. In July 2004, DEFRA published a new draft Animal Welfare Bill (www.defra.gov.uk) and it is now open for discussion. The most novel feature of this draft Bill is that it will impose upon animal owners a duty of care to ensure the welfare of animals based upon existing good practice. In other words, it will no longer be necessary to base a prosecution on proof that suffering has occurred; it will be possible to prosecute on the basis that animals were being kept in such a manner that suffering is likely to occur. This acknowledges the principle enshrined in *Animal Welfare Law in Britain* (Radford, 2001), namely that 'Ownership incontrovertibly carries with it *a positive, continuing, non delegable, legal duty to exercise reasonable care and supervision in order to prevent the animal suffering unnecessarily*' (his italics). A law that makes 'failure to ensure animal wellbeing' a criminal offence would be completely unworkable. However, it should be possible through the new Animal Welfare Bill to make it an offence to keep (or breed) animals in a manner that would be considered by a competent and compassionate individual to be likely to cause avoidable suffering. This would, at last, address Ruth Harrison's grim paradox, namely that 'if one person is unkind to an animal, it is considered to be cruelty, but where a lot of people are unkind to a lot of animals, especially in the name of commerce, the cruelty is defended and, once large sums of money are involved, will be defended to the last by otherwise intelligent people' (Harrison, 1964).

11.3 The politics, philosophy and economics of animal welfare: what *should* be done and what *could* be done

When we address the problem of animal welfare as perceived by the animal itself we can operate within relatively straightforward and non-contentious rules of engagement. Although we can never be sure how they feel, we can, through a combination of well-designed scientific experiments, careful observation and unsentimental empathy, build up a competent and compassionate picture of their physiological and behavioural needs; what things matter, how much they matter, what they seek and what they avoid. This problem can be considered in a 'scientific' manner because it can be focused on a single target, the animal itself. If the answers to the two questions 'Is it fit?' and 'Is it happy?' are both 'Yes' then there are no further questions. If either answer is 'No' then we can follow the rules of the Five Freedoms to identify the specific welfare problem, make provision to address the problem and seek to prevent its recurrence.

When we consider animal welfare as a responsibility of society it all gets much more complicated. This is not just because values are involved, it is because different parties are involved: all the animals and all the people, indeed the whole living environment. In Chapter 1, I introduced the concept of the ethical matrix (Table 1.4). This identifies the parties whose values are worthy of respect: consumers, producers, 'animals used by man' and the living environment. It gives special emphasis to our moral duty to the animals and the environment because these parties do not enjoy built-in protection from 'the invisible hand of the market'. It also outlines the ethical principles that should govern respect for all parties. These are *beneficence* (do good and avoid harm for the greatest possible number), *Autonomy* (respect the rights of each individual ('Do as you would be done by')) and *Justice* ('be fair'). This implies, in almost all cases, an acceptance of compromise.

The principles of beneficence, autonomy and justice offer a serenely wise set of moral rules from which to offer guidance, in the abstract, as to what *should* be done. In real life, however, moral philosophy has to operate within the constraints of politics and economics. This section, the PPE (politics, philosophy and economics) of animal welfare, considers the ways whereby we can work to persuade society that what *should* be done, *could* be done. Useful stepping stones *en route* towards a society that offers a fair deal to the sentient animals include:

- awareness
- reason and respect
- politics by decree
- politics by other means.

11.3.1 Awareness

The usefulness of this book is inherently limited by the fact that almost everybody who reads it will have been a recruit to the cause of animal welfare before they begin. If you read books like this all the way through, then you should also be a well-informed recruit. However, a concern for animal welfare does not necessarily require an education. It arises from the simple acceptance that the animals we use for our own purposes are sentient creatures who have the capacity to experience suffering and pleasure. Having accepted the principle of sentience, it becomes a matter of common justice to care for these animals in such a way as to offer them a reasonable quality of life and a quiet death. In other words, as soon as we give any thought at all to animal welfare, our responsibilities become obvious. However, the big problem, worldwide, is that most of the people think about (or feel for) animal welfare not at all, or hardly at all, or (which is worst) only in circumstances where it makes them feel comfortable. An extreme example of someone who does not think about welfare at all is the slaughterman secretly filmed by Compassion in World farming (CIWF) who suspends five live lambs from hooks by their Achilles tendons, then goes off for a smoke before returning to kill them. He was probably not acting cruelly by his own standards (i.e. wilfully causing unnecessary suffering) because it simply had not occurred to him that the lambs had the capacity to suffer. I repeat, this is an extreme case, but one has only to watch many traditional practices carried out during the transport, slaughter or routine mutilation of animals in many regions of the world to conclude that the operators involved have simply not given a thought to the concept of animal suffering.

An even bigger problem of lack of awareness lies much closer to home. I accuse, above all, those whose 'love' of animals amounts to no more than a spasm of sentimental self-indulgence, to be turned on and off at a whim; those who will say 'Aaaah' at the sight of lambs in a field, weep at a film like Bambi, cheer at a film like Babe but give not a thought to the provenance of the meat they buy in the supermarket (or worse, simply switch their minds off as they reach for the chicken nugget). The sentimentalists who cannot bear too much reality contribute not a jot to the cause of animal welfare. Supermarkets who have a vested interest in maximising their sales are all too aware of this soggy majority and tend to present most of their meat products in a way that avoids any association with the live animal for fear of putting people off. Reassuringly, many traditional family butchers have recognised that one way to compete with the bland and deliberately mindless image presented within the supermarkets is to cater for those who value food produced to high standards of welfare (etc.) by emphasising the provenance of their meat and providing details of how the animals were reared.

Those who campaign sensibly for improved standards of farm animal welfare (e.g. CIWF, RSPCA) place great emphasis on linking the image of meat, eggs and dairy products to that of sentient animals whose lives we have controlled and whom we have killed to serve our own needs. These images are sometimes unfair (but they are in the business of polemic). They may drive some people to become vegetarians or vegans (although maybe not for life) and this may reduce the total number of animals that are born only to suffer and die. On a worldwide basis this impact is likely to be marginal since it will apply only in those areas where vegetarians (by choice rather than by necessity) constitute a significant proportion of the population. The worldwide trend in consumption of meat and animal products climbs ever upwards as more and more people become able to afford these things. To achieve the greatest good for the greatest number of animals on a worldwide basis, it is necessary to recognise this as a fact of life and seek to promote an increasing awareness of the nature of sentience in farm animals, and the responsibilities that this brings. This is not intended as a patronising admonition from the affluent to the poor. It should be obvious from what has been written already (e.g. Chapter 5) that industrial agriculture in the developed world has been responsible for the most widespread abuses of farm animal welfare. Moreover, by divorcing most of the people from the realities of animal farming it has permitted them the luxury of not having to think about the problem at all. In a society where most of the people have some direct involvement in food production and where that involvement involves direct daily contact between man and animals, then it is impossible to be unaware of animal welfare. It may not always be a very competent or compassionate awareness, but the option of simply shutting one's mind to the whole thing is simply not available. Application of the principles of good husbandry based on increased awareness of animal sentience, supported by judicious financial incentives, could allow those in the developing world who still live close to their animals and value their animals to progress towards improved, humane, sustainable systems of farming without passing first through the purgatory of machine-driven, drug-dependent, factory farming of animals unfit for purpose.

11.3.2 Reason and respect

Action for the animals only becomes right action when it is effective. There are three basic steps to this process, all of them essential. One needs first to identify a problem, then draw attention to the problem, then devise a workable solution to the problem. Steps one and three, the identification and resolution of problems of animal welfare, require professional competence, sweetened with compassion;

in short, good husbandry. They also require an acceptance of political reality; a recognition that, for very good moral reasons, the aspirations of any one group should not be allowed to trample all others under foot. However, nothing effective will ever be accomplished without step two. It is an inescapable fact that action for change in regard to matters of animal welfare would not have been achieved without the contribution of those whose active campaigning has kept the issue on the front page. Inevitably, such an emotionally charged campaign has attracted the anarch, the hooligan and the very silly 'What do we want? Eden! When do we want it? Now!' Nevertheless, the majority of those who campaign for animal welfare, those who put the passion into compassion, are as essential to the movement as the most dedicated welfare scientist or politician. In a democratic, listening society, one should never underestimate the impact of the angry little old lady with nothing to lose. I remind you of the response of USA President Harry Truman to a reasoned argument from a lobby group: 'I am persuaded that you have a very good case. Now go out and put pressure on me'.

11.3.3 Politics by decree

Let us now consider some of the approaches to working for improved welfare through political action. The area that is most amenable to progress through politics by decree involves those industrialised systems of animal production (battery hens, broiler chickens) where welfare problems intrinsic to the system are largely independent of the quality of stockmanship within the system. Because these systems are so standardised they are particularly amenable to legislation to improve minimum standards. Moreover, as indicated in Table 1.5, the cost to the consumer of legislation to enforce improved standards across an entire economic community can be very small. While only a relatively small proportion of the community may be prepared to pay 50% more money for high-welfare food marketed as a specialist line, very few would seriously complain if compelled by legislation to pay 5% more for food if the outcome was better farm animal welfare. Most of us will concede that sometimes we need the help of the state to make us into better people.

What then are the principles that should govern the progress of animal welfare through political decree? At a recent congress of the British Veterinary Association, I was asked to debate the question 'Should you compromise the animal welfare of this country for politics?' My answer to this was an unequivocal 'Yes and No'. In most circumstances, the answer has to be 'Yes' for the good reason that one must seek a fair deal for all concerned parties:

- Animals: on the farm, in the laboratory and in the home.
- Society: the rich and poor, the healthy and the sick; those whose livelihood and contribution to society requires them to 'do things' to animals, the farmers and scientists.
- All other creatures who make up the living environment.

Avoidable suffering

'No' is the obvious answer in reference to those acts and omissions that are recognised as criminal in law. It can also be 'No' for those acts that are currently permissible within existing law but where the case for a repeal of the law and the will of the people in support of that case become sufficiently strong to persuade politicians of the need for change. I have already given two examples where the legal justification for current practices is studded with internal inconsistencies and repeat them here in the context of the present argument.

The first relates to religious slaughter (Chapter 7). Schedule 12 of the Welfare of Animals at Slaughter (1995) Act exempts those licensed to practise Halal or Shekita slaughter from the regulation that 'no person engaged in the movement, lairaging, restraint, stunning, slaughter or killing of animals shall cause any avoidable excitement, pain or suffering to any animal'. The excitement, pain and suffering intrinsic to these methods may, through an act of sophistry, be deemed 'necessary' to the religious observances, but these things are *avoidable*. The aim of all who work to improve animal welfare by any political means should be to minimise avoidable suffering. I repeat therefore my recommendation that Schedule 12 of the Welfare of Animals at Slaughter Act should be repealed and amended to read: '*Whenever it is deemed necessary, on the grounds of established religious practice, to consume meat from animals that have been killed by exsanguination without experiencing prior physical damage, then the animals should be rendered unconscious and insensitive to pain by methods that do not cause physical damage*'.

The other exploitable anomaly in current UK and EU law relates to the production of eggs from hens confined in conventional battery cages. In 2012 it will become unacceptable in law for producers within the European Community to produce eggs from hens kept in cages that fail to meet minimal standards for animal welfare. Since anyone who sells such eggs will be guilty of a criminal offence, it should follow that anyone who buys them should also be guilty of an offence. Some painful but accurate analogies may be drawn here. It is illegal to purchase ivory on the basis that it promotes the suffering of elephants. It is illegal to purchase child pornography on the basis that it permits the suffering of children. The law says that all these are unacceptable practices. However, in the case of hens, but not elephants or children, it permits us (retailers and customers) to profit from these practices so long as they are carried out in a far-off country of which we know little.

Changing the 'accepted standards'

The next category of welfare problems that can be addressed by political action involves those systems that may be defined at any one time as 'accepted agricultural practice' but where 'accepted standards' can be made to change. The most conspicuous of these are those originally identified by the Brambell Commission in 1965, namely the rearing of veal calves in crates, pregnant sows in stalls and laying hens in battery cages. All these practices have been subject to legislation to improve minimum standards. However, it would be dangerously complacent to assume that things were now all right. Compassion in World Farming (CIWF) has made it its policy to challenge existing law by bringing prosecutions against companies on the basis of systematic disregard for animal welfare. In the 1980s CIWF unsuccessfully prosecuted a white veal production unit for rearing calves in the extreme confinement of individual crates and without access to the fibrous food necessary to support normal rumen development. In 2003 it prosecuted (equally unsuccessfully) a broiler breeding company for breeding birds unfit for purpose based on a high prevalence of leg disorders and an appetite inconsistent with the need to sustain fitness. Both cases were lost on the grounds that, in each case, this was 'accepted agricultural practice'. In the case of veal production, the law has now changed, first in the UK (1990) and later throughout the EU (from 2006). The law now accepts that CIWF was right in its assertion that extreme confinement of calves in individual crates without access to the fibrous food constitutes a systematic failure to provide minimum standards to promote animal welfare. Thus in this case CIWF lost the battle but helped to win the war. It is therefore perfectly realistic to predict that the defence of the broiler industry on the basis that it is 'accepted agricultural practice' may also be overcome by the force of public opinion.

Poultry meat production has so far escaped judgement by political decree not, I believe, because there is less evidence of welfare abuse in poultry meat production than in other intensive systems but because nobody has come up with an effective, enforceable recommendation for legislation. It was easy to legislate for improved minimum housing standards for sows, laying hens and veal calves since it involved nothing much more complicated than taking the animals out of cages. Some of the worst welfare problems for broilers and turkeys can be addressed by careful attention to the standards for feeding and housing laid down by the Codes of Welfare and it may be argued that it would not achieve a great deal more if these standards were given the force of law. However, the most serious welfare abuse (addressed by the CIWF prosecution) has been the breeding of animals that are unfit for purpose. Since the international broiler industry is dominated by less than five breeding companies who supply over 80% of the world market, it would not be difficult in practice to achieve an overall improvement in broiler welfare through a ban on the wholesale commercial production of any strain of bird that failed to meet defined standards with regard to the prevalence of leg disorders or cardiac failure. This could only be enforced after thorough and careful independent tests and it would be absurdly Draconian to pass a law that rendered a major international strain of broiler chickens illegal overnight. Nevertheless I see no difference in principle between a law that requires egg producers to provide within ten years a cage to new, improved specifications, and a law that requires broiler breeders to produce within ten years a bird to new improved specifications. In 1992 the Farm Animal Welfare Council (FAWC) stated:

The Council considers that the current level of leg problems in broilers is unacceptable. We recommend that steps should be taken to ensure that there is a significant reduction in the number and severity of leg problems. It will be the responsibility of the industry to achieve this objective and the Council intends to look at this aspect of broiler production in five years time, when significant improvements should be apparent. If no reduction in leg problems is found, we may recommend the introduction of legislation to ensure the required improvements.

The broiler breeders have taken some action in response to this pronouncement and have presented the results of their actions to FAWC and DEFRA although the evidence is not yet within the public domain. I am informed by FAWC that any decision to 'recommend the introduction of legislation to ensure the required improvements' is still under review, after twelve years! If we can achieve legislation to improve minimum standards for provision of resources, there is no good reason why we cannot achieve legislation to improve minimum standards for provision of a phenotype that can cope with the resources we provide. This would be a blessing, both for the animals and for the farmers who have to work ever harder to promote the welfare of animals phenotypically unfit for purpose.

Control of new technology

Some of the most pressing demands for action by political decree arise in relation to the application of new technology to animal production. Although it is still customary for politicians and civil servants to state that judgements in these matters should be based 'strictly on the scientific evidence', the debate usually centres on questions of ethics. Table 11.1 uses the ethical matrix to review three technology-driven alternatives to conventional animal production. The first is the use of regular injections of recombinant bovine growth hormone (or somatotropin, BST) to increase the production of 'normal milk' from cows. The second is the creation of genetically modified animals that can synthesise commercial amounts of a biologically active compound such as α-1-antitrypsin, which can restore health to

Table 11.1 Ethical evaluation of three applications of technology to animal production: bovine growth hormone (BST), production of pharmaceuticals in milk from genetically modified animals (GM milk) and production of oestrogen in pregnant mares' urine (PMU).

	BST	**GM milk**	**PMU**
Manufacturers	Profitable	Risky	Profitable
Animals: fitness	Loss of condition Reduced life expectancy	Increased value	Few problems
Animals: behaviour	Exhaustion, discomfort	No problem	Restricted
Farmers	'Forced choice'	Potentially good	Satisfactory
Human welfare	No effect	Potentially good	Good

individuals with inherited disorders of metabolism. The third category, included for comparison although it is not particularly technology driven, is the production of pregnant mares' urine to supply oestrogen for use as hormone replacement therapy.

The regular injection of cows with BST is permitted in the USA but banned in the EU. In both cases the decision has nominally been made on the basis of scientific evidence with regard to 'quality, safety and efficacy' where 'safety' is interpreted in terms of the safety for humans of milk from BST-treated cows. When the evaluation is made strictly on the basis of these three criteria alone then it is difficult to argue against the USA decision. The product is consistent in quality, it works and the milk carries no more or less risk to man than any other. However, it does compromise cow fitness by exacerbating her already extreme metabolic load and increases the risk that she will suffer prematurely from exhaustion, loss of body condition and the physical injuries to which the exhausted and emaciated are prone, especially when expected to rest on concrete. Farmers did not need BST, but when it came onto the market they were forced into the choice. 'Spend money and drive your cows harder or fail to compete.' The financial benefits to the consumer are negligible (Table 1.5). Moreover, since milk from BST-treated cows carries no label, consumers cannot easily exercise their right not to buy. Thus everybody but the manufacturers stands to lose. This seems to be a much more honest reason for extending the EU ban indefinitely, rather than persisting with the present moratorium 'pending further scientific evidence'.

The creation through genetic modification of animals that can produce specific drugs essential to keep certain people alive has the potential to make a significant contribution to the welfare of society. The surgical procedures necessary to create the line of genetically modified animals may be prolonged and carry a significant welfare cost. However, once the line is established, the animals themselves can enjoy the benefits of being very expensive individuals and expect to be pampered like racehorses. The most serious constraint to this application of biotechnology is the reluctance of the pharmaceutical companies to embark on such risky investments. It is proper that any commercial application of genetic modification in animals should be subject to ethical analysis and prohibited whenever there is a real risk that it might cause harm to any of the sentient parties involved. When there is no apparent risk, then government should be reluctant to stand in the way of progress. However, some risks only become apparent when a new process has been operating for several years with a large number of animals. I repeat my suggestion from *Eden I* that such procedures should be controlled by a two-stage licensing process. An initial provisional licence would allow the commercial exploitation of the new technology to proceed. Subsequently (after approximately five years) a full licence may be granted dependent on proof (acquired at the manufacturer's expense) of quality, safety and efficacy in relation to its application to human health and welfare, and safety and humanity in regard to animal welfare.

I have included, for comparison, the rearing of mares for the production of pregnant mares' urine (PMU); a cheap and effective source of oestrogen used mostly for hormone replacement therapy in menopausal and post-menopausal women. The efficacy of this product is not in doubt, nor its net contribution to human happiness. The production of urine containing a high concentration of oestrogen during pregnancy is as natural as the production of milk during lactation. In this sense it is not an application of new technology. However, so far as the mares are concerned it does involve unnatural practices; prolonged constraint in tie-stalls, long-term harnessing and chronically indwelling urethral catheters. There is a slight risk of infection, but the most serious welfare concern relates to the denial of the freedom to express normal patterns of behaviour. I do not believe that this is a case for special legislation. However, it should be regulated by a strict Code of Practice, stricter than that which currently seems to apply in the misleadingly titled 'ranches' for the production of PMU in Canada.

Approaches to compromise: the badger dilemma

So far, I have presented examples of improvements to animal welfare where the decision enforced by political decree can be definitive and clear cut. Some people might not like a decision to ban the conventional battery cage, or ban the exsanguination of a fully conscious animal, but at least the reasons can be made clear. Political action to resolve a welfare problem becomes much more difficult when there is real conflict between the legitimate needs of the concerned parties and compromise becomes inevitable. In this case, compromise becomes the moral path, provided that it gives proper respect to the legitimate needs of all concerned parties. However, it is seldom easy. As an illustration, let us consider one of the most serious and intractable animal health and welfare problems of the moment in the UK, namely the control of bovine tuberculosis (bTB) in cattle and badgers. This presents a massive problem even for those who consider that animal welfare is more important than anything else, since it involves a conflict between the welfare of the badger and the welfare of the cow. It is an offence in law 'wilfully to kill a badger, to interfere with a badger sett, or to disturb a badger when occupying a sett' (Protection of Badgers Act 1992). The State Veterinary Service has a statutory duty to eradicate bTB in cattle. In many areas of the UK bTB is endemic in the badger population and (despite any pious hopes to the contrary) it is an inescapable fact that cattle are much more likely to contract bTB from infected badgers than from any other species of wild animal. The statutory duty of the State Veterinary Service to eradicate bTB from British cattle would be greatly aided by a Draconian policy of killing all badgers in areas where the disease was endemic. The statutory duty of society to refrain from killing a badger or disturbing a badger sett wilfully ignores a major problem in public health. The two instruments of policy cannot coexist and something has to give.

Figure 11.1 explores options for control through application of the HACCP principle (Hazard Analysis at Critical Control Points). The central aim is to min-

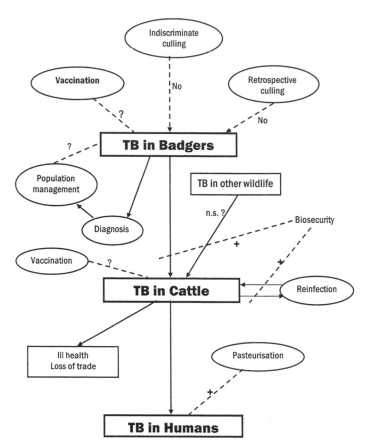

Figure 11.1 Control of tuberculosis in badgers and cattle: hazard and control analysis. *n.s.* Not significant.

imise the incidence of bTB in cattle. In the first decades of the twentieth century this was the most important zoonotic disease in the UK. In the 1920s, 40% of dairy herds were infected with bTB and thousands of people, mostly children, contracted tuberculosis as a result of drinking infected milk. This route of infection has been effectively controlled by pasteurisation. There is still a small risk to humans drinking unpasteurised milk or working in direct contact with infected cattle, but bTB is now essentially a cow problem. In the interests of improving the health and international trading value of the British cattle population it became from 1950 the policy of the State Veterinary Service to eradicate bTB from the national dairy herd through a compulsory policy of routine diagnostic 'tuberculin' testing, slaughter of infected animals and restriction of movement of cattle on infected premises. In the early 1980s it appeared that the eradication process was close to complete success (infection present in less than 0.4% of herds). However, in the last 20 years the situation has been deteriorating at an alarming and accelerating rate, particularly in areas such as South-West England where there has also been a very large increase in the population of badgers, many of whom are infected with bTB. This is not the place to review and criticise the disintegration of the bTB eradication policy for cattle. What is and is not known about the association with bTB in badgers is well covered by the Krebs report (1997). My aim here is only to explore how political priorities for action to recover control of this complex problem may be set on the basis of what is realistic and what is fair.

The options for control of bTB through the culling of badgers include massive pre-emptive culling, retrospective culling or no culling at all. The total elimination of badgers in areas where there is a high incidence of bTB in cattle has been shown (in trials conducted over relatively small areas) to be effective. However, the general implementation of this solution is not acceptable to society (or indeed the badgers). Retrospective culling of badgers diagnosed to have bTB has recently been shown to make the problem of bTB in cattle worse (worse indeed than a 'no culling' policy) partly because the diagnostic techniques are inadequate and partly because the selective culling of badgers in infected areas destabilises the population, leading to more movement and more cross-infection. A proactive, selective process of culling that effectively managed the badger population in stable groups but in smaller overall numbers than now would stand a reasonable chance of success but is currently illegal under the terms of the Protection of Badgers Act (1992). The most effective and humane approach to control would, in theory, be through a policy of vaccination. Unfortunately there is no immediate prospect of an effective vaccine for either species. A partially effective vaccine (e.g. 75% effective) is unlikely to be welcomed by the cattle industry and Ministry vets on the grounds that it would complicate the policy of eradication and compromise international trade. The counter argument to this is that the current eradication policy is not working either. A 75% effective vaccine for badgers, administrable by the oral or aerosol route, could be very effective since it is not essential to eradicate the disease in badgers. It would be a great help simply to achieve a major reduction in its prevalence.

There is no doubt that the cattle industry could do a great deal more to reduce the risk of infection or reinfection in previously 'clean' herds through greater attention to biosecurity. This should include a policy to ensure that any purchased cattle are tuberculin tested and pronounced clear of bTB before arrival on the farm. It should also include measures designed to keep badgers and cattle apart. This is easier said than done. Cattle may become infected by inhalation of bacteria from badger urine and faeces, which means that all cattle at pasture are at some risk. However, badgers do tend to concentrate their excretion in latrines and most good countrymen know where these latrines are. There is probably a greater risk from badgers that get into the farm buildings and infect cattle feed in store or in the mangers. It is theoretically easier to keep badgers out of farm buildings than off pasture. However, it is not *that* easy and on most farms would require considerable capital investment. A new, balanced policy for control of bTB in badgers and cattle is essential, if only to rein in the runaway costs of the existing control programme. This should be as sympathetic to the costs of improving biosecurity as to the costs of developing new vaccines.

This discussion of the control of bovine tuberculosis might appear to be an unnecessary digression at this late stage of the book when both reader and author are approaching saturation. I justify its inclusion as a timely illustration of one of my central themes; namely the proposition that animal welfare is important but not all-important and has to be accommodated within an ethical and political framework that respects all parties. The extrinsic value of the cow is greater to the farmer and to the physical needs of most of society than the badger. The badger carries a greater extrinsic value than the cow in relation to the emotional needs of some of society. In this context the badger is akin to the tiger. Most of us will never see a live one in the wild and would not wish to bump into one on a dark night. Neither species is of any use to us, but we would feel the world to be a poorer place without them. This is, of course, still an expression of the relative extrinsic value to us of the badger, the tiger and the cow. The intrinsic value of the badger is no greater or less than that of the tiger, the cow or, indeed, Cordelia the rat.

11.3.4 Politics by other means

Legislation as a vehicle for the progressive improvement of animal welfare carries many attractive features. It is, at least in theory, enforceable and should benefit all the animals, rather than the minority that may be involved in value-added, nominally high-welfare schemes like organic, free-range egg production. Moreover, when it compels us to pay more to sustain higher standards of animal welfare, it helps us to be better people. Nevertheless, there are clear limits to that which can be achieved through the conventional political process. It is possible to legislate for improved minimum standards for caged hens or commercial broiler production because the production systems and the animals used within those production systems have become extremely standardised. One large successful broiler unit is very much like another. However, when we come to consider more traditional family farming systems, whether in the developed or developing world, legislation is not really appropriate in relation to anything beyond the most basic standards of animal welfare because different individual farms have different individual problems and these require specific solutions (Chapter 4).

The other problem with politics by decree is what David Fraser calls 'Demosclerosis'. Anyone who has sat for any time on committees drafting new legislation or Codes of Practice for animal welfare will have suffered from the slow erosion of good intentions through expedience. 'Must' becomes 'Should'. 'Should' then becomes 'Should, unless'. At times like this, action through politics by other means becomes particularly attractive. I am not here referring to banner and megaphone diplomacy. I discussed this briefly under 'Reason and respect' (Section 11.3.2). What I am referring to is action aimed directly at those who have the most power to promote or enforce higher standards of animal welfare. These are, of course, not the farmers but the major retailers who, on the one hand, already demand standards of quality assurance from the producers who supply their goods and, on the other hand, are themselves absolutely dependent on quality assurance to maintain market share in an environment where the consumer has freedom of choice.

McDonald's, the burger barons, having vigorously defended but lost a prosecution for failure to ensure animal welfare, made the company decision to instigate improvements in animal welfare, particularly at the point of slaughter that go far beyond that required by legislation. It may be that McDonald's had become morally aware of the need for beneficence. They may also have been commercially aware that a large sector of their market is made up of young people who have an emotional concern for the welfare of farm animals and may, when McDonald's are getting a bad press, choose to buy their burgers elsewhere. In either event, it is clear that McDonald's were pressed into action by the force of public opinion. When a company that claims to sell 67 million burgers per day acts to improve its welfare standards, life or, at least, death, is made a little better for a very large number of animals.

In Britain, the public demand for free-range eggs has radically altered the buying habits of the supermarkets and this has fed through to the producers. As I discussed in Chapter 5, the jury is still out as to the welfare pros and cons of free range v. the enriched cage for laying hens. The interval between the publication of the Brambell Report (1965) and the phasing out in the EU of the conventional battery cage for laying hens (2012) will be 47 years! The growth of free-range egg production, driven by the force of public opinion acting directly upon the retailers, has simply driven straight through the slow march of the legislators.

'Real' farms, where animals form an integral part of biologically sustainable systems for working the land, are more likely to prosper through 'politics by other means' than through legislation. The aim here is for farmers to work with the retailers to supply premium food products to consumers seeking added value, whether defined by high welfare, 'organic' sustainability, local produce or any combination of these three. For this approach to succeed, the customer must first be persuaded by the claim for added value, whether perceived in terms of food quality (e.g. tasty, healthy) and/or production methods (e.g. high welfare, organic). The customer must also be prepared to trust the assurances of quality expressed by the producers and retailers. It is unrealistic to expect that every discerning customer will make it his or her business to discover what goes on within every farm, or even read all the small print on the Quality Assurance (QA) leaflets. All of us have to take most things on trust, simply because we have other things to do with our lives. However, that trust should be based on the knowledge that we can, if we wish, get access to the truth. This could involve direct access, a personal visit to production units or, more realistically, trust in the competence and honesty of an independent inspector acting on our behalf.

In Chapter 4, I outlined protocols for farm-specific programmes of quality control based on independent assessment of standards of husbandry provision and welfare outcome, coupled to a policy that insists upon action to resolve specific welfare problems. These programmes are designed to promote better animal welfare on two fronts: by improving husbandry on the farm, and by increasing customer demand for high-welfare products within the supermarket. However, QA costs money, to cover the costs of both the inspection process and the actions needed to address welfare problems as they arise. It is therefore completely unrealistic to assume that QA schemes can achieve significant improvements in animal welfare unless the customers are prepared to pay a significant premium. This, unfortunately, means that nationwide, 'red tractor' or similar farm assurance schemes are unlikely to have much effect upon standards for the simple reason that any system that is universal cannot, by definition, carry a premium. 'When everyone is somebody, then no one's anybody'.

For a QA scheme to succeed it has to be written by 'the invisible hand of the market'. In other words, it must benefit all the stakeholders. The main driver for welfare-based QA schemes has to be the major retailers because they are overwhelmingly the most powerful individual players in the game and so can set the rules. The potential benefit to the retailer, be it a major supermarket or a local butcher, of QA schemes in general and welfare-based QA schemes in particular is that they will appeal to the customers, and so attract them into the shop. The local butcher may seek to keep his customers out of the supermarket by offering meat from local farms. The supermarket may attract the concerned customer by the offer of 'Freedom Food' high-welfare bacon in the expectation that she will also buy baked beans. In both cases, the aim of the retailers is to persuade customers to select *their* shop.

Trust in a high-welfare QA scheme requires proof of the full package of quality control: compliance with the provisions of good husbandry, independent assessment of welfare outcomes and enforcement of action to resolve specific problems. It is very difficult to establish that proof unless the control policy is carried out at the local level. Local farmers (e.g. in the UK and EU) can benefit from a welfare-based QA scheme because it can give them a competitive advantage with respect to imports from countries where such rigorous standards of quality control cannot be assured. I suggest that farmers in the UK may have a better long-term prospect of profiting from high-welfare schemes than from organic production. At present, supermarkets appear to have little difficulty in buying and selling imported food that meets approved standards for organic production. This becomes much more difficult when quality assurance requires independent proof of welfare outcomes.

While it should benefit the retailers to initiate and drive high-welfare QA schemes, and while it should benefit traditional farmers to participate in such schemes, their success, in the final analysis, will depend entirely on whether or not the consumers (the people) are sufficiently impressed by the claims of added value to buy into the scheme. 'Freedom Food' free-range eggs have been a conspicuous success in the UK. This apart, the impact of other high-welfare products on the food-buying habits of the general public has been disappointing. For this, one cannot blame the supermarkets. Many have advertised and stocked their shelves with high-welfare lines of poultry, pork and bacon, only to withdraw them after months of trying due to lack of demand. Unfortunately 'high-welfare' does not begin to compete with 'organic' as a brand name. Animal welfare is an essential element of standards for organic farming, but these standards, of course, are much broader in scope and incorporate a concern for the overall sustainability and welfare of the living environment. I would like to believe that the greater appeal of organic produce was a true reflection of this broader environmental concern. It is difficult, however, to escape the conclusion that many people buy organic food in the hope or belief that it is less likely to harm them. Our actions are in strict accord with the model of motivation and behaviour in sentient animals, illustrated in Figure 3.1. Motivation to buy organic food in *Homo sentiens* can occur as the result of a strictly emotional interpretation of incoming signals with little or no cognitive involvement whatever. Inevitably therefore, organic food tends to be promoted on the basis that it is somehow safer or tastier. This may sometimes be cynical, sometimes innocent (and very occasionally true). There is plenty of evidence (enough for another book) to show that the composition of meat, milk and eggs can be influenced by the ways animals are fed and reared, and that these effects can affect taste, texture and the impact of diet on health.* Nevertheless I believe that it is fundamentally dishonest to market high-welfare, organic or any other sort of food on the basis of health claims unless they are very well founded. Animal welfare and the sustainability of the living environment should be recognised for their own values. It should not be necessary to promote these virtues through exploitation of ignorance and fear; which assertion leads naturally into the final and perhaps most important element of my entire argument, namely the case for education.

11.4 Education in animal welfare

Education is one of the great virtues. It helps us to understand our perceptions and the emotions they arouse. In so doing it helps us to cope as we seek to meet our needs. It also helps us to understand the needs of others (of all species) as they too struggle to cope. The word education is derived from *e ducare*, the process of 'leading out' the mind of each individual to prepare that person for experience and guide him or her through experience to achieve the information and understanding necessary to become a competent, compassionate and interesting person. All

* Two important examples are saturated v. unsaturated fatty acids and n-3 v. n-6 polyunsaturated fatty acids.

education should be a lifetime experience and the more the better, but any education, in my belief, is a good thing. It is often (too often) said that 'a little knowledge is a dangerous thing'. This cliché can only apply to knowledge without education, since one of the first aims of a proper education is to instil the awareness of how much we do not know and how little we truly understand. This provides a shield against both wrong belief and wrong action. Knowledge and education concerning the husbandry and welfare of animals kept in the service of man can shield us from irrational belief in propaganda from any source, be it industrialists, politicians, welfare lobbyists or simple nutters. Knowledge and education should also restrain our own impulses to wild assertions.

In the confident assumption that all education in animal welfare is a good thing and the more the better, I identify three levels at which this education should be pursued:

(1) awareness;
(2) education for the public good;
(3) education of the professional.

I have already identified increased awareness of the nature of animal sentience as the single most effective step towards increasing the sum of human compassion. This can be instilled early in life. Children can be brutal because the principle of 'Do as you would be done by' does not appear to be innate. However, children are motivated to love their pets. From this excellent starting point they can, with some effort, be motivated to care for their pets and, from this, motivated towards a compassion for all sentient animals. Adults, even in the most brutalising environment of the abattoir, can be moved to treat animals better simply by bringing the matter to their attention. I am very impressed by the following notice written over the point of entry of animals to a Scottish abattoir: 'Quality control starts here. Animals should be treated with care and compassion at all times'. If such a sign had been present 20 years ago it would almost certainly have ended with the word care. Simple awareness of the need for compassion addresses the moral virtue of respect for autonomy.

Education for the public good is that which is necessary to guide the actions of those who are aware of animal sentience and animal suffering; who benefit from animals but do not actually work with them. The first step in this process is to seek the closest possible match between how people feel about problems of animal welfare and how the animals feel about these things themselves. This will help to ensure that action for animal welfare with response to public demand will, in fact, be right action. This addresses the moral virtue of beneficence. The next step is to acquire knowledge and education with respect to the benefits we derive from the animals and how these benefits to us may be achieved at least cost to them. This addresses the moral virtue of justice. As always, such education cannot be enforced simply through the didactic presentation of 'facts' to be learned and accepted. Didactic teaching can only be justified as a method for preparing the mind to interpret personal experience. If children are to understand matters of animal welfare on the farm or in the laboratory they need to encounter this form of directed self-education in what goes on and why. This means that farms and laboratories have to make themselves open to the public, especially school children, to a degree constrained only on the grounds of health, safety and proper respect for the need to earn a living without constant interruption. It also means that education authorities should provide the funds and the time within the curriculum to meet this essential element of education in citizenship.

The third category is education of the professionals, those who make their living by working in direct contact with animals and are, thereby, most directly responsible for their welfare. Every student who embarks on an education in agriculture, animal care, veterinary science or medicine should have formed some impression of what is meant by animal welfare. All members of the Royal College of Veterinary Surgeons commit themselves on oath to promote the welfare of all animals committed to their care. In most of these cases it may be possible to take compassion for granted. Here the goal is professional competence.

It should be self-evident that the subject of animal welfare is an integral part of all education in agriculture and veterinary science. The essence of these vocations – good husbandry and the diagnosis, prevention and treatment of disease – is critical to ensuring that animals are fit and happy. However, the traditional structure of the agriculture and veterinary curricula that deals with production and health seldom, if ever, includes all that is necessary to give students proper knowledge and understanding of the science and values that should underpin a professional career in animal care. One of the first essential messages to convey to senior (older) academics in agriculture and veterinary colleges is that animal welfare, a discipline based on sound science and sound ethics, is as essential to the veterinary curriculum as a programme in pathology or surgery.

11.5 A curriculum for animal welfare

A programme for education in animal welfare should include the following elements:

- Definitions of welfare, sentience and suffering:
  - Elements of good and bad welfare: the 'Five Freedoms'
  - Elements of good husbandry: resources, records and stockmanship.
- An ethical framework that incorporates animal welfare concerns within a matrix of respect for human values.
- Animal welfare science:
  - The physiology of stress and adaptation to stress
  - The neurobiology and ethology of animal perception, emotion, cognition, motivation and behavioural response to environmental stimuli
  - The recognition and motivational basis of abnormal behaviour in animals
  - The human–animal bond.

- Animal welfare laws and regulations.
- The practical implementation of good husbandry and welfare:
  - Elements of stockmanship
  - Welfare problems associated with the 'unnatural' breeding and rearing of animals to serve human needs for food, medicine, etc.
  - Assessment of husbandry provisions and welfare outcomes on farms, laboratories and other animal-rearing establishments
  - Causes and consequences of cruelty to animals: actions and omissions likely to cause unnecessary suffering.

This outline contains the elements necessary for a full programme of study in animal welfare within a degree course for veterinarians. A course for degree and diploma students in agriculture and animal science would need to give attention to most (but not all) of these elements. They would probably devote relatively less time to (e.g.) neurobiology and more to stockmanship. The teaching methods should involve a combination of formal lectures, practical experience and directed self-education. At Bristol we teach our veterinary students the elements of welfare and husbandry in Year 1 through formal lectures reinforced by practical classes in stockmanship. We also introduce them to ethical principles and how animal welfare may be incorporated within a proper set of human values. The 'Five Freedoms and Provisions' form the basis for Year 1 teaching of welfare and husbandry. Ethical values are taught within the structure of the 'ethical matrix' (Table 1.4) which identifies the parties worthy of respect (animals, consumers, producers and the living environment) and examines how a proper balance of respect may be achieved according to the moral principles of beneficence, autonomy and justice.

Animal welfare science is taught largely in Year 2 and is founded on the classical scientific disciplines of physiology and ethology. These convey an understanding of how animals feel. The diagnosis and prevention of production diseases in farm animals and behavioural problems in pet animals are formally taught in the third and fourth years within clinical modules organised mostly according to species. Our final (fifth) year is lecture-free and students are required to acquire practical clinical skills on the farm and in the surgery through directed self-education. We use this approach to develop their skill and confidence in the assessment and resolution of animal welfare problems and the recognition and proper description of circumstances that might be considered to constitute unnecessary suffering.

It is for individual universities and colleges to decide how best to deliver the syllabus. The problem in the past has been that many teachers in veterinary and agricultural colleges were not sure what the syllabus should contain. The World Society for the Protection of Animals (WSPA), in association with the Veterinary School at the University of Bristol, have produced an excellent syllabus, 'Concepts in Animal Welfare', that is computer based and designed for distance learning. It is sufficiently comprehensive and flexible to form the basis for a wide range of programmes for teaching and examining animal welfare at the level of the veterinary graduate, the agriculture graduate, the veterinary nurse and the animal care technician in a scientific laboratory. The syllabus is comprehensive because it gives regard to science as the route to the proper understanding of animals, ethics as the route to proper respect for animals, and professional training as the route to converting right thoughts into right action. I am confident that it will make a significant contribution to improving the teaching of animal welfare worldwide. This will be good for the animals too.

11.6 Finally, but not in conclusion

And so to bed. This is the end, not of a journey; merely a very long day on a journey that has no end. In *A Cool Eye Towards Eden*, I was able to set down guidelines for the understanding of animal welfare based on the study of how it feels to be an animal. I was then able to progress to careful polemic; a constructive approach to the problem of man's dominion over the animals. Much of this could be considered in an abstract and academic sort of way because, at the time, the journey had scarcely begun. Now we are well into our journey and limping a little because the going is hard. It was relatively easy, and very satisfying, to pronounce on what should be done in the interests of animal welfare. It is harder, and more frustrating, to make real progress within a world of messy realities and conflicting objectives. This is therefore a tale of work in progress and work that will still be in progress long after I am gone. As such it would not, I think, be fitting to conclude with a phrase as exalted as that with which I closed *A Cool Eye*, namely Albert Schweizer's assertion that 'Until he extends the circle of his compassion to all living things, man will not himself find peace'. Embarked upon an endless journey, the hopeful traveller needs something more downbeat. '*The path of duty lies in what is near.*' We may never expect to see our final destination, but, for those who are prepared to open their eyes, the immediate horizon is full of promise.

Further Reading

Albentosa, M.J., Kjaer, J.B. & Nicol, C.J. (2003) Strain and age differences in behaviour, fear response and pecking tendency in laying hens. *British Poultry Science*, **44**, 333–44.

Animal Procedures Committee (2003) *Consultation Paper on the Statistics of Scientific Procedures on Living Animals in Great Britain*. APC, London, www.apc.gov.uk.

Assured British Pigs (2001) *Standards Manual*. Assured British Pigs, Stourport on Seven.

Banner, M. (1995) *Committee of Enquiry into the Ethics of Emerging Technologies in the Breeding of Animals*. HMSO, London.

Bartussek, H. (1999) A review of the Animal Needs Index (ANI) for the assessment of animals' well being in the housing systems for Austrian proprietary products and legislation. *Livestock Production Science*, **61**, 179–92.

Bateman, A., Singh, A., Kral, T. & Solomon, S. (1989) The immune-hypothalamic-pituitary axis. *Endocrinology Reviews*, **10**, 92–107.

Bateson, P. (1991) Assessment of pain in animals. *Animal Behaviour*, **42**, 827–40.

Beattie, V.E., O'Connell, N.E. & Moss, D.W. (2000) Influence of environmental enrichment on the behaviour, performance and meat quality of domestic pigs. *Livestock Production Science*, **65**, 71–9.

Beauchamp, T.L. & Childress, J.F. (1994) *Principles of Biomedical Ethics*. Oxford University Press, Oxford.

Boivin, X., Lensink, J., Tallet, C. & Veissier, L. (2003) Stockmanship and farm animal welfare. *Animal Welfare*, **12**, 479–92.

Bradshaw, E.L. & Bateson, P. (2000) Welfare implications of culling red deer (*Cervus elaphus*). *Animal Welfare*, **9**, 3–24.

Brambell, F.W.R. (1965) *Report of the Technical Committee to Enquire Into the Welfare of Livestock Kept Under Intensive Conditions*. HMSO, London.

Broom, D. & Johnson, (1993) *Stress and Animal Welfare*. Chapman and Hall, London.

Brunk, C.G., Haworth, L. & Lee, B. (1991) *Value Assumptions in Risk Assessment: A Case Study of the Alachlor Controversy*. Wilfred Laurier University Press, Waterloo, Canada.

Burns, Lord (2000) *Report of Committee of Inquiry into Hunting with Dogs in England and Wales*. HMSO, London, www.archive.official-documents.co.uk.

Butterworth, A. (1999) Infectious components of broiler lameness: a review. *World Poultry Science Journal*, **55**, 327–52.

Clarkson, M.J., Downham, D.Y., Faull, W.B., *et al.* (1996) Incidence and prevalence of lameness in dairy cattle. *Veterinary Record*, **138**, 563–7.

Commission of the European Communities (CEC) (1983). *Abnormal Behaviour of Farm Animals.* A report of the CEC expert group, Farm Animal Welfare, August 1983. CEC, Brussels.

Compassion in World Farming (2002) *Farm Animal Genetic Engineering and Cloning.* CIWF Trust, Petersfield.

Cooper, J.J. & Nicol, C.J. (1991) Stereotypic behaviour affects environmental preferences in bank voles *Clethrionomys glareolus. Animal Behaviour*, **41**, 971–77.

Crawley, J.N. (2000) *What's Wrong with my Mouse? Behavioural Phenotyping of Transgenic and Knockout Mice.* Wiley Liss, USA.

Danbury, T.C., Weeks, C.A., Chambers, J.P., Waterman-Pearson, A.E. & Kestin S.C. (1999) Self-selection of the analgesic drug carprofen by lame broiler chickens. *Veterinary Record*, **146**, 307–311.

Dawkins, M.S. (1980) *Animal Suffering: The Science of Animal Welfare.* Chapman and Hall, London.

Dawkins, M.S. (1990) From an animal's point of view: motivation, fitness and animal welfare. *Behavioural and Brain Sciences*, **13**, 1–61.

Dawkins, M.S. (1993) *Through Our Eyes Only? The Search for Animal Consciousness.* Freeman, Oxford.

Dawkins, M.S. (2001) How can we recognise and assess good welfare? In: *Coping with Challenge: Welfare in Animals Including Humans* (ed. D.M. Broom), pp. 63–76. Dahlem University Press, Berlin.

DEFRA (Department of the Environment, Food and Rural Affairs) (2003) *Revised Codes for the Welfare of Pigs, Laying Hens, Meat Poultry and Dairy Cattle.* HMSO, London (www.defra.gov.uk).

DEFRA (Department of the Environment, Food and Rural Affairs) (2003) *Report on the Welfare of Farm Animals at Slaughter or Killing: Part 1 Red Meat Animals.* HMSO, London (www.defra.gov.uk).

Duncan, I.J.H., Slee, G.S., Kettlewell, P., Berry, P. & Carllisle, A.J. (1986) Comparison of stressfulness of harvesting broiler chickens by machine and by hand. *British Poultry Science*, **27**, 109–114.

Edney, A. (1989) Killing with kindess. *Veterinary Record*, **124**, 320–322.

El-Lethy, H., Aerni, V., Jungi, T.W. & Wechsler, B. (2000) Stress and feather pecking in hens in relation to housing conditions. *British Poultry Science*, **41**, 22–8.

Farm Animal Welfare Council (FAWC) (1991) *Report on the European Commission Proposals on the Transport of Animals.* DEFRA, London.

Farm Animal Welfare Council (FAWC) (1992) *Report on the Welfare of Broiler Chickens.* DEFRA, London.

Farm Animal Welfare Council (FAWC) (1993) *Second Report on Priorities for Research and Development in Farm Animal Welfare.* DEFRA, London.

Farm Animal Welfare Council (FAWC) (2001) *Interim Report on the Animal Welfare Implications of Farm Assurance Schemes.* DEFRA, London.

Foley, C.W., Lasley, J.F. & Osweiler, G.D. (1979) *Abnormalities of Companion Animals*. Iowa State University Press, Iowa.

Fraser, D. (1995) Science, values and animal welfare: exploring the inextricable connection. *Animal Welfare*, **4**, 103–117.

Fraser, D. (2003) Assessing animal welfare at the farm and group level: the interplay of science and values. *Animal Welfare*, **12**, 433–44.

Fraser, D. & Broom, D.B. (1990) *Farm Animal Behaviour and Welfare*. CAB International, Wallingford, Oxon.

Fraser, D. & Duncan, I.J.H. (1998) 'Pleasures', 'pains' and animal welfare: toward a natural history of affect. *Animal Welfare*, **7**, 383–96.

GeneWatch UK (2002) *Genetically Modified and Cloned Animals. All in a Good Cause?* GeneWatch UK, www.genewatch.org.

Gentle, M.J. & Tilston, V.L. (2000) Nociceptors in the legs of poultry: implications for potential pain in pre-slaughter shackling. *Animal Welfare*, **9**, 227–36.

Grandin, T. (ed.) (1993) *Livestock Handling and Transport*. CAB International, Wallingford, Oxon.

Grandin (1998) Cattle handling. In: *Animal Welfare and Meat Science* (N. Gregory). CAB International, Wallingford, Oxon, pp. 42–63.

Greenough, P.R. & Weaver, A.D. (1997) *Lameness in Cattle*, 3rd edn. W.B. Saunders, Philadelphia.

Gregory, N.G. (1998a) Physiological mechanisms causing sickness behaviour and suffering in diseased animals. *Animal Welfare*, **7**, 293–305.

Gregory, N.G. (1998b) *Animal Welfare and Meat Science*. CAB International, Wallingford, Oxon.

Gregory, N.G. & Wilkins, L.J. (1989) Broken bones in domestic fowl: handling and processing damage in end of lay battery hens. *British Poultry Science*, **30**, 555–62.

Gross, W.B. & Siegel, H.S. (1983) Evaluation of the heterophil:lymphocyte ratio as a measure of stress in chickens. *Avian Diseases*, **27**, 972–8.

Halverson, M.K. (2002) *Farm Animal Health and Wellbeing*. Technical Working Paper. State of Minnesota Generic Environmental Impact Statement on Animal Agriculture.

Harris, R. (1998) *The Physiological Response of Red Deer (Cervus elaphus) to Prolonged Escape Exercise Undertaken During Hunting*. Unpublished report from Joint Universities Study on Deer Hunting.

Harrison, R. (1964) *Animal Machines*. Stuart, London.

Haslam, S.M. (2003) *The development of a unitary index for the assessment of welfare in broiler chickens*. PhD Thesis, University of Bristol.

Hawkins, P. (2002) Recognising and assessing pain, suffering and distress in laboratory animals: a survey of current practice in the UK with recommendations. *Laboratory Animals*, **35**, 378–95.

Home Office (2000) *Guidance on the Operation of the Animals (Scientific Procedures) Act 1986*. HMSO, London.

Honeyman, M.S., Roush, W.B. & Penner, A.D. (1998) *Pig crushing mortality by hut type in outdoor farrowing.* Iowa State University Farms Reports, ISRF 98-10, 16-18. Iowa State University.

House of Lords Select Committee (2002) *Animals in Scientific Procedures.* HMSO, London.

Houston, A.I. (1997) Demand curves and animal welfare. *Animal Behaviour*, **53**, 983–90.

Iggo, A. (1984) *Pain in Animals.* Universities Federation for Animal Welfare, Wheathampstead, Hertfordshire.

Jensen, P. (2001) Motivation and coping. In: *Coping with Challenge: Welfare in Animals Including Humans* (ed. D.M. Broom), pp. 123–34. Dahlem University Press, Berlin.

Jones, J.B., Webster, A.J.F. & Wathes, C.M. (1999) Trade-off between ammonia exposure and thermal comfort in pigs and the influence of social contact. *Animal Science*, **68**, 387–97.

Jones, R.B., McAdie, T.M., McCorquodale, C. & Keeling, L.J. (2002) Pecking at birds and at string enrichment devices by adult laying hens. *British Poultry Science*, **43**, 337–43.

Kendrick, K.M. (1998) Intelligent perception. *Applied Animal Behaviour Science*, **57**, 213–31.

Kestin, S.C., Knowles, T.G., Tinch, A.E. & Gregory, N.G. (1992) Prevalence of leg weakness in broiler chickens and its relationship with genotype. *Veterinary Record*, **131**, 191–4.

Kestin, S.C., Gordon, S., Su, G. & Sorensen, P. (2001) The relationship between lameness in broiler chickens and liveweight, growth rate and age. *Veterinary Record*, **148**, 195–7.

Kirkden, R.D., Edwards, J.S.S. & Broom, D.M. (2003) A theoretical comparison of the consumer surplus and the elasticities of demand as measures of motivational strength. *Animal Behaviour*, **65**, 157–78.

Knierem, U. & Gocke, A. (2003) Effect of catching broilers by hand or machine on rates of injuries and dead-on-arrivals. *Animal Welfare*, **12**, 63–73.

Knowles, T.G. (1998) A review of the road transport of slaughter sheep. *Veterinary Record*, **143**, 212–19.

Krebs, J.R. (1997) *Bovine Tuberculosis in Cattle and Badgers.* Independent Scientific Review Group. HMSO, London.

Kyriazakis, I. & Emmans, G.C. (1991) Diet selection in pigs: dietary choices made by pigs following a period of underfeeding with protein. *Animal Production*, **52**, 337–46.

Lorenz, K.Z. (1966) *On Aggression.* Methuen, London.

Main, D.C.J., Whay, H.R., Green, L.E. & Webster, A.J.F. (2003) Effect of the RSPCA Freedom Food scheme on dairy cattle welfare. *Veterinary Record*, **197**, 227–31.

Manser, C.E. (1992) *The Assessment of Stress in Laboratory Animals.* RSPCA, Horsham, Sussex.

Martin, P. & Bateson, P. (1993) *Measuring Behaviour: An Introductory Guide.* Cambridge University Press, Cambridge.

Mason, G.J., McFarland, D. & Garner, J. (1998) A demanding task: using economic techniques to assess animal priorities. *Animal Behaviour*, **55**, 1070–75.

Matthews, L.R. (1993) Deer handling and transport. In: *Livestock Handling and Transport* (ed. T. Grandin). CAB International, Wallingford, Oxon.

McFarland, D. (1989) *Problems of Animal Behaviour*. Longman, Harlow.

McFarlane, J.M., Curtis, S.E., Shanks, R.D. & Carmer, G.G. (1989a) Multiple concurrent stressors in chicks. 1. Effects on weight gain, feed intake and behaviour. *Poultry Science*, **68**, 501–9.

McFarlane, J.M., Curtis, S.E., Simon, J. & Izquierdo, O.A. (1989b) Multiple concurrent stressors in chicks. 2. Effects on haematologic, body compositon and pathologic traits. *Poultry Science*, **68**, 510–21.

McFarlane, J.M. & Curtis, S.E. (1989c) Multiple concurrent stressors in chicks. 3. Effects on plasma corticosterone and the heterophil/lymphocyte ratio. *Poultry Science*, **68**, 522–7.

McInerney, J.P. (1998) The economics of welfare. In: *Ethics, Welfare, Law and Market Forces: The Veterinary Interface* (eds A.R. Michell & R. Ewbank). UFAW, Wheathampstead, Hertfordshire.

McNally, P.W. & Warriss, P.D. (1996) Recent bruising in cattle at abattoirs. *Veterinary Record*, **138**, 126–8.

Medway Report (1979) *Report of a committee to investigate welfare aspects of shooting and angling*. RSPCA, Horsham, Sussex.

Mendl, M. & Paul, E.S. (2004) Consciousness, emotion and animal welfare: insights from cognitive science. *Animal Welfare*, **13**, S17–25.

Mepham, B. (1996) Ethical analysis of food biotechnologies: an evaluative framework. In: *Food Ethics* (ed. B. Mepham), pp. 101–19. Routledge, London.

Moloney, V., Kent, J.E. & Robertson, I.S. (1993) Behavioural response of lambs of three ages in the first three hours after three methods of castration and tail docking. *Research in Veterinary Science*, **55**, 236–45.

Moloney, V., Kent, J.E. & Robertson, I.S. (1995) Assessment of acute and chronic pain after different methods of castration of calves. *Applied Animal Behaviour Science*, **46**, 33–48.

Morton, D.B. & Griffiths, P.H.M. (1985) Guidelines on the recognition of pain, distress and discomfort in experimental animals and a hypothesis for assessment. *Veterinary Record*, **116**, 431–6.

Newberry, R.D. & Wood-Gush, D.G.M (1986) Social relationships of pigs in semi-natural units. *Animal Behaviour*, **34**, 1311–18.

Nicol, C.J., Davidson, H.P.D., Harris, P.A., Walters, A.J. & Wilson, A.D. (2002) Study of crib-biting and gastric inflammation and ulceration in young horses. *Veterinary Record*, **151**, 658–62.

Odberg, F.O. (1992) Bullfighting and animal welfare. *Animal Welfare*, **1**, 3–12.

Ossent, P. & Lischer, C. (1998) Bovine laminitis; the lesions and their pathogenesis. *In Practice*, **20**, 415–27.

Overmeir, J.B. (2002) On learned helplessness. *Integrative Physiological and Behavioural Science*, **37**, 4–8.

Povinella, D.J. & Vonk, J. (2003) Chimpanzee minds: suspiciously human? *Trends in Cognitive Sciences*, **7**, 157–60.

Pryce, J.E., Veerkamp, R.F. & Simm, G. (1998) Expected correlated responses in health and fertility traits to selection on production in dairy cattle. *Proceedings of the 6th World Congress on Genetics Applied to Livestock Production*, Australia, pp. 383–6.

Radford, M. (2001) *Animal Welfare Law in Britain: Regulation and Responsibility.* Oxford University Press, Oxford.

Raj, A.B.M. (1996) Aversive reactions of turkeys to argon, carbon dioxide and a mixture of carbon dioxide and argon. *Veterinary Record,* **138,** 592–3.

Rawls, J. (1972) *A Theory of Justice.* Oxford University Press, Oxford.

Rifkin, J. (1993) *Beyond Beef: The Rise and Fall of the Cattle Culture.* Dutton Books, Washington, DC.

Roberts, M (1998) *The Man Who Listens to Horses.* Ballantyne Books, USA.

Roitblat, H.L. (1987) *Introduction to Comparative Cognition.* Freeman.

Rollin, B. (1982) *Animals' Rights and Human Morality.* Prometheus, Buffalo.

Rose, J.D. (2002) The neurobehavioural nature of fishes and the question of awareness and pain. *Reviews in Fisheries Science,* **10,** 1–38.

Royal Society (2001) *Response to the call for evidence by the House of Lords Committee investigating the use of animals in scientific research.* Royal Society, London, www.royalsoc.ac.uk.

Russell, W.M.S. & Burch, R.L. (1959) *The principles of humane experimental technique.* Methuen & Co., London.

Ryder, R.D. (1998) *The Political Animal: The Conquest of Speciesism.* McFarland.

Sandoe, P., Christiansen, S.B. & Appleby, M.C. (2003) Farm animal welfare: the interaction of ethical questions and animal welfare science. *Animal Welfare,* **12,** 469–78.

Schwartz, S. (2003) Separation anxiety syndrome in dogs and cats. *Journal of American Veterinary Association,* **222,** 1526–32.

Selye, H. (1950) *Stress.* Acta, Montreal.

Shettleworth, S.J. (1998) *Cognition, Evolution and Behaviour.* Oxford University Press, Oxford.

Simpson, A., Webster, A.J.F., Smith, J.S. & Simpson, C.A. (1978) Energy and nitrogen metabolism of red deer (*Cervus elaphus*) in cold environments; a comparison with cattle and sheep. *Comparative Biochemistry and Physiology,* **60,** 251–6.

Singer, P. (1990) *Animal Liberation: A New Ethics for our Treatment of Animals.* Avon, New York.

Smith, A. (1776) *The Wealth of Nations.* Reprinted 1990. Penguin Classics.

Sneddon, L.U., Braithwaite, V. & Gentle, M.J. (2003) Do fishes have nociceptors? Evidence for the evolution of a vertebrate sensory system. *Proceedings of the Royal Society of London Series B,* **270,** 1115–21.

Sodian, B., Hulsken, C. & Thoemer, C. (2003) The self and action in theory of mind research. *Consciousness and Cognition,* **12,** 777–82.

Stolba, A. & Wood-Gush, A.D.M. (1989) The behaviour of pigs in a semi-natural environment. *Animal Production,* **48,** 419–25.

Tannenbaum, J. (1961) Ethics and animal welfare: the inextricable connection. *Journal of the American Veterinary Medical Association,* **198,** 1360–76.

Thurstone, L.L. (1927) A law of comparative judgement. *Psychological Reviews,* **76,** 31–48.

Uystepruyst, C.H., Coghe, J., Dorts, T.H., *et al.* (2002) Optimal timing of elective Caesarian section in Belgian White and Blue breed of cattle: the calf's point of view. *The Veterinary Journal,* **163,** 267–82.

Vermunt, J.J. & Greenough, P.R. (1996) Sole haemorrhages in dairy heifers managed under different underfoot and environmental conditions. *British Veterinary Journal*, **152**, 57–73.

Wahlsten *et al.* (2003) In search of a better mouse test. *Trends in Neuroscience*, **26**, 132–6.

Wall, P.D. & Melzack, R. (1994) *Textbook of Pain*. Churchill Livingstone, London.

Webster, A.J.F. (1984) *Calf Husbandry, Health and Welfare*. Collins, London.

Webster, A.J.F. (1990) Housing and respiratory disease in farm animals. *Outlook on Agriculture*, **19**, 31–6.

Webster, A.J.F. (1992) Problems of feeding and housing: their diagnosis and control. In: *Livestock Health and Welfare* (ed. R. Moss), pp. 293–333. Longmans, London.

Webster, A.J.F. (2002) Effects of housing practices on the development of foot lesions in dairy heifers in early lactation. *Veterinary Record*, **151**, 9–12.

Webster, A.J.F. & Main, D.C.J. (eds) (2003) Proceedings of the 2nd International Workshop on the Assessment of Animal Welfare at Farm and Group Level. *Animal Welfare*, **12**(4).

Webster, A.J.F., Chlumecky, J. & Young, B.A. (1970) Effects of cold environments on the energy exchanges of young beef cattle. *Canadian Journal Animal Science*, **50**, 89–100.

Webster, A.J.F., Tuddenham, A., Saville, C.A. & Scott, G.B. (1993) Thermal stress on chickens in transit. *British Poultry Science*, **34**, 267–77.

Webster, J. (1993) *Understanding the Dairy Cow*, 2nd edn. Blackwell Scientific Publications, London.

Webster, J. (1994) *Animal Welfare: A Cool Eye Towards Eden*. Blackwell Science, Oxford.

Weeks, C.A., Danbury, T.D., Davies, H.C., Hunt, P. & Kestin, S.C. (2000) The behaviour of broiler chickens and its modification by lameness. *Applied Animal Behaviour Science*, **67**, 111–25.

Weiss, J.M. (1971) Effects of coping behaviour in different warning signal conditions on stress pathology in rats. *Journal of Comparative Physiology and Psychology*, **77**, 1–13.

Wemelsfelder, F., Hunter, E.A., Mendl, M.T. & Lawrence, A.B. (2001) Assessing the 'whole animal': a free-choice profiling approach. *Animal Behaviour*, **62**, 209–20.

Whay, H.R., Waterman, A.E., Webster, A.J.F. & O'Brien, J.K. (1998) The influence of lesion type on the duration of hyperalgesia associated with hindlimb lameness in dairy cattle. *Veterinary Journal*, **156**, 23–9.

Whay, H.R., Main, D.C.J., Green, L.E. & Webster, A.J.F. (2003a) Animal-based measures for the assessment of welfare state of dairy cattle, pigs and laying hens: consensus of expert opinion. *Animal Welfare*, **12**, 205–17.

Whay, H.R., Main, D.C.J., Green, L.E. & Webster, A.J.F. (2003b) Assessment of dairy cattle welfare using animal-based measurements. *Veterinary Record*, **153**, 197–202.

Whay, H.R., Main, D.C.J., Green, L.E. & Webster, A.J.F. (2003c) An animal-based welfare assessment of group-housed calves on dairy farms. *Animal Welfare*, **12**, 611–17.

Wiseman, M.L., Nolan, A.M., Reid, J. & Scotte, M. (2001) Preliminary studies on owner-reported behaviour changes associated with chronic pain in dogs. *Veterinary Record*, **149**, 423–4.

Index